PEACEBUILDING STARTS AT HOME

HOW YOU CAN MAKE IT HAPPEN

CHARLES HAUSS

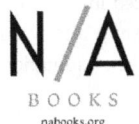

BOOKS

nabooks.org

Copyright © 2025 by Charles Hauss

All rights reserved.

No part of this book may be reproduced in any form or by any electronic or mechanical means, including information storage and retrieval systems, without written permission from the author, except for the use of brief quotations in a book review.

❦ Formatted with Vellum

To the memory of Dick O'Neill

CONTENTS

1. Start Where You Are — 1
2. Reality Tells Me What to Do — 23
3. Let It Begin With Me — 55
4. Peace Is a Verb — 89
5. The Peacebuilding Pivot — 120
6. Spreading Ideas Worth Spreading — 155
7. Redesigning the Room Where It Happens — 195
8. Charting Our Own Evolution — 225
    Study Guide — 243

    Acknowledgments — 247

CHAPTER 1
START WHERE YOU ARE

The future of our country is in your hands.

ROBERT PUTNAM

Peacebuilding Starts at Home is an invitation masquerading as a book.

I will not be inviting you to come over to my house for a gourmet dinner or to be a plus one on a trip to some exotic and exciting vacation spot. Instead, I will be asking you to join me and the people you will meet in these pages in turning this country around.

By deciding what we want our country to be like.

By redefining peace as peacebuilding which will turn it into a powerful tool that we all can use to begin changing life here at home.

By helping you find your own personal on-ramp for a journey that I want us to take together and that we need to take together.

By creating a movement that pulls the United States out of the rut that it is in.

You don't need me to tell you that we face unprecedented social, economic, and environmental challenges.

Or that the experts are predicting that most of them are only going to get worse.

Or that we are more polarized than we have been at any time since the Civil War.

Or that trust in our institutions and the men and women we have chosen to run them is plummeting, whoever you voted for.

Or that there is a mismatch between the problems that we face and the tools we are using to solve them.

Or that for the moment at least, the problems seem to be winning.

This book is based on some simple but challenging assumptions about what can be done about those problems.

We aren't locked into the status quo.

We have alternatives.

We can all work on them together.

And I do mean *all* of us.

This book charts one path out of the mess that we are in that starts with peacebuilding. Peace and peacebuilding have been a part of my life since I attended my first demonstration protesting the launch of a nuclear submarine while I was in high school in New London CT.

I've learned a lot in the sixty years since then, working mostly on problems facing the rest of the world. That includes realizing that I am a peace builder and not just a peace advocate.

I'm not playing with words here.

Peacebuilding means more than putting down the guns or stopping the screaming—although you do have to do that, of course.

It means tackling all of the problems that got us into trouble in the first place.

It means combining peace and building into something approaching an all-purpose tool—sort of like a Swiss army knife—for addressing many if not all of our problems.

It means pivoting away from complaining about what we are against toward building what we are for.

It means adapting what my colleagues have learned in places like South Africa and South Sudan so that our fellow Americans can make life better in the South Bronx, South Dakota, South Park, and everywhere in between.

It means helping people like you create a movement that changes the way most Americans solve most of their problems most of the time.

I'll be the first to admit that the odds are not in our favor. But as I did the research for this book, I discovered just how much progress the people you will meet have already made and how easy it would be for us to speed things up—even given the headwinds we are facing in the middle of our century's version of the roaring twenties.

So, I wrote *Peacebuilding Starts at Home* to make it as easy as possible, as enjoyable as possible, and as rewarding as possible for you to do your part in producing the paradigm shift in human relations that has been at the heart of my work since I first read Thomas Kuhn's *Structure of Scientific Revolutions* as a college sophomore in 1966.[1]

We are not going to create some sort of heaven on earth in which everyone gets along. No such society has ever existed. No such society will ever exist.

But, to use a phrase I will keep coming back to, we can build a society in which most people solve most of their problems most of the time without the use of force or violence.

That can only happen if you join me and the thousands of other Americans who have already accepted their version of the invitation (which didn't come from me, by the way). In the rest of this book, I will introduce you to more than forty organizations, all but two of which I have personally worked with. They—and the hundreds of others I didn't have room to squeeze in—have begun building the "scaffolding" for the more peaceful United States that so many Americans think is beyond our reach.

There will be a few glitzy examples. Daryl Davis is a Black blues and boogie woogie pianist who has led more than two hundred people out of the Ku Klux Klan. John Mackey built Whole Foods Market into a juggernaut and has become the most visible champion of what he calls conscious capitalism. Each year, John Hunter's fourth graders "solve" fifty of the world's most troubling problems and reach world peace. Emily Post's great-grandchildren have updated her book on etiquette

---

1. Thomas Kuhn, *The Structure of Scientific Revolutions*. (Chicago: University of Chicago Press, 1961).

to help twenty-first century citizens navigate the uncertainties that all humans encounter whenever and however they interact with each other. A sword-swallowing doctor and statistician will even make a cameo appearance (but you have to wait until the second half of chapter 8 to find out who he is and why he is worth learning about—it has nothing to do with his sword swallowing skills).

Most of the people you will meet are average citizens who are doing amazing things that are often hiding in plain sight. Some are members of service clubs like Rotary. Some are high school students. Some are health care providers. Some live in red states in the heartland. Others, like me, live in one of the blue states concentrated on the coasts.

They are the heroes of this book. I will use my career as a thread to tie everything together. But this book is not about me. It definitely is not my blueprint to get us out of the crises we face.

That's the case for one simple reason. However much the people I profile may have accomplished, they—and we—have only just begun. In the words of the evolutionary biologist David Sloan Wilson whose work will feature prominently in the final three chapters, the most I can say is that they have created tiny islands that together form a scattered archipelago of social change initiatives in a vast ocean of problems.

That's why I will be asking you to join them and me in creating new "islands," adding "landfill" to the ones that already exist, and building "bridges" to connect them all across that "ocean." If we do that, we can turn what are now fledgling initiatives into large, unified, and powerful movements that can reshape our troubled country. Sooner rather than later.

That said, I know that making lasting progress on the issues dividing our country will be an uphill struggle. I watch the news. I live and work inside the (in)famous Washington DC beltway. In other words, I'm under no illusion that success will come easily.

We face daunting challenges that demand the best from all of us, including you and the people you know. Therefore, my book-long invitation will include plenty of entry points you can choose from as you find your own "route" to my "party."

At the same time, I'm also enough of a realist to know that I shouldn't ask for your RSVP yet. I will use the rest of this first chapter to outline my case before asking you to decide if, when, or how you will show up to this life-long non-party that I am throwing.

PEACEBUILDING DOES START AT HOME

As is often the case, it took a while before this book "found" its title. Those early days in a book's history are rarely worth mentioning—other than, perhaps, to the author's therapist (who will appear briefly in the pages to come). In this case, however, my original title does tell you a lot about what our journey together will be like.

At first, I wanted to call it *Peace is a Verb*. Of course, I know that peace is a noun, always has been a noun, and will forever be a noun. In every language I know of.

Unless you want to drive what Anne Curzan calls your inner grammarian crazy, you cannot get away with using "to peace" as an infinitive or put your foot down in the middle of an argument and scream that "I peace."[2]

But by adding the helping verb build to peace-as-a-noun, a new world of peace-as-a-verb possibilities open up. Peace becomes something you and I do. And keep doing.

We may never get to peace-as-a-noun, but if you do peace-as-a-verb long enough and well enough, you can make progress, learn from your successes and failures, make more progress, learn some more, and make some more progress. Ad infinitum. Until we get close to creating a society in which most of the people peacefully solve most of their problems most of the time—and you get tired of my (over)using that phrase.

As much as I loved it, that title went out the window one day in January 2024. Liz Hume, the Executive Director of the Alliance for Peacebuilding (AfP) invited my wife, Gretchen Sandles, and me to a

---

2. Anne Curzan. *Says Who?: A Kinder, Funner Usage Guide for Everyone Who Cares About Words*. (New York: Crown, 2024). Her book has *nothing* to do with peacebuilding, but it made me laugh and taught me a lot about writing during the depressing 2024 presidential election campaign.

meeting to help the organization set its priorities for the upcoming year. AfP had been created in 2002 to help American-based peacebuilding NGOs work together. I was asked to join its board of directors in 2005 and remain on it to this day in an emeritus capacity, while also serving as its Senior Fellow for Innovation.

In my twenty years on its board and staff, AfP has become one of the world's leading peacebuilding networks with about two hundred fifty member organizations at work in 181 countries. Early on, just about all of that work took place in those other 180 countries, not the United States. For good or ill, while AfP grew, conditions in the United States kept deteriorating. As early as 2014, it had become clear to our team that existing groups—including AfP's member organizations—were not doing enough to address the problems here at home.

Things did not get any better over the course of the next decade. That led Liz to call that meeting because she knew that AfP would have to up its game with that year's presidential election looming on the horizon. She invited us because she knew that I had completed a very rough first draft of *Peace is a Verb* and wanted me involved in whatever we ended up doing.

Toward the end of the meeting, she threw me for a loop when she suggested that AfP should use peacebuilding starts at home as its tag line for whatever we decided to do in the United States. Liz gladly admitted that peace is a verb would be a great book title or t-shirt logo (I was wearing mine that day). But, she pointed out that it would not be a good phrase to build a movement around. She was right. Before I left the office, I had changed the title so that this book could help build the movement that we decided to create that morning and vice versa, although I did salvage peace is a verb as the title for chapter 4.

By the time I got home, I had fully embraced the new title because I realized that its very words take you quickly and surprisingly deeply into both what this book and our movement are all about—including why you should join us. To see why, consider the four main words in what ended up as my title.

Peace. Spell checkers routinely reject the word peacebuilding. Long before I started this book, I had had to train mine to not insert red squiggly lines whenever I typed p-e-a-c-e-b-u-i-l-d-i-n-g, which I did a lot.

But to show you where this book is heading, I decided to let Microsoft Office declare a (temporary) victory because the two words peace and building lend themselves to different ways forward at this stage in our peacebuilding (or do I mean peace building?) journey together.

Peace is one of our most cherished goals. How can you be against it? Even when we go to war, our leaders tell us that we are fighting in order to restore peace.

Yet, it is also one of our most elusive goals. In the sixty years that I've worked for peace, I've lost track of the number of times that someone has called me a pie-in-the-sky idealist or worse.

Often deservedly so.

Still, I'm convinced that times have changed.

Building. We combined building with peace twenty years ago as we started coming to grips with the most powerful lesson we learned from our work abroad. Successful peacebuilders did more than just end wars. Sure, we have to stop the fighting—in Vietnam in my youth or in Ukraine, Israel/Gaza, or Sudan today.

But we also learned that no troubled society can definitively leave its conflict behind unless and until it addresses all of the issues that gave rise to its troubles in the first place.

And I do mean all of them. It is hard to imagine anything resembling a peaceful United States that hasn't addressed climate change, all forms of inequality, social isolation, the challenges facing senior citizens (like me) or its youth (like my grandchildren).

Adding building to peace also gets us closer to peace-as-a-verb. It turns peace into something I do. Just like a home or office, peace can be built metaphorical brick by metaphorical brick.

Last but by no means least, peace building is a skill that anyone can learn. In places as different as South Africa, East Timor, Northern Ireland, and the Western Sahara, we have worked with people from all walks of life who held all sorts of political opinions and all learned how to do peace.

All of this leads to some obvious questions. Why can't we build peace in the world's strongest and wealthiest country? Where the problems actually aren't as menacing as those faced by people in places like Ukraine, Gaza, Israel, or Sudan? But whose implications ripple around the world until we do something about them?

Starts. I don't want to mislead you. We will always disagree. So will our children and grandchildren. And their children and grandchildren.

All we can do is start building a country and a world in which getting to my three "mosts" becomes the rule rather than the exception. And then keep at it because practice won't make us perfect, but it can make us a lot better.

The first step involves adopting a new kind of strategy which I would not expect you to accept until I have made a lot more of my case. Unlike the social movements of my youth, this one can be built from the inside out. Rather than starting at the extremes as we did in the 1960s, we can start with mainstream America today because just about everyone is frustrated with the status quo. To that end, you will be meeting Rotarians, high school students, therapists, and entrepreneurs—among others—rather than just some version of my generation's counterculture.

At home. As you will see throughout this book, I chose this title because the word "home" has two distinct meanings. Both are at the heart of what I am inviting you to do.

When I was asked to join AfP's board in 2005, I was a lone wolf because I wanted it to work on issues facing the United States, precisely because it was our home country. I didn't get very far until Michael Brown was killed by police officers in Ferguson MO in 2014. Shortly thereafter, we convened a meeting with some of our more prominent members to see if and how what we had learned from our work around the world could help Americans deal with racism and other problems here at home. A number of the organizations represented in the room had offices in Maryland and seemed more than a bit reluctant to add American domestic disputes to their agenda. So, after a frustrating hour or so, I blurted out:

> *How dare we tell people in Burundi or Bosnia or Brazil that we can help them solve their problems if we can't do it in Baltimore?*

Since then, I've asked a version of that question hundreds of times. Wherever I've gone, I've used that city's first letter and the name of a country in the global south that also began with it. It turns out that it works just about everywhere. "Q" is a problem since you have to pair Qatar with Queens which is technically a borough of New York City. My only utter failure is "x." There is no country to go along with Xenia OH.

It didn't take us long to realize that equating home with the entire United States was not going to be enough. We also have to include the word's other meaning—our literal home. Here, I will take home to mean not just the places where you and I live but also our workplaces and neighborhoods as well as the literal homes that we share with our families.

Indeed, if we have learned anything from our decades of work around the world, it is that the most effective peacebuilding efforts start as close to this second meaning of home as possible. It is hard to change countries or even companies unless the people who are their heart and soul change first.

GETTING STARTED: THREE IDEAS AND SOME HOMEWORK

I wrote *Peacebuilding Starts at Home* because I know that the people and organizations you will meet in its pages can't get the job done on their own. They will need people like you to join them.

Not just people like you.

Literally you.

In other words, I want you to do more than nod your head when you agree with what I have to say or shake it when you don't. To help you get beyond the head nodding stage, I've included homework exercises in each chapter that build on the three that I am am about to ask you to do.

Having written more than my share of college textbooks in political science and peacebuilding, I know that readers rarely do assignments like these. I also have to confess that I usually skip them when they appear in books that I am reading.

In this case, please do what I say, not what I do.

For once, it will be worth it.

I have done my best to make the exercises short, fun, and provocative. More importantly, if you do them all, you will have developed not just your own personal peacebuilding agenda but you will also have outlined a strategy for building peace here at home in all senses of that term by the time you finish chapter 8.

Each assignment in this chapter takes off from short videos which do not explicitly deal with peacebuilding. Nonetheless, each blew me away and left me asking all sorts of difficult questions about what peace-as-a-noun and peacebuilding-as-a-verb were all about. Answering them helped me write this book. As you do them, you will also, *de facto*, begin RSVPing to my invitation.

I've included transcripts of each of them. However, they are far more inspiring if you watch the original video. If you are reading *Peacebuilding Starts at Home* electronically, clicking on each title will take you to its YouTube page. If you are reading the old-fashioned way, you will have to retype the link which is in the footnote that appears at the end of the relevant sentence. Or search for it yourself.

The homework assignments should not take you more than ten minutes each. You will find them in boxes at the end of the sections on each of the three videos. Each subsequent chapter will have versions of each of them designed to deepen your understanding and clarify the ways you can contribute to peacebuilding at home yourself. Hold on to them, because you will keep adding to your responses when you get to the exercises in the chapters to come.

If you do them, I'll be glad to react to (but not grade) your responses. You can begin handing them in when you send me your RSVP at the end of this chapter.

America reMADE. The polls don't lie. More Americans are more disappointed with their leaders than they have been at any time since the first public opinion surveys were conducted in the 1930s. There is also next to no chance that we can turn things around unless most of us unite around a credible alternative to the status quo.

As the corporate world keeps reminding us, simply having a mission statement does not guarantee success. You also have to have a goal or North Star to head toward which you could get close to reasonably soon, even if what I mean by the words "goal" and "soon" remain more than a bit fuzzy at this point.

I spent years looking for such a statement that might galvanize potential peacebuilders but nothing quite clicked. Then, in late 2023, Gretchen and I attended a discussion led by Kelly Corrigan who, by the way, gave me the second assignment. We were put in a breakout room with Lily Spencer who told us about the project she then worked for, Australia reMADE. We had never heard of it but we decided to check it out, if for no other reason than we liked Lily and wanted to get to know her better.

It turns out that the organization had an origin story that I could relate to. Like the United States, Australia has had more than its share of protest movements that call for sweeping change on specific issues. By the late 2010s, some of their leaders had come to the conclusion that they weren't connecting with enough average Australians.

So, they decided to do something that might seem obvious in retrospect, but was a radical departure at the time. They went on a listening tour to find out what average Australians wanted their country to be like.

A single common denominator quickly popped out of their data. The vast majority of Australians want to live in a country in which everybody thrives. What's more, most of them had at least an inkling that all of the individual issues that activists worked on were interconnected.

Once they had digested all of the transcripts from all of the meetings, they turned what they had learned into a compelling short video about an ordinary paradise that just about all of the Australians they met wanted to live in.[3]

---

3. https://www.youtube.com/watch?v=dm8GR2soFGE&t=18s (Accessed June 4, 2023.)

Imagine waking up in the country of your dreams.
What is it like? This place?
What does it look like?
Feel like?
Because we've been through an awful lot lately.
And we think it's time to ask, "who are we now?"
What do we want for ourselves? Our future? Our families? Our whole country?
What do we want to see more of in the world?
What sort of legacy do we want to leave?
There is a power in ideas. We get to ask. To challenge. To renegotiate.
Dreaming itself propels us forward.
We get to focus on what we do want.
Not just what we don't want.
When we do, we realize that deep down, we all basically want the same thing.
This country that we dream of, this ordinary paradise.
It's entirely possible. Common sense, even.
We start by naming it.
In order to remake it.
Dream big. Start here.

That led them to create Australia reMADE which now serves as an umbrella organization that builds support for social change that would make the country look more like that ordinary paradise. Lily served as its communications director until mid-2024 when she moved on to create her own progressive media company.

Make no mistake. Lily and her colleagues are not happy with their country's leaders and their policies. Still, the video they made is a vivid, constructive depiction of what a new Australia could look like which average Australians could rally around. To use another line that I have already introduced and will return to repeatedly, it focuses on what they are for, not what they are against.

Peacebuilding Starts at Home, of course, is about the United States, not Australia. Once again, Lily came to the rescue. It turns out that she was born and raised here, decided to go to college in Australia, and never left. She had already shown the video to her American friends and relatives who wanted to learn what she was up to. They had loved it.

So, I started showing it to other Americans. They loved it, too, and had no trouble realizing that it would be terrific if we could create an America reMADE of our own.

Later rather than sooner, it dawned on me that the video and its vision had to be part of both Peacebuilding Starts at Home, the movement, and *Peacebuilding Starts at Home,* the book.

So, imagine how you would react if it had an American narrator? Wouldn't she be describing an ordinary paradise that most Americans would love to live in or work for?

EXERCISE 1.1: AMERICA REMADE

I assume that you don't have either the time or the money to conduct the kind of listening tour that Australia reMADE went on or make a video as compelling as this one.

However, you can use their video as a jumping off point for building your own vision of an America reMADE that could serve as a launching pad for peacebuilding here at home. So, take no more than ten minutes and jot down some features of your own ordinary paradise. Who are we now? Who could or should we be, given the fact that we've been through a lot lately? Once you've done that, dream big.

Nailing it. I want you to do more than just dream. I want you to get out of your chair and do something. And keep doing it until things do change.

Here, too, I stumbled across a video. On April 29, 2020, Gretchen and I sat down to watch the PBS NewsHour.[4] We were about six weeks into the pandemic. Almost everything had shut down, and almost everyone was depressed—or worse. Just before the end of the broadcast, Judy Woodruff announced that Kelly Corrigan would give her humble opinion on what a post-COVID world might be like if we had nailed it.[5]

I am not a fan of the Humble Opinion segments and had never heard of Corrigan. But since we were stuck at home, I resisted the temptation to change the channel or hit the mute button. Within seconds, I was transfixed because she spoke about how to turn lofty dreams like Australia reMADE's into action.

> KELLY CORRIGAN: *Sometimes, when I feel outmatched by the thing in front of me, I do a little mental exercise.*
> *I tell myself the story of what happened, as if it's over and I nailed it.*
> *This morning, I waited for 54 minutes to check out from the Safeway. The woman behind me, whose hair and makeup were perfect, had seven bottles of Martini & Rossi Vermouth. That's it.*
> *And the guy in front of her had a full-face double ventilator gas mask. And I felt outmatched by the thing in front of me.*
> *So, right there, I told myself the story of the 2020 pandemic and how we nailed it.*
> *My success fantasy went like this. At first, it was awful, nothing but bad news on top of bad news. But then we rose up. We made soups and stews for old people and dropped them off, so they felt included and secure and nourished.*
> *We read books to children over the Internet. We stepped outside at the end of the day and played music and clapped, so that each of us knew we were not alone.*

---

4. PBS aficionados will know the show was known as the PBS NewsHour without a space between news and hour at the time. It became the News Hour with a space when it moved into a new studio in 2024.

5. https://www.youtube.com/watch?v=BJCs89wQXrA (Accessed October 25, 2023.)

We sent pizzas and Chinese food to ERs to sustain both our hospitals and our restaurants.

We called old friends and told them things we'd forgotten to say: I miss you. I still think of you. Remember that time?

We turned up, all of us, on our screens to keep businesses afloat. And in so doing, we're exposed to the more tender elements of our colleagues' lives. Pets and children were now, to our mutual benefit, in the frame.

People figured out they don't need fancy equipment to exercise. We stopped flying around and jumping in cars for no reason. Everyone planted things they could eat. We played cards with our families. We had long conversations.

We identified what kind of learning can be delivered online. We discovered that teaching is the most complex, high-impact profession known to man, and we started compensating our teachers fairly for their irreplaceable work.

Everyone voted after coronavirus. Kids who lived through the virus valued science above all. They became researchers and doctors, kicking off the greatest period of world positive discovery and innovation the planet has ever seen.

We came, finally and forever, to appreciate the profound fact of our shared humanity and relish the full force of our love for one another.

JUDY WOODRUFF: Thank you, Kelly Corrigan. And wouldn't it be wonderful if all of that came true?

George Floyd was still alive when the segment aired. We hadn't yet sunk to the polarized depths that culminated in that fall's election, the insurrection on January 6, 2021, and everything that has happened since. Even as conditions worsened, I found myself wanting to make my own peacebuilder's version of what had happened as if it's over. And we had nailed it.

EXERCISE 1.2: NAILING IT

You can't make your own version of this video either.

But you can do the mental exercise that Corrigan put herself through at the Safeway that morning. Don't do it about the pandemic unless it still touches your life. Rather, pick something else that keeps you up at night. It doesn't have to be a big global issue; it can be something that has your community or your family stuck in a rut. Then, think about what it would take for you to nail it. That could be something(s) that you do on your own. And/or with others. And/or something done wholly by others. As with the first exercise, take no more than ten minutes and jot down what comes to mind when you think about nailing it. As with the America reMADE exercise, hold on to what you came up with.

A lunch pail f***king job. The journey I want you to go on will have to start with small and simple steps that you can can dream up in your equivalent of Corrigan's Safeway moment. At the same time, I also know that I am inviting you to start what will be a long and convoluted trek.

That was driven home by one last video—the monologue Jon Stewart delivered when he returned to the Daily Show in February 2024.[6] The first nineteen minutes are typical Stewart which I enjoyed but weren't insightful or funny enough to include here.

Then, in the last two minutes, he got dead serious as he set the stage for the upcoming election campaign.

> *You're gonna get inundated with robocalls, and push polls, and real polls, and people are gonna tell you to rock the vote, and be the vote, and vote the vote, and finger-bang the vote, and it's all going*

---

6. https://youtu.be/NpBPm0b9deQ?si=xXKEEXdSphXZiwfh (Accessed January 22, 2025.)

to make you feel like Tuesday, November 5 is the only day that matters.

And that day does matter, but man, November 6 ain't nothing to sneeze at, or November 7. If your guy loses bad things might happen, but the country is not over, and if your guy wins, the country is in no way saved.

The work of making this world resemble one that you would prefer to live in is a lunch pail f***ing job, day in and day out, where thousands of committed, anonymous, smart and dedicated people bang on closed doors and pick up those that are fallen and grind away on issues until they get a positive result, and even then have to stay on to make sure that result holds.

EXERCISE 1.3: A LUNCH-PAIL F**KLING JOB

Like me, you may not know exactly what Stewart had in mind when he talked about "a lunch-pail f***king job."

Still, I was drawn to this video because I agree that nailing your version of America reMADE will be one, whatever Stewart actually meant.

So, take about as much time as you did with each of the first two exercises and sketch out what it would take to complete your version of his task.

Don't worry about the specifics of how we'll get it done. We'll get there. For now, it's enough for you to sketch out a basic strategy that you—and the rest of us—could follow.

OUR JOURNEY TOGETHER

You can think of the rest of this book as a general strategy for peacebuilding here at home that will also let you find your own pathway onto our journey together. When corporate and military leaders talk about strategy, they do not have a detailed step-by-step plan for reaching a specific goal in mind.[7] That's OK. As you will see in the next chapter, the world is too complex and too fluid for anyone to develop any such plan that has any chance of succeeding.

Instead, think of this as a general strategy or overarching framework for pulling off a paradigm shift in the way Americans deal with each other which I will develop through the Peacebuilding Starts at Home Loop, a version of which will appear in the chapters to come. Each step will build off the one that came before it and lead to the one that comes next with as few flashbacks and flash-forwards as possible. And, to use a term I used earlier and will also keep coming back to, it is the scaffolding that provides the framework and only the framework around which a peace "building" can be constructed.

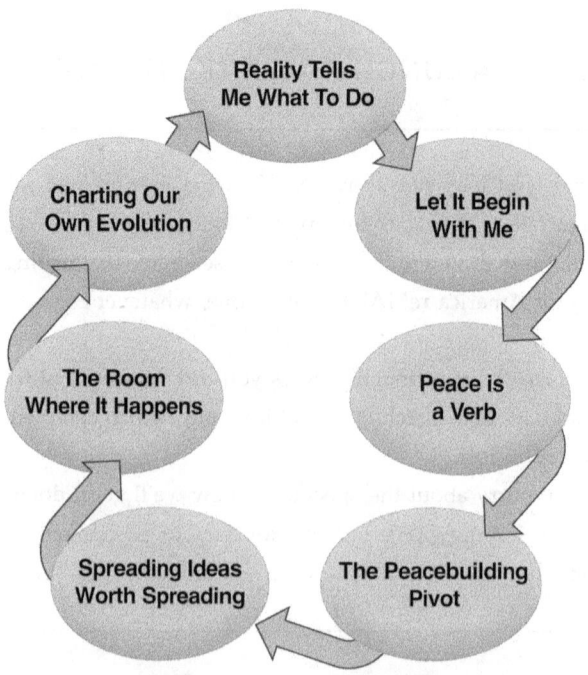

Figure 1.1: The Peacebuilding Starts at Home Loop

---

7. Seth Godin, *This is Strategy*. (New York: Authors Equity, 2024).

My colleagues and I are asking you to do something that has never been done before because it has never been possible to do it before for reasons that I will begin laying out in the next chapter. I can't guarantee that we will succeed. All I can say with any degree of certainty is that a paradigm shift that enables most of us to solve most of our problems peacefully most of the time is possible.

I also know that the Alliance for Peacebuilding and its partners will not be able to make it happen on their own. Although I've dedicated the last twenty years of my life and a good bit of my money (including the royalties from this book) to AfP, I will be the first to admit that we don't have all the answers. So, I will spend the bulk of my time exploring work that others are doing. It should already be clear that I will take you far beyond most conventional understandings of what peace and peacebuilding are all about, which is why I included people like Daryl Davis, John Mackey, and John Hunter.

And, as is the case with any loop, you won't be done with it after you've finished this book and cycled through the whole thing once. Instead, like me, you will find yourself regularly repeating your "trip" around its circuit. If I'm right, as more and more Americans work their way through some version of this loop, we will come close to pulling off a paradigm shift.

IT'S RSVP TIME

Every non-fiction author knows that it is a bad idea to ignore a chapter's title and epigraph until the end. I couldn't avoid doing so here, because you had to read something like the first eighteen pages before either statement might make sense.

Robert Putnam. Start with the epigraph. Gretchen and I had taken a course from Robert Putnam when we were PhD students and he was a young political science professor at the University of Michigan. At the time, I was getting ready to do my doctoral thesis on the new left in France and wasn't thinking in terms of peacebuilding now that the Vietnam war was winding down. Putnam was putting the finishing touches on a pair of books on political elites. It would be another decade before he got interested in the social conditions that sustain democracy, which led to his most famous book, *Bowling Alone*.[8]

As is often the case with former professors and their students, Bob, Gretchen, and I occasionally saw each other at political science meetings at which we mostly smiled at each other and engaged in professional chit chat. In the last twenty years, however, we ended up spending more time together after I started working on peacebuilding here at home. By that point, he was already a rock star whose opinions about making democracy work were sought by leaders on both sides of the Atlantic.[9]

In 2022, a mutual friend introduced Gretchen and me to Pete Davis, who lived in the same small suburban town that we do. Although that wasn't why our friend wanted us to meet, we quickly learned that Pete had been in Bob's last undergraduate seminar at Harvard and was finishing a documentary on his work, *Join or Die*, which is now available on Netflix and I will feature in chapter 6.[10]

Pete invited us to the film's DC premier in October 2023. Because we had seen several versions of the rough cut, we only decided to go because Bob was going to be there to help facilitate a discussion after the screening.

At the end of the Q and A, Bob stood in front of the crowd of Georgetown students and uttered the words that begin this chapter. "The future of our country is in your hands."

I wrote them down because it was obvious that they would help frame what became this entire book. Then, I looked around me. Most of the people in the audience were nodding in agreement. As everyone was filing out of the auditorium, I asked a few of the head nodders if they were doing anything to actually put the future of our country in

---

8. Robert Putnam, *Bowling Alone: The Collapse and Revival of American Community*. (New York: Simon and Schuster, 2000).
9. I chose these exact words because they are the title of a book Bob wrote on democracy in Italy in the 1990s that actually goes a lot farther than any of his later books on the United States. Robert Putnam, *Making Democracy Work: Civic Traditions in Modern Italy*. (Princeton: Princeton University Press, 1994).
10. www.joinordiefilm.com (Accessed September 3, 2024).

their own hands. Most shrugged their shoulders and said something like "why bother" or "what's the use?"

They are not alone. Many—maybe most—Americans have drawn a powerful but paralyzing lesson from the stories that fill their news feeds. They have convinced themselves that average everyday people can't make much of a difference.

On one level, I agree. None of us can (re)shape the future of our country on our own. Or overnight. Or easily.

But do take Bob's version of my invitation seriously. As you will also see, you don't really have a choice.

Start where you are. Then there is this chapter's title. All authors of a book like this one face a dilemma. We write our books because we want our readers to get involved. Yet, as authors, we don't know anything about them, including you.

While the RSVP will give us an opportunity to meet each other and for me to help you figure out which on-ramps work best for you, all I can do at this point is to try to write for anyone and everyone who picks up a copy of *Peacebuilding Starts at Home*. Luckily, I stumbled across the expression "start where you are" and realized that it is the best single piece of advice that I could possibly give to readers I know nothing about.

No one knows for sure where the phrase comes from. I first encountered it as the title of a best selling book by Pema Chödrön.[11] As a Buddhist nun, her understanding of the world starts with the assumption that what is happening today is the only reality that we can influence. That isn't to say that history or therapy or anything else that helps us understand the past is irrelevant.

But Chödrön (and your therapist) got one thing right. You may not like the world we live in. I certainly don't. However, ruminating on the past alone will never make things better.

Besides, when you get right down to it, all you can really change is yourself. Starting where you are. Your impact can ripple out into your

---

11. Pema Chödrön, *Start Where You Are: A Guide to Passionate Living*. (Boston: Shambhala Press, 2001).

household and beyond until it reaches the "rooms where it happens." But it starts at home. And it starts now.

I am not one of those peace activists who claim that we can change the world if we just meditate long and hard enough. Nonetheless, as you will see, I am convinced that peacebuilders are at their best when they become as self-aware as possible and they act in ways that make sense given their immediate environment, which for most of us means our home, our community, and our workplace. In other words, everything else we do—including supporting an organization like AfP or any of those others you will meet—works best when and if we all start where we are.

It's time to RSVP. On p. 1, I said that I would give you until the end of this chapter before asking you to RSVP. Well, here we are.

I wanted to wait this long so that you could see more about "the ask" and could make an informed decision about whether or not to take me up on my offer to do peacebuilding at home, become part of our growing team, learn a lot, enjoy yourself (because peacebuilding can be fun), and help change the world.

The easiest way to "come on board" (and send me your homework) is to send me an email at hauss@allianceforpeacebuilding.org. You can also get in touch with me and the AfP team through this book's website, www.peacebuildingstartsathome.us.

Whichever you choose, someone will get back to you within a day or so. Meanwhile, you can explore the issues covered in these pages in more detail and see that we intend each to be a one stop shop that can help you find your own on-ramp toward building peace here at home, however you choose to define it. More importantly, because AfP will be a hub for the Peacebuilding Starts at Home initiatives that I will be describing, we will serve as a kind of digital help desk that can connect everyone who gets in touch with us to peacebuilding projects that fit their interests, skills, location and needs.

Actually, If you really want to, you can procrastinate. You can keep reading and come on board at any point.

But remember that in my teaching days, I took a third of a letter grade off per day if students handed in any assignment late.

CHAPTER 2
REALITY TELLS ME WHAT TO DO

The real voyage of discovery comes not in seeking new lands but in seeing with new eyes.

MARCEL PROUST

I was tempted to leap right into a discussion of those "islands" in the peacebuilding "archipelago" here at home. That's what excites me. I also assumed you would be eager to learn about peacebuilding options that you could explore.

Before we get there, however, I want you to think through some big ideas, but not because I'm a recovering academic who loves theory. Rather, coming to grips with concepts like interdependence, complexity, the accelerating rate of change, and systems thinking will help you see that there is a mismatch between the problems we face and the tools we try to solve them with, while also showing you that we need to do more than just tinker with the status quo.

As a result, your trip along the Peacebuilding Starts at Home Loop has to start with those general concepts as viewed through the lens of this chapter's title and epigraph which I will use to start rather than end it with.

That said, I doubt either of them made sense to you.

What does it mean for reality to tell me what to do? Why should you pay any attention to a quote from a French novelist whose work is all but impenetrable? How could either of them help us build peace?

Trust me.

They do.

Both are filled with implications for how we could and should build peace here at home. By the end of this chapter, it should become clear that seeing the troubling realities of life in the 2020s through Proust's "new eyes" points us toward concrete steps that I will spell out in the six chapters to come.

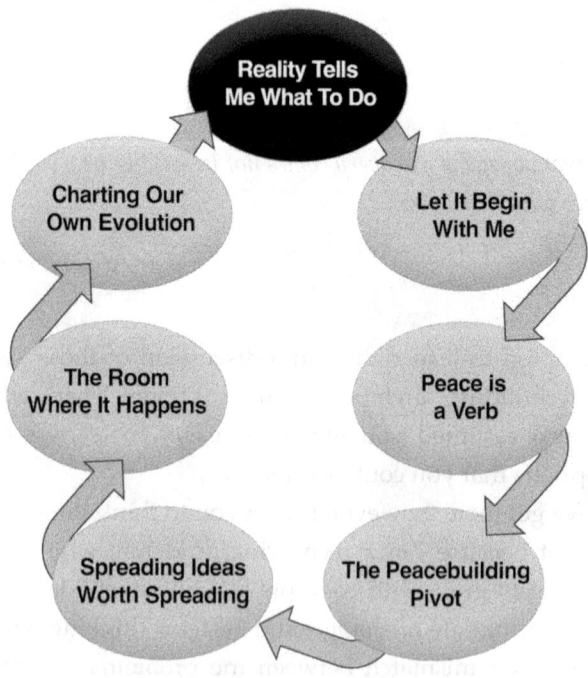

Figure 2.1: The Peacebuilding Starts at Home Loop

A STRANGE INVITATION

I first encountered both the title and epigraph at the 1987 Beyond War national leadership seminar that was held at its lovely retreat center in the foothills overlooking Santa Cruz CA. Beyond War itself is long gone. Someone else owns the retreat center.

Still, that seminar started me on what has been a forty-year-long journey that redefined what peace meant to me and ultimately led to this book. To use the phrase I now use as the title of my Substack, I came to see the value of connecting the dots in new and far more productive ways because seeing the world through broader, Proustean eyes made a huge difference in my life.

But I'm getting ahead of myself.

When the 1980s began, I could not have imagined being at a leadership workshop on anything to do with peace. I had spent the second half of the 1970s establishing my academic career. Activism was not on my personal or professional agenda. On those rare occasions when I looked for a way to rekindle the political commitments of my student days, I assumed it would be as an environmentalist.

Then, an utterly unpredictable chain of events changed my life. I had just gotten tenure at Colby College and was beginning to think about the rest of my career, including how the next phase of my research could address social and political paradigm shifts. I was on sabbatical when the college decided that the next fall's freshmen would read Jonathan Schell's *The Fate of the Earth* as part of the orientation program in 1983.[1] Unexpectedly, the head of the planning committee had to go on medical leave, and the president of the college asked me to step in. Although I would never have chosen Schell's book, I agreed.

The job seemed easy enough. Call Schell and offer him a few thousand dollars to come to campus, give a talk to the incoming class, and meet with interested students. I would organize faculty-led discussion groups that all freshmen would attend right after his presentation.

It got complicated when I finally scrunched up the courage to call Schell. He said something like, "I write books. I don't give talks." All of a sudden, my simple task wasn't so simple after all. I had a pile of money and no speaker. So, on the spur of the moment and undoubtedly with some panic in my voice, I asked Schell what he would do if

---

1. Jonathan Schell, *The Fate of the Earth*. (New York: Knopf, 1982).

he were in my shoes. He suggested using the money to bring a series of less expensive speakers to campus during the course of the academic year for talks that would be open to the entire Colby community, which is what I did.

One day early in the spring semester, a colleague in the physics department asked me to invite a couple who had just moved to Maine to get the Beyond War movement off the ground in northern New England. My first reaction was "no, who needs another peace movement." But Gene and Donna Richeson were willing to come to campus for free and take me out for dinner, too.

So, I agreed.

And learned that the cliché that there is no such thing as a free lunch (or dinner) was true.

Minutes after they arrived at my office, my doubts began melting away. It turns out that Gene Richeson had designed the payload for the first geosynchronous satellite when he was in graduate school. Then, he founded ROLM, the first successful digital telecommunications company, which IBM had just bought for $1.5 billion—an astronomical (pun intended) sum in those days. He and Donna had decided to move to Maine at their own expense to volunteer full time for Beyond War for at least two years.

As someone who had used computers a lot in college and grad school and was helping Colby figure out how to enter the world of personal computing, I was fascinated. As a veteran of the 1960s new left, however, Silicon Valley or the corporate world in general had never crossed my mind as a place to find peace activists or as a home for political movements that focused on self-awareness and taking personal responsibility for social change. Any lingering skepticism turned to curiosity when Gene took my office telephone apart to see if it had any of the state of the art switching devices that his company made. We did not.

By the time we left for dinner, I was hooked.

Beyond War appealed to me precisely because it wasn't a conventional peace movement, many of which seemed overly committed to the kind of new left politics that was running out of steam even for people like me who had built its powerful but evaporating protest movements. It had been created earlier that decade as an outgrowth of Creative Initiative, a spiritually based movement that helped its members take charge of their everyday lives. At the heart of its curriculum were core principles that aided participants in putting the issues of the day, like renewed tensions between superpowers, in the broadest possible perspective.

Fast forward to 1987. I had begun teaching courses in peace studies and was spending as much time as I could leading Beyond War's efforts in Maine. We held regular "orientations to a world beyond war" in people's living rooms and gave talks to local service organizations. We also organized flashy public events, including "space bridges" in which we used the then-radical satellite television technology to convene people around the world for our annual awards ceremony.

Because there weren't many social scientists in its ranks, I had already been asked to spend 1988 on its national leadership team while on my second sabbatical. I would spend the year getting Beyond War established on campuses and write a book about the movement.

So, I was not surprised when I found an invitation to its national leadership seminar in my inbox one morning.[2] In fact, if I hadn't had an unusually heavy teaching schedule that semester, I would have been on the team that organized it.

I *was* surprised to discover that it came with a six-word agenda—reality tells me what to do.

That was it.

I snickered after I read and reread the message, wondering how we could spend an entire weekend exploring something that seemed so obvious.

I snickered some more when I walked into the room and saw Proust's sentence on a flip chart. At the time, I did my academic research on French politics. As a budding Francophile, I had bought Proust's seven volume novel, *Remembrance of Things Past*, in both French and English. I knew I should read it. It was a classic. I was an

---

2. If you are of a certain age and know anything about the Internet, you might have doubts about using email in 1987. It was rare but was widely used in some circles even before the Internet as we know it today was created. Both Beyond War and Colby College were early adopters of email and other online technologies.

intellectual. Yet, I had never made it past page five in the first volume in either language because I couldn't follow either his prose or his plot line.

I stopped snickering as soon as the facilitators explained what we would be doing over the weekend.

As they saw things, Beyond War had to rethink its mission now that Cold War tensions were fading. None of them expected the superpower rivalry to end before the decade was over. Nonetheless, they knew that Beyond War would no longer be able to center its pitch solely on the threat of nuclear war. It would have to pivot. The national leadership wanted the organization's most active local activists to use the weekend to take a step back from the issues of the day, revisit the organization's roots, and see the "reality" of our work by defining our version of Proust's "new eyes."

Far from wasting my time, the weekend gave me a title and a tagline that I refer to any time when my colleagues or I need to pivot.

Like now.

PROUST'S EYES

Since then, I've been to dozens of workshops and read dozens of books that have used Proust's statement. None of them bothered to track down the original—presumably because they didn't have the patience to read his novels either. Because my copy editor is a stickler for accuracy, I knew I would have to be able to provide her with a source.

So, I tracked it down and learned that it appears in the middle of volume 5, *The Captive*.[3] In good Proustean fashion, the original sentence is more ornate and convoluted than the poorly translated version that has become a fixture at corporate retreats. Since the original statement is also more telling for the purposes of this book, I've included it here—with my translation.

---

3. At least in the Vintage translation which still sits unread on my bookshelf. For what it's worth, I use Ecosia as my search engine. It uses the revenue it gets from ad sales to plant trees and combat climate change.

> *Le seul véritable voyage, le seul bain de Jouvence, ce ne serait pas d'aller vers de nouveaux paysages, mais d'avoir d'autres yeux, de voir l'univers avec les yeux d'un autre, de cent autres, de voir les cent univers que chacun d'eux voit, que chacun d'eux est.*
>
> *The only real voyage, the only bath in the Fountain of Youth, will not come from seeking new lands, but from using new eyes to see the universe, from seeing that universe through another's eyes, from hundreds of others' eyes and from seeing the hundreds of universes that each of them sees, that each of them is.*

As Proust (probably) saw things, the value of any journey—including ours toward peacebuilding in the United States—does not lie in the physical roads it takes you down. Rather, as his repeated use of the words eyes and see attests, it's how you interpret what you encounter along the way that matters. And what you learn from what others see as they travel down the same roads and take the same pathways. Even the phrase *nouveau paysages* is worth noting, because it is best translated as new landscapes rather than new lands—at least if by lands you mean something like modern nation states.

Interdependence. The Beyond War team chose that particular sentence because they wanted us to use our new eyes as we grappled with two social and economic trends—interdependence and change. Both were inching their way into our lives, and the seminar organizers assumed that they would only become more important in the years to come in ways that we would have to take into account in our work in the post-Cold War world.

They were right. Even then, the often abstract trends we dealt with that weekend became the scaffolding around which I developed much of my approach to peacebuilding. If anything, those developments matter even more today because that new understanding of reality we explored still tells us what to do.

As the Beyond War team saw it, the threat of nuclear war was just the clichéd tip of a clichéd iceberg. Most of the other issues we faced at the time also had global implications. Some came with dangers like the threat of nuclear war while others brought opportunities for more international cooperation—as was the case with the Montreal Protocol to protect the ozone layer, which was approved a few months after we met.

Not many people used the term globalization in those days. Instead, we spoke of interdependence and the fact that our lives were increasingly intertwined. In the seminars and workshops that we hosted around the country, we asked participants to take the simple statement "we are one" seriously and then deal with the fact that we rarely act as if it were true. The two hundred volunteers who made it to California that weekend took a much deeper dive into those interconnections, their implications, and the fact that next to no one acted as if that was the case.

Interdependence may have been an outside-of-the-box idea in 1987, but it is all but a truism today, albeit a controversial one. My point here is not to make the case that globalization and interdependence are either a blessing or a curse as they are so often portrayed in political campaigns. They are simply a fact of life.

We can see glimpses of how interdependent our world has become in the spread of the Internet, cell phones, or even the popularity of the NBA. We may not be within six degrees of separation of everyone on the planet as the meme about the actor Kevin Bacon would have it. Still, we are directly or indirectly tied to growing numbers of people and all living systems around the world. The fact that those links exist also means that the impact of our actions ripples out in ways our grandparents could never have imagined.

We also decided that it was time to emphasize the lessons we drew from a video that was already included in our orientation curriculum. *No Frames/No Boundaries* features words spoken by Russell Schweickart to describe how he felt when he was the first Apollo astronaut to go on a space walk.[4] We watched it again that weekend. This time, we figured out how to use it to help the people we met reconsider its implications for a world that no longer had the threat of a nuclear holocaust at the top of its collective agenda.

The only version of the video that I could find online is a grainy

---

4. https://www.youtube.com/watch?v=7y7O_9WB3ZU. Accessed, January 4, 2025.

copy of the original VHS cassette. Nonetheless, its message comes through more clearly there than it does in this transcript.

> *You go around it in an hour and a half and you begin to recognize that your identity is with that whole. And that makes a change. You look out and you can't imagine how many borders and boundaries you have crossed. Again and again and again. And you don't even see 'em. And you see it. This thing as a whole. It's so beautiful. You recall standing out there looking at the spectacle right there before your eyes. Because you're no longer inside something with a window looking out at a picture. Now you're out there. There are no limits. There are no frames. There are no boundaries.*
>
> *And you think about what you are experiencing and why. Do you deserve this? Are you separated out here to have some experience here that other men can't have? <u>The answer to that is no.</u> You know very well at that moment, it comes through to you so palpably, that you are the sensing element for man.*

That is not how most Americans thought about interdependence then. But what if we think about it this way today?

EXERCISE 2.1: AMERICA REMADE (FROM SPACE)

No one reading *Peacebuilding Starts at Home* is likely to see the earth from space the way that Rusty Schweickart did. You can, however, repeat what the attendees at our retreat were asked to do.

You can visualize what an earth—or a United States—would be like if we acted as if there were no frames and there were no boundaries.

In short, take another five to ten minutes and update your vision of an ordinary paradise once you have thought about the world as a single, interdependent whole.

The challenge of change. The weekend's organizers also encouraged us to zoom out and put the problems of the 1980s in a broader perspective as Creative Initiative had done before it launched Beyond War. We were asked to think of history as a succession of crises which humanity had overcome because our ancestors met what it called the challenge of change.

That story began not with the world of Silicon Valley tech companies where most of them worked but with something Heraclitus allegedly said some 2,500 years ago. Change is the only constant.

There is no way of knowing if his words were accurate when he made that statement. They certainly are today.

We live in a time of rapid and accelerating change. Technology. Culture. Globalization. Travel. Fashion. The arts.

Given Beyond War's roots in Silicon Valley, we explored change-is-the-only-constant through a technology lens that weekend. At a time when personal computers were still rare and the Internet as we now know it today did not exist, their use of Moore's Law took most of us at the workshop by surprise.

In 1965, Gordon Moore was the founding CEO of Intel and thus preoccupied with computer chips. As he tried to make sense of his rapidly growing industry, he realized that engineers had been able to double the number of semiconductors that fit on a computer chip while cutting the cost of making them in half every eighteen months. He also predicted that those trends would continue indefinitely, which held true beyond his death in 2023 and shows no sign of ending any time soon.

The two halves of Moore's Law can be expressed mathematically in the exponential functions, $n=x^2$ (speed) and $n=x^{-2}$ (cost), respectively. If you remember your high school algebra, the graph of any exponential curve builds slowly until it reaches what Malcolm Gladwell famously called a tipping point and then takes off as depicted below.[5] Because

---

5. Malcolm Gladwell. *The Tipping Point: How Little Things Can Make a Big Difference.* (New York: Little Brown, 2000). See also his updated reconsideration of the idea which I found even more fascinating because his argument was more nuanced. Malcolm Glad-

Moore's law has 2 as the exponent, it yields this series when taken to the fifteenth power—2, 4, 8, 16, 32, 64, 128, 256, 512, 1024, 2048, 4096, 8192, 16,394, 32,768, 65,584. If the exponent is larger than 2, the growth is even more stunning. Taking three to the fifteenth power yields 14,348,907. Ten to the fifteenth power is a lot easier to calculate but a lot harder to get your intellectual arms around—1,000,000,000,000,000.[6]

That is not how most Americans thought about interdependence or the rate of change then.

But what if we think about them this way today?

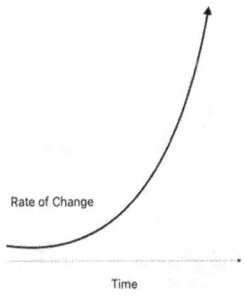

Figure 2.2: Exponential Change

Combining the two—with telephones. We also discussed a second law from the tech world that helped us see how interdependence and accelerating change feed off each other. The more interdependent the world becomes, the more rapidly it changes. Exponentially again.

Robert Metcalfe is not as well-known as Gordon Moore, but that doesn't make his insight any less eye-opening. Shortly after finishing his PhD in computer science in 1973, he took a job at Xerox's famous Palo Alto Research Center (PARC) which produced many of the technological breakthroughs that made modern computing and the internet possible. Within months of arriving in Silicon Valley, he had

---

well. *The Revenge of the Tipping Point: Overstories, Superspreaders, and the Rise of Social Engineering.* (New York: Little, Brown 2024).

6. If you are tempted to experiment with other examples, you don't have to do the calculations by hand. There are dozens of websites that will do them for you.

co-invented ethernet which many of us still use to connect electronic devices in our homes and offices. By 1980, he had founded a telecommunications company and developed his own "law" about how networks grow. Given where and when he worked, Metcalfe's law is usually presented using pictures of rotary telephones in a network connected by physical wires, which were all we had in those days.

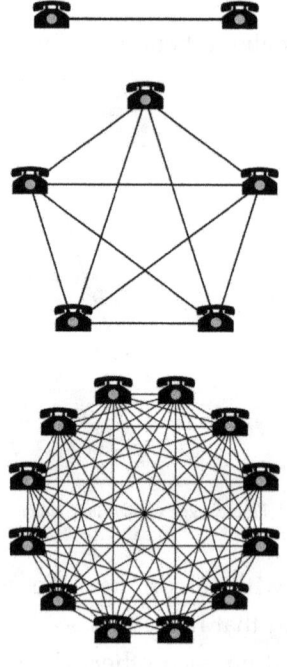

Figure 2.3: Metcalfe's Law

If you are in a network with two telephones, you can only talk to the person at the other end of the line. But, if you add four more phones, ten different conversations can take place (three-way calls were not an option in those days).

Now, if you add five more phones for a total of ten, the number skyrockets to forty-five following the formula:

$$N=n(n-1)/2$$

where N is the number of possible connections and n is the number of telephones. This equation yields a graph that is all but identical with the one for Moore's law.

Obviously, no one on any network ever talks to everyone in their orbit. Nonetheless, the number of real-world connections has grown exponentially, although perhaps not as smoothly as figure 2.2 might suggest.

And remember that Metcalfe's Law applies to any network, not just those involving today's smart phones. Just think about how quickly the COVID-19 virus spread in 2020.

That is not how most Americans thought about interdependence and networks then.

But what if we think about it this way today?

PROUST'S EYES MEET REALITY

Think again about the two sentences you just read—which I used three times in the previous section. To put it in the bluntest possible terms, we haven't adjusted our Proustean eyes so that we can see and begin to figure out how to react to those stark new realities.

We didn't get very far in doing so that weekend either. It wasn't completely our fault, because the points I make in this section had not made their way into what even a group of highly educated thought leaders could have been expected to be familiar with. While some of us knew a bit about systems theory, only a handful of cutting-edge scientists were thinking in terms of either complexity science or wicked problems at the time. Now, we can take those three ideas together as a set of Proustean trifocal lenses that could "adjust our vision" to those realities and then help us change the world.

Systems theory. Until surprisingly recently, most scientists assumed that they learned the most by breaking any phenomenon down into its component parts. They focused on the micro level, such as the individual voter in political science, firm in economics, or cell in biology. Meanwhile, the way the overall government, economy, or organism functions tended to get short shrift.

In the late 1920s, a handful of scientific outliers started paying more attention to the macro side of things. The Austrian biologist Ludwig van Betalanffy, for example, made the case that any living thing is an interconnected whole whose component parts directly or indirectly affect the entire organism. Then, during World War II, weapons designers added feedback to the loop—at which point modern systems theory was born.[7]

By the time we met in California, the word ecology, which literally means the study of whole systems, had become part of everyday language. Similarly, the scientists who designed new technologies that allowed us to do things like send Rusty Schweickart and his colleagues into space discovered that they had to think in terms of the ways entire systems operate. Sometimes we learned that lesson too late and some seemingly trivial mistake led to catastrophe as happened the year before when the Space Shuttle Challenger exploded barely a minute after liftoff because a simple O-ring failed.

As far as I know, Beyond War was the first major peace movement to help its members see that systems theory was the best tool we could use for understanding what reality was telling us to do. Forty years later, almost all AfP members base their work on some version of it and everything else that follows in this chapter. In fact, when we started working in the United States, we were surprised to discover that few of our colleagues who worked on polarization and related issues used systems theory—which led me to stress it here.

---

7. The best general introductions remain Donella Meadows. *Thinking in Systems*. (White River Junction VT: Chelsea Green, 1998) and Peter Senge, *The Fifth Discipline: The Art and Practice of the Learning Organization*. (New York: Currency, 1990), and Cynthia Rayner and François Bonnici. *The Systems Work of Social Change: How to Harness Connection, Context, and Power to Cultivate Deep and Enduring Change*. (Oxford: Oxford University Press, 2021).

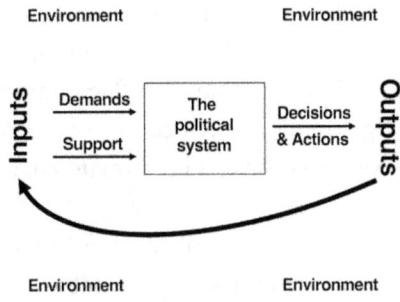

Figure 2.4: The Political System

I had begun using systems theory as the organizing framework for everything I did as a political scientist before I graduated from college. So, I started using this bare boned outline of a political system in my Beyond War work as well and still use it to outline any system's basic dynamics today.

Because systems are loops, deciding where to start describing one is arbitrary. Social scientists, however, usually start with its "environment," the jargon term they use to describe everything that lies beyond its formal boundaries. While you can think of what theorists call closed systems, every cell or city or economy or government is shaped to some degree by what happens elsewhere. The environment does, of course, include our natural surroundings but extends to the social, economic, transportation, and other forces which don't typically make their way into the political science curriculum.

Choosing where to begin your analysis once you move inside a system is arbitrary, too. Not surprisingly, people in a democracy usually start with the impact of people like themselves.

Citizens use "inputs" to show their support for and/or place demands on the government and other key decision makers. Those actions—including a decision not to act—have their roots both in enduring cultural norms and what we think about the issues of the day.

Decision makers inside and outside of government turn those inputs into the "outputs" or policies that shape our lives. Some regulate what we can and cannot do. You can't drink alcohol (legally) until you are twenty-one. Others (re)distribute resources as is the case with tax and health care policy. Still others are symbolic—here just think of how often we drape things in American flags. Important, too, are the decisions that don't get made, which can most easily be seen today in our failure to take concerted action on climate change or enact immigration reform.

Systems theory's most useful contribution to our understanding of just about anything comes from its use of feedback loops. They can get very complicated very fast. Still, the basic idea is simple.

In political systems, whatever our leaders do now has an impact that can be felt far into the future. For the purposes of this chapter, it is enough to note that people's actions can lead them to adopt new cultural norms or change the supports and demands they later place on decision makers. Thus, adding feedback turns what might otherwise look like a snapshot of the status quo into the equivalent of an extended play video that helps us understand how any system changes over time.

Feedback also gives new meaning to the phrase that what goes around comes around. What happens anywhere has at least a small impact everywhere.

That's as true for average citizens like you and me as it is for national leaders. To be sure, our impact will be tiny compared to theirs. Nonetheless, it does exist. If I'm right and if you follow the steps along the Peacebuilding Starts at Home Loop, your ability to (re)shape the system(s) that matter to you will grow—again, exponentially.

Systems theory also leads us to add a new dimension to conventional definitions of power in ways that will shape the rest of this book. If, for example, I exert power over you, you are not likely to be happy with the outcome. You will probably lick your wounds, resent what I've done, and begin figuring out how to get back at me. On the other hand, if I treat you well, I can trigger an entirely different dynamic through which what goes around comes around can lead to different and more constructive outcomes. In that sense, I can empower you so that we can solve the problems we face together.

With that in mind, note that systems can change in three basic ways. Dysfunctional ones deteriorate and, if things keep getting worse, collapse. This is what the first generation of political scientists who used these models were most worried about. Instead, they looked for ways to keep a system stable in much the same way that a thermostat regulates the temperature in your house. They did not pay much attention, however, to the ways that the awkwardly labeled eufunctional systems improve over time because their "members" find ways of making the whole become truly greater than the sum of its parts.

A eufunctional system is also one in which everyone's interests get met, at least over time. No one individual or group can run roughshod over anyone else. We seek and find find common ground when we address climate change, race relations or economic inequality together. Everyone's voice matters to the point that all end up getting a growing piece of a growing pie.

Not always. But to reuse one of my favorite expressions, a eufunctional system is also one in which most people solve most of their problems peacefully most of the time.

That is what Australia reMADE has in mind when they work to build an ordinary paradise. It is also what Ezra Klein and Derek Thompson were thinking of when they entitled their new book *Abundance*.[8]

Complexity science. Even in 1987, we knew that reality was a lot more complicated than simple models like mine suggest. At that time, scientists were beginning to write about a version of system theory known as complexity science that took those realities into account. Their insights had two overlapping intellectual roots. Some physicists, computer scientists, and engineers began organizing intense theory-building exercises at places like the Santa Fe Institute. Meanwhile, research on topics like climate change uncovered complex systems that seemed to shift dramatically all but overnight in unpredictable ways which were, of course, a far cry from the apparent simplicity of the diagrams I drew on classroom blackboards.[9]

Global peacebuilders got to see both sides of complexity over the

---

8. Ezra Klein and Derek Thompson, *Abundance*. (New York: Simon and Schuster/Avid Reader, 2025).
9. M. Mitchell Waldrop. *Complexity: The Emerging Science at the Edge of Order and Chaos*. (New York: Simon and Schuster, 1992, reissued in 2019).

course of the next decade because they started using systems-based approaches when designing new projects. They did not start with a preconceived model like mine. Rather, facilitators like Rob Ricigliano wanted the people they worked with to "map" the system so that they could better understand the systems they wanted to change.[10] Typically, Rob or his colleagues arrive at the NGO's conference room with stacks of sticky notes and a bunch of markers. They ask members of the team that was planning the project to put each idea that came to mind onto a single sticky note. After spending a few minutes writing, the participants put their slips of paper up on a wall and group them into clusters. Then, they draw arrows connecting them and go on to talk about how each "x" led to each "y" on a crowded wall. Unfortunately, the resulting map would be a lot more complicated than figure 2.4 and more often led to reactions like "oh s***" rather than "aha, here's what I can do to make this system work better."

It wasn't just peacebuilders. In 2005, I was invited to give a keynote talk at a conference at the Special Operations Command (SOCOM) headquarters in Tampa shortly after the war in Afghanistan reached one of its many stalemates. Before I took the stage, they presented the first version of what has come to be called the Spaghetti Map.

SOCOM's planners use more sophisticated analytical tools than sticky notes and markers, but the underlying logic behind their mapping exercise was the same as the one we peacebuilders used. So was the map's impact. Everyone in the room could see why toppling the Taliban government in late 2001 was not going to be enough to bring peace to that troubled country. And when I spoke to them privately, there were plenty of "oh s***" reactions, too.

---

10. Robert Ricigliano, *Making Peace Last: A Toolbox for Sustainable Peacebuilding*. (London: Routledge, 2011).

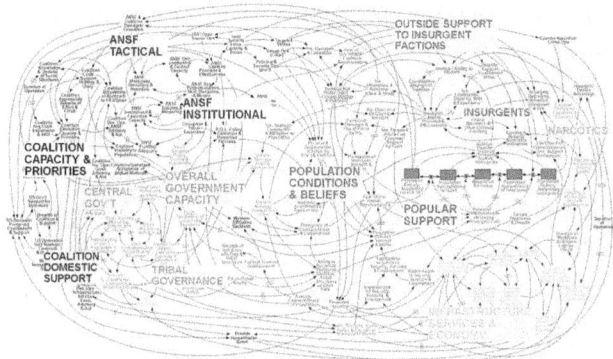

Figure 2.5: The Afghanistan Spaghetti Map

Don't worry if you can't read the fine print. The words were impossible to decipher even when the colonels projected them onto the largest screen I had ever seen. It is enough to see that the topics in capital letters represent the hub of a sub-system and that each of them affects all of the others in a maze of indirect and often unintended consequences. Thus, the narcotics trade helped fund the Taliban (insurgent behavior) in the upper right-hand corner which, in turn, contributed to declining support for the American-backed government which is as far away as possible on the chart. Many of the causal connections, feedback loops, and side effects are indirect because they pass through economic and other social conditions and the way the country was governed at the provincial and national level.

The fact that the connections are so circuitous reinforces the point that everything matters and that what goes around comes around. In this case, the Spaghetti Map actually understates the complexity because the map itself kept changing as American and Afghan policy makers watched those feedback loops evolve over the next fifteen years until the Taliban regained power in 2021. And even though American troops are gone, the conflict is far from over. And the map keeps changing.

The spaghetti map itself may have been new to most people in the room that day in Tampa. The general problem it depicted was not.

Thought leaders in the military world already knew that the situation in Afghanistan was far from unique. A few years earlier, faculty members at the United States Army War College, for example, had coined a term to describe situations like the one in Afghanistan. They are VUCA, for Volatile, Uncertain, Complex, and Ambiguous.

VUCAness isn't just a military problem. The dynamics underlying climate change, economic inequality, or the COVID-19 pandemic are just as mind numbingly complex and would yield a spaghetti map that would be at least as convoluted as this one.

That brings to mind another one-liner attributed to Heraclitus:
You can never step into the same river twice.[11]

Because its current keeps the water flowing, a river changes from one moment to the next.

So, too, does the metaphorical rhythm of our lives whether in Kabul or Kansas City.

Wicked problems. As if this discussion weren't already depressing enough, I need to add one more concept that captures the severity of the situation we find ourselves in. In the early 1970s, the urban planners Horst Rittel and Melvin Webber found themselves frustrated both with the deteriorating conditions in American cities and the war in Vietnam and realized that both had turned into what they called wicked problems.[12]

They didn't pick that term because the problems were themselves evil. Rather, they thought of them as problems whose causes and consequences are so inextricably intertwined that they cannot be solved quickly, easily, or separately—if they can be solved at all.

Like VUCA and complexity in general, the idea of wicked problems has gained a following in academic and corporate circles in the last generation. In his book on the wicked problems that destroyed the flight training, shoe manufacturing, and computer industries in Binghamton NY, Guru Madhavan defined them as having:

---

11. Denise Blanc takes off from Heraclitus' line in her book on personal relationships and conflict resolution, *River Logic: Tools to Transform Resistance and Create Flow in all of our Relationships.* (Lavergne TN: Ingramspark, 2022).
12. Horst Rittell and Melvin Webber. "Dilemmas in a General Theory of Planning." *Policy Sciences.* 4(1973): 155-169. In a curious twist of fate, Webber's granddaughter is one of my favorite young colleagues who introduced me to somatic approaches to peacebuilding.

vexing staying power; working like franchises, with premieres and prequels, remakes, reissues, reboots, sequels, spin-offs, and streaming on demand. One can't opt out, log off, autocorrect, unsubscribe, block, mute, cancel, or shut down wicked problems. Nor can we click and clear them like browser history. As their forms change, so do their formulations.[13]

Seeing that we live in a world of wicked problems and spaghetti maps drives home Jon Stewart's conclusion, albeit with less graphic language. There are no quick fixes. There is no magic wand we can wave that will solve our problems over night.

EXERCISE 2.2: NAILING IT

Return to your notes from the nailing it exercise in chapter 1.

Given what you have learned so far about interdependence, systems theory, complexity science, and wicked problems, how would you change your plans for nailing it? If, not surprisingly, your battle plan (pun intended) has gotten more complex, now what do you think could be done to improve things in ways that go beyond tinkering with the system?

NEW EYES AND PARADIGM SHIFTS

The Beyond War seminar also was a game changer for me because I could suddenly see how my renewed activism could lead to a paradigm shift in the ways we handle what reality is telling us to do. Until then, I had mostly used Thomas Kuhn's understanding of paradigm shifts as a classroom tool to help students see that history is

---

13. Guru Madhavan, *Wicked Problems: How to Engineer a Better World.* (New York: W. W. Norton, 2024) 6.

filled with what I inelegantly called large-scale social change.[14] Now, I began to see that his ideas had real world implications, too.

Kuhn was a physicist and scientific historian who understood something that non-scientists often miss. His research showed that major progress comes when scientists make a major new breakthrough that lets them come a lot closer to answering big but befuddling questions. Why do we get sick? What keeps planets in their orbits? What is intelligence?

Along the way, he undermined the conventional wisdom about how scientists make discoveries that revolutionize entire fields. Of course, they toil away in their labs and pore over their data. However, Kuhn became famous because he realized that scientists only make quantum leaps forward when they adopt a new framework or paradigm that solves those big and befuddling problems. That process starts with the kind of creativity that only comes when a scientist—or anyone else—takes a step back and reframes the facts in a dramatically new way.

It was Kuhn's discovery that paradigm shifts go through three main stages that is most useful here. The first one starts once scientists begin uncovering what he called anomalies, which is a fancy term for saying that their research produced results that were at odds with what their theories led them to expect. An occasional anomaly is one thing. However, once their number mounts, the paradigm ceases being a reliable guide for conducting scientific research. Progress slows down and may even stop altogether. At those moments, we end up with the scientific equivalent of political gridlock. The research community may be at an impasse, but no one considers alternatives to the current paradigm because everyone "knows" that it is "true."

Until, that is, the second phase begins, when someone proposes a new paradigm that unblocks the gridlock. This only happens after a long period when pioneering scientists connect the evidentiary dots in a new way and come up with a new theory that keeps what the old

---

14. Thomas Kuhn, *The Structure of Scientific Revolutions*. (Chicago: University of Chicago Press, 1962).

one explained well *and* helps solve the problems that gave rise to the anomalies. In short, they have created a new set of Proustean eyes.

Third, Kuhn also knew just how rare and difficult these transitions were when he chose to call them scientific revolutions rather than paradigm shifts. He also showed that they almost never happen in one fell swoop. Rather, they typically include power struggles in which supporters of the old paradigm refuse to give way. Indeed, a paradigm shift's game changing implications may not be clear until the "insurgents" have won.

Kuhn is best known for illustrating how all of this happens through the history of the Copernican revolution. In the early sixteenth century, just about everyone in the Western world "knew" that the earth was the center of the universe. As telescopes and other new inventions revealed anomalies, observers developed the idea that the planets and stars followed epicycles or what amount to looping, curlicue-like trajectories in their orbits because everyone took for granted the "fact" that all celestial bodies revolved around the earth.

Then, Nicolaus Copernicus and a handful of other outsiders looked at the evidence through a new mental lens. In their heliocentric (suncentered) model, moons still revolve around planets. Now, however, the planets revolve around the sun in a solar system that is, itself, a tiny part of a much larger universe. It is only a bit of an oversimplification to say that Copernicus was able to make his breakthrough because he was willing to "see" the movement of heavenly bodies through new "eyes."

Yet, as compelling as the evidence was, it didn't immediately convince the powers that be. Copernicus chose not to publish his findings during his lifetime because he feared persecution by the Catholic Church, which rejected anything that challenged its teaching that the earth was at the heart of everything. He had good reason to be afraid. A century later, Galileo Galilei spent the last decade of his life under house arrest because he refused to recant his own writings that showed that the heliocentric interpretation was correct. It was only in 1822 that the Church allowed books about heliocentrism to be published and removed Galileo's work from its list of banned books.

I subjected you to this crash course in scientific history because paradigms are also an important part of how we all conduct our daily lives even if we tend to use other terms to describe them like mindsets, world-views, or cultural norms. In 1987, the Beyond War team wanted us to see their importance because they had been at the heart of Creative Initiative's work in the 1970s and they assumed that it would be again in the post-Cold War world.

Social paradigms are never as all encompassing as, say, the chemists' periodic table, nor do they ever have anything approaching universal approval. Nonetheless, we rely on personal and social paradigms. What's more, major progress in social life occurs when (and if) we adopt new ones.

The Beyond War team wanted us to see how desperately the world needed a paradigm shift that extended far beyond the ways the superpowers dealt with each other. As was their wont, they tried to inspire us by using two statements made by Albert Einstein, who is not widely seen as a great source for one-liners.[15] Both apply to any moment in time when "we" (however you choose to define we) are stuck in a rut.

First:

> *The definition of insanity is doing the same thing over and over again and expecting different results.*

I can't speak for Einstein. However, I have watched too many of my fellow peacebuilders—including myself—rely for too long on a tried-but-not-so-true toolkit for solving issues as different as the tensions between Palestinians and Israelis, climate change, and the legacy of racism in the United States with relatively little to show for their efforts.

Second:

> *You can never solve a problem on the same level you created it.*

In choosing the term level, Einstein undoubtedly had something like a

---

15. He never included either of them in anything he published. As a result, you will find other authors using slightly different versions of both of them.

paradigm in mind. Einstein should not be taken to task for his word choice because the term paradigm only took on its current meaning as an overarching and widely accepted worldview with the publication of Kuhn's book seven years after Einstein died. Nonetheless, everything about Einstein's scientific career as well as his writing on the dangers of nuclear weapons reflected his awareness that we can only solve tough, vexing, wicked problems by first seeing them through something like Proust's new eyes and then acting accordingly.

WHAT REALITY TELLS US TO *DO*

You could and should be skeptical about what you've read up to this point. Other than a couple of vague hints, this chapter hasn't been a call to action.

I do, of course, have the rest of *Peacebuilding Starts at Home* to help you put your to-do list together. Still, let me use the rest of this chapter to outline three guidelines that you can use to convert these general principles into broad strategies, if not specific things reality is telling us to do. Lists like this one will appear in some of the other chapters to come. Taken together, they will amount to more than any one individual can do. Even me. And I do peacebuilding full time.

Think of them as the mental equivalents of the sliders you use to edit a photo on your favorite social media app. If my experience is any indication, you will frequently find yourself moving them all up and down to reflect the importance any of these activities has in your life at the moment.

The homework assignments are designed with that metaphor in mind. The Peacebuilding Starts at Home team is also ready to help you determine which—if any—of the initiatives I will describe offer the best fit, given your interests, skills, and circumstances. If none of them work for you, we will help you find other ones.

The whole system matters. The first pathway may not seem all that action oriented. However, peacebuilding projects around the world have shown that it is hard to do good work unless and until you map the system and see how all of its component parts intersect. If you want to create a new system, you first have to understand how the current one works or, as the strategist Seth Godin put it, we have to make the whole system visible so that we can attack it (non-violently, of course) in its entirety.[16]

That starts by defining something that may not have been obvious in the examples I used in this chapter—your North Star or long-term goal. It has to be clear and plausible enough to motivate people, which is why I decided to use Australia reMADE as a jumping off point even though it is not about the United States. At the same time, it has to be concrete enough that you can measure, assess, and adapt your progress—including the lack thereof—toward nailing it.

Once you've defined your North Star, the best way to proceed is to get a stack of sticky notes and draw your own version of what the system looks like. Even a crude map will give you a sense of the causal links that are at the root of our wicked problems and political gridlock. And, you should also begin to see subsystems which seem easiest to reshape, something that the military planners in Afghanistan whom I met that weekend never succeeded in doing.

There will never be a direct route or simple path toward a North Star in any complex system that has its share of wicked problems. There will always be plenty of twists and turns and lots of setbacks. Nonetheless, a North Star and basic system map do give us something to constantly aim for, whatever tactics we adopt in the short run, in ways that I will begin exploring in the next chapter.

Build virtuous circles, not vicious cycles. Even if you had never encountered systems theory before you started this chapter, you would have had plenty of experience dealing with one of its most important and discouraging concepts—vicious cycles. We've all seen families fall apart and companies teeter toward bankruptcy, seemingly unable to stop their downward spiral. Many argue that our political, social, environmental, and economic systems are in one today.

If so, it is time to think differently so that we can do something that has not found its way into most Americans' everyday language—we can build virtuous circles. That means focusing on something that got lost in the intellectual shuffle when systems theory was introduced to

---

16. Seth Godin. *This is Strategy*. (New York: Harper Collins, 2024).

my home field of political science sixty years ago. Not all systems get worse. Sometimes, individuals, organizations, and even governments buck those trends and perform better over time.

Successful peacebuilding work around the world has also shown us that building virtuous circles and systems whose performance improves over time and are also based on a new kind of activism. I came of political age in the new left of the 1960s and then went to graduate school to learn how to build more effective social movements. In those days, my mentors assumed that successful movements had to start on the social and ideological fringes and gradually work their way toward the center. Most also assumed that they would have to use force if they wanted to succeed, although I never went that far.

Now, the combination of today's reality and Proust's new eyes are steering us toward a different pathway toward peace and social change in general that builds from the inside out. Just about everybody is unhappy with the status quo. As you will see, it's no longer just young radicals like the teenage me who want something akin to a paradigm shift. So, too, do plenty of Rotary Club members and corporate executives, and we can start with them as well as with today's equivalents of my college-aged self.

In a world in which everything that goes around comes around, demonizing the "enemy" with chants like "hey, hey LBJ, how many kids did you kill today" in the 1960s or engaging in "cancel culture" today deepens divisions but rarely leads to constructive or lasting change. The same could be said for conservatives who branded antiwar protesters as unpatriotic in the old days or react with fear and anger while making worst case assumptions about "wokeness" today.

Instead, I am drawn to Loretta Ross's suggestion that we call people in rather than call them out.[17] She starts with the assumption that it is all but impossible to convince people to change their minds if you start by attacking them.

She draws on those parts of Martin Luther King's version of nonviolence that are also at the heart of modern peacebuilding including

---

17. Loretta Ross, *Calling In: How to Start Making Change with Those You'd Rather Cancel.* (New York: Simon and Schuster, 2025).

empathy, compassion, self-awareness, mindfulness, and the like. She goes even farther and suggests that it is our obligation to take the first step to turn toward the people we disagree with, starting wherever they are in Pema Chödrön's terms.

When you call people in and use the other tools that I will describe in the rest of this book, you can find ways to use the fact that what goes around comes around to build virtuous circles. Thus, Peacebuilding Starts at Home will forge coalitions through which we can address problems like racism or climate change that affect us all, whatever issues preoccupy us. To anticipate a point I will come back to in the last three chapters, this is something some corporate leaders have understood for decades when, for instance, they talk about "both and" rather than "either or" solutions to the challenges that their companies face.[18]

Probe. Sense. Respond. Because complex systems can't be changed in their entirety quickly, I will end this set of action guidelines with one last concept from one last authority. Unlike Gordon Moore and Robert Metcalfe, David Snowden doesn't have his own law. Nonetheless, his Cynefin (Welsh for habitat and pronounced *canaven*) framework is just as important for our purposes because it lays out a general strategy to use especially when you are just beginning to deal with a wicked problem.[19]

Snowden developed Cynefin when he was chief scientist for IBM in the United Kingdom. For the last twenty-five years, he has been applying it in social settings—including peacebuilding—in ways that pull together most of the threads I have raised in this section.

As you can see, he thinks in terms of five types of systems. We can ignore disorder which is at the center of the chart because Snowden is

---

18. There are literally hundreds of books to turn to here. This phrase comes from Wendy Smith and Marianne Lewis, *Both/And Thinking: Embracing Creative Tensions to Solve Your Toughest Problems*. (Boston: Harvard Business School Press, 2022).
19. Most books published on Cynefin are too dense for most readers. Snowden's website is therefore the best place to start. https://thecynefin.co/about-us/about-cynefin-framework/?srsltid=AfmBOorFFXMjBM1RfhNREZh-2ZHQrYxHghuoVnEx0qA-QkRS83hW1tTi (Accessed February 13, 2025.)

convinced that no system is truly disordered but can only appear that way to us because we can't figure out how to make sense of it.

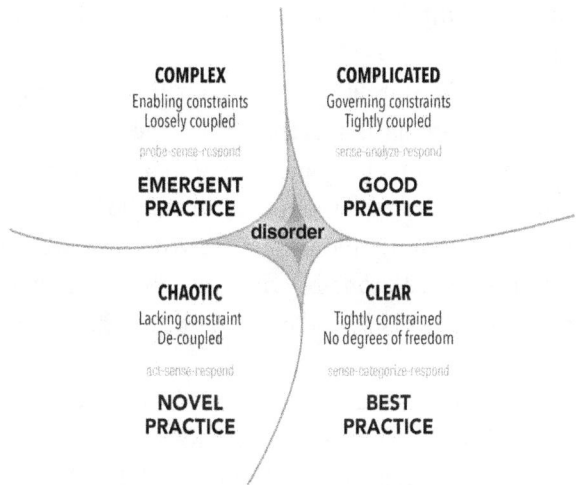

Figure 2.6: The Cynefin Framework

In the real world, systems fall into the main types outlined in the chart's quadrants.

We can ignore the first or chaotic systems, too, because there aren't any important human systems that have no underlying structure.

We can almost do the same with the situations he calls clear, because they are not much of a challenge. Since I like to cook, I am drawn here to recipes. Once I decide what I want to make and have all the ingredients and utensils I need, I can go about making even the most sophisticated version of, say *blanquette de veau*, quite easily. I just have to faithfully follow the steps in Julia Child's *Mastering the Art of French Cooking*, because she has defined the best practices for making that scrumptious veal dish with a cream sauce, mushrooms, and pearl onions. It also doesn't take a lot to adapt her recipe for vegetarians (blanquette de tofu) though I will admit that a vegan blanquette would be quite a culinary challenge.

The same logic applies to complicated systems. Thus, when President Kennedy announced that we would send a man to the moon by the end of the 1960s, we knew more or less what it would take to do so even if we still had to figure out how to build the rocket, spacesuits, and lunar landing module. Similarly, we don't need to break new intellectual ground in order to get better at playing chess, including the mind-numbingly complicated Five-Dimensional Chess with Multiverse Time Travel.[20]

As is the case with simple systems, your first challenge in dealing with complicated systems is to sense what the system is like. Here, however, you have to analyze the situation and learn how best to handle it. But there is no equivalent of Julia Child to turn to. Instead, you have to pick from a number of guides who provide good insights about your path forward, none of which can be considered definitive. In fact, part of your job is to define how to go about getting the job done.

Last but by no means least are complex systems which include the kinds of predicaments peacebuilders face today. Although he is by no means alone in saying it, Snowden forces us to focus on the fact that they are qualitatively different from the systems we were trained to work in and on. If reality today is defined by clusters of overlapping and interlaced networks and if it is therefore dramatically different from anything that came before, our response to those problems has to be radically different, too.

His probe-sense-respond terminology points us toward the kinds of collective action I will explore in the next six chapters. As was the case for the generals in Afghanistan, it is hard to chart a plan of action when the system is as complex as the one they faced and that also keeps changing in unpredictable ways. Under those circumstances, Snowden suggests starting out by probing the system. You should try something that you think might work, find out what happens, make sense of those emerging patterns, and change what you do next on the basis of

---

20. There really is such a game. My then fifth grade grandson made me learn to play it. Even though you play simultaneously on five boards, players can move from one to another, and they can move backward (but not forward) in time. There are rules that you can master, and if you follow them you can win. If, heaven forbid, you are interested, https://store.steampowered.com/app/1349230/5D_Chess_With_Multiverse_Time_Travel/ (Accessed June 14, 2023).

what you've learned. In other words, you should create situations in which you can learn from feedback.

As peacebuilders have always known and the military leaders in Afghanistan quickly learned, you can't blithely probe, sense, and respond when there are lives at stake. As a result, a lot of people who have tried to apply Snowden's principles to high-risk situations talk about the need to fail quickly or do everything you can to make a minimum viable product so that you can learn as much as you can as fast you can.

You may not find that satisfactory given the high stakes and urgency of the crisis the United States finds itself in today. Still, it is one way to start.

That got driven home for me in an unexpected way when I read Lizzie Wade's surprisingly upbeat book—at least given its title—*Apocalypse*. Her historical reporting found that humans always find ways to respond to the worst things that happen to their communities. Sometimes, things even get dramatically better. As she put it in ending her book:

> *The adaptations our ancestors have made from the very beginning of our species drive home the notion that people have already faced challenges as dangerous as most of those looming over our horizon, and we can learn from what they carried forward and what they were willing to let go. Learning to see human history through the lens of apocalypse teaches us that our past is a story of survival, transformation, and reinvention, often in the face of tragedy, loss, and individual and collective pain.*[21]

---

21. Lizzie Wade. *Apocalypse: How Catastrophe Transformed Our World and Can Forge New Futures.* (New York: Harper-Collins, 2025), 253.

EXERCISE 2.3: LUNCH PAIL F***ING JOB

This is the first—but not the last—chapter in which the third exercise comes at the very end.

That's the case because everything you saw so far in this book builds toward the first steps you could take in what will be the long slog of building peace at home.

In this case, the key is to start with your North Star. If it hadn't emerged clearly in your mind from the two previous exercises, define yours now. Then, at least roughly outline the system of interconnected parts that keeps us from getting closer to it. Finally, pick a bright spot or two in that system and design a set of constructive projects you could use to probe it and get the kind of information you could use to take the next set of steps that would bring you closer to your so-far elusive goal.

CHAPTER 3
LET IT BEGIN WITH ME

> *God, grant me the serenity to accept the things I cannot change; courage to change the things I can; and wisdom to know the difference.*
>
> REINHOLD NIEBUHR

It's time to switch gears, get you out of your head, start where you are, and help you find (or expand) one or more on-ramps onto your peacebuilding starts at home journey.[1]

Literally you.

And literally where you are.

And literally right now—or at least once you've finished reading this chapter.

To see why, let me emphasize one more point from Beyond War's six-word invitation.

Reality is telling *me* what to do. And you.

---

1. I do find the metaphors of journey and exploration compelling. See Alex Hutchinson, *The Explorer's Gene: Why We Seek Big Challenges, New Flavors, and the Blank Spots on the Map.* (New York: Mariner Books, 2025).

Stressing "little old me" might seem counterintuitive. After all, our country is in deep trouble, and I just finished asking you to adopt an entirely new world view that includes just about everything. Yet, here I am, claiming that peacebuilding starts with you? Or as my AI program asked after it turned this chapter into a podcast. "Me, a peacebuilder?"[2]

I am not suggesting that what you or I do on our own will ever come close to being enough. I do want to make the case, however, that starting peacebuilding as close to home as possible is the first active step you can take along the Peacebuilding Starts at Home Loop.

So, let me be blunt.

Unless you and I do this part of what reality demands of us, there is next to no chance that the paradigm shift will occur. I can't guarantee that one will take place if you do what follows in the rest of this chapter or the rest of this book. But in the terminology of undergraduate logic courses, doing what reality tells me to do is a necessary but not sufficient precondition for anything resembling a paradigm shift.

Note that what follows flies in the face of much of what I learned in my first twenty years as an activist and political scientist. But even before the Richesons introduced me to Beyond War, I had begun to see that any strategy that stressed building political movements from the outside in was not our best option. That is even more the case in the mid-2020s when so many Americans are convinced that average citizens like themselves can't make a difference.

But you can. At least if you figure out how to answer the questions that follow, which will help you develop your personal peacebuilding skills so that you can easily "create space" for your friends, relatives, neighbors, and co-workers to do the same.

What if you could identify steps that you could take right now without disrupting your life that could make a difference where you live or work?

What if those actions could turn into baby steps on a longer journey

---

2. I used Notebook LM to fine tune *Peacebuilding Starts at Home*. Among other things, it creates remarkably good "deep dive" podcasts using two remarkably real-sounding artificial voices. The "podcasts" are so good that you can find them on www.peacebuildingstartsathome.us.

through which your influence expands to include more of your community, your country, and your planet?

Could that help you get over some of the pessimism that contributes to gridlock?

The lack of trust?

The polarization?

And empower yourself?

Coming to grips with questions like these will help you turn the new "eyes" I just gave you into the equivalent of a pair of bifocal glasses. Chapter 2 helped you see the new reality from a global perspective by improving the equivalent of your distance vision. This one will do the same by giving you a second "lens" that sharpens your ability to see things that are right in front of your metaphoric eyes so that you can do something about them. Then, I will use the rest of the book to show how you *might* be able to make those sweeping changes possible (emphasis very much on might).

But, you will already have become the peacebuilder my AI ended up deciding that anyone could be after it "read" and "processed" this chapter.

Before digging into that material, consider one more metaphor. I wanted Chapter 2 to show you that we need the equivalent of a Swiss army knife that can do at least a little bit of everything because peacebuilders have to deal with just about everything. Peacebuilding that starts at home could become that kind of handy device for our social change toolkit. It may never reach the standard set by the Victorinox Swiss Champ Swiss army knife with its thirty-three utensils, but it can come close.

The original Swiss army knife only had a single blade and three other tools when it was introduced in 1890, but it still amounted to a paradigm shift in what soldiers could do with any single utensil. This chapter, too, will start small and just introduce a first set of tools you can pull out from your virtual Swiss army knife, knowing that there will be more to come. By the end of the book, you will be able to use the equivalent of your knife's corkscrew, can opener, nail clippers, pliers, fish scaler, and saws until we are able to create a movement that is strong enough to do what most Americans think is impossible today —change the entire system.

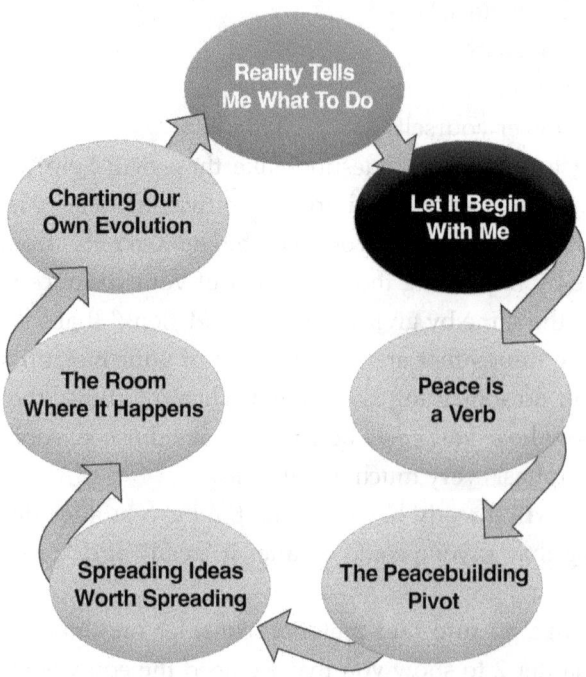

Figure 3.1: The Peacebuilding Starts at Home Loop

To see where I'm heading, consider the next figure which will reappear twice more in slightly different form in later chapters. Perhaps because I've been obsessed with startups since I first met the Richesons and Beyond War, I started worrying about how we could take our work to scale long before most of my peacebuilding colleagues did. Over the years, I've come to realize that we can't just copy what startups have done to reach unicorn status.

We have to begin by going to scale inwardly and changing ourselves. We will get to the other two dimensions later. But once again, I don't want to get ahead of myself.

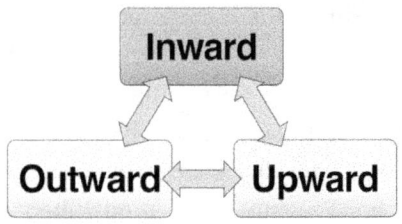

Figure 3.2: Going to Scale Inward

TWO MORE AHA MOMENTS FROM THE 1980S

In addition to attending the Beyond War leadership seminar, two other things happened that spring that drove home the importance of personal growth as the first step in any peacebuilding journey. At the time, both events only changed the way I taught. Since then, their "lessons" have found their way into everything I've done and now serve as core building blocks for the entire Peacebuilding Starts at Home initiative.

In those days, I team-taught Colby College's introduction to comparative politics course. Because my usual colleagues were on leave that semester, I was teaching it with two visiting professors who did not enjoy teaching the course and did not share my quirky classroom style. To make a long story short, by the time we got to the last week of classes, we couldn't even agree on questions to ask on the final exam.

Somehow, the two of them let me take the academic coward's way out. At the start of the final lecture, I asked the students to suggest essay questions, and we would then pick the best one(s) to include on the test.

As we were filing out of the lecture hall, a student I didn't know because he was in one of my colleagues' discussion sections came up to me and said:

Chip, it's obvious. The world is f***ed up. Discuss.

He was right. That's what the course was all about.

So, after my colleagues got over their qualms (and, maybe, I pulled a bit of rank), I walked into the room a few days later, handed out the bluebooks, and wrote those six words on the blackboard. Without the asterisks. After a few audible gasps and giggles, they dove into the assignment with more enthusiasm than I had ever seen at exam time.

I stayed up all night grading what turned out to be the best set of exams I had ever read. The students demonstrated an uncanny understanding of the course's concepts which they illustrated with evidence about Great Britain, the Soviet Union, Nicaragua, Japan, and Tanzania with more skill than I would have expected from graduate students.

And then I got depressed.

I did not go into teaching to help my students see what was wrong with the world. Especially now that I had rediscovered my activist roots through Beyond War, I wanted to help them see solutions that they could get behind.

A few weeks later, I attended the first national conference of the Peace and Justice Studies Association. In his presidential address, Notre Dame's George Lopez admonished the hundred or so professors in the room for teaching courses that stressed what he called Doom and Gloom 101. Having read that remarkable set of final exams just a few weeks earlier, I had to nod my head in agreement.

And then I got depressed again.

I realized that I had to change what I did in the classroom and in my peacebuilding work. I decided to give the people I worked with what I called a rational basis for hope in the first article I published on peace studies.[3] I have continued doing so (without that rather pompous title) in every venue and with every audience I have worked with since then. Culminating in this book.

And I stopped being depressed by what happened in my classrooms, workshops, and other meetings. I started living up to the goals I set for myself when I became an activist and an academic—helping my students and everyone else I work with see that paradigm shifts are possible, but only if we all do our part.

---

3. Charles Hauss, "A Rational Basis for Hope." In Linda Rennie Forcey, ed. *Peace: Meanings, Politics, Strategies*. (New York: Praeger, 1989), 203-218.

FROM PROUST TO NIEBUHR

Whenever I say something like that, most people in the audience want to get right to work. At that point, I tap on the mental brakes and remind them that it helps to think through what reality is telling them to do—and not to do—first.

There is no need to become an expert on such topics as emotional intelligence, self-awareness, or empathy and other personal skills that would help you contribute to turning the new paradigm into reality. In my experience, however, when people skip the going to scale inward step, they either don't accomplish a lot or they burn out. Or both.

To see what I mean, consider Reinhold Niebuhr's Serenity Prayer that begins this chapter. It is best known today because it is recited at the end of all twelve-step meetings.

Niebuhr was not thinking about addiction when he wrote the first version of this twenty-six word prayer in 1932. He was inspired, instead, by his commitment to pacifism and social justice. A decade later, the founders of Alcoholics Anonymous discovered the prayer, which millions of men and women have used to help keep themselves in recovery.

In neither guise are they words that one typically hears from activists who are appalled by what their government is doing. If anything, most people I work with bristle when they first hear that they should accept the things that they cannot change.

But be careful with the word "accept."

Christian leaders like Niebuhr or Buddhists like the Dalai Lama draw a sharp distinction between accepting and agreeing with something. How could it have been otherwise for a nation's spiritual leader who was forced into exile or a socialist and pacifist pastor who came of age as the Nazis were coming to power in the country where his parents were born?

In its twelve-step version, acceptance simply means coming to grips with an unpleasant, unwanted, and stubborn habit that has become a central part of your reality.[4] Acknowledge that you are

---

4. James Clear, *Atomic Habits: An Easy and Proven Way to Build Good Habits and Break Old*

addicted to alcohol or drugs or gambling. Or that your beloved Tibet is occupied by the Chinese. Or that your family's country of origin is ruled by Nazis.

Then, figure out what you can do about the situation you find yourself in. That starts by acknowledging that there are things that you cannot change. As wonderful as it might be, you cannot rerun history and erase centuries of systemic racism in the United States. Similarly, even though I know plenty of people at fairly high levels in the United States government, I can not single handedly change American public policy.

Nor can you.

Once you've accepted the things you cannot change, you can begin exploring the things you can do to begin moving us away from the status quo—whether that is a personal addiction to alcohol or a society-wide addiction to a dysfunctional political system. Whatever success you enjoy can go on to further empower you and the people you work with. And that can spark even more changes that touch even more people, some of whom might be able to reach people "at the top."

At the same time, remember that Niebuhr did not ignore the things you can't control. How you deal with them matters, too.

In other words, reality is telling me that everything I do—and don't do—matters. I have spent a lot of time learning about conflict resolution. Despite those years of training and practice, I know that I can't solve every conflict that comes my way. Neither can you. You certainly can't do so quickly. Similarly, you can't control how a person you are in conflict with behaves. Still, you do have leverage over how you deal not just with conflict but with every relationship you are a part of. In other words, how you deal with the things you cannot change matters, too.

Ones. (New York: Avery, 2018) and Charles Duhigg, *The Power of Habit: Why We Do What We Do in Life and Business.* (New York: Random House, 2012).

FOLK SONGS AND KINDERGARTENERS

So, that leads to some obvious questions.

What are the things you can change?

Where do you find the wisdom to know the difference between places where you can make a difference and those where your actions amount to little more than tilting at windmills?

What are the things you can do that will also keep you going on a journey that will take far longer than the time it will for you to finish this book?

That's where this chapter's title and personal paradigms come into play. My AI is, in fact, right. Anyone can learn how to use Niebuhr's prayer as a North Star to guide their lives. Each of us will go about doing so differently, given the personal backgrounds, skills, and resources that we bring to the metaphoric table which can turn you into a peacebuilder that my AI would be proud of.

Still, there are some core principles that can help get you started. Unlike chapter 2, I am not going to challenge you with sophisticated and abstract concepts—although everything that follows has roots in a host of recent scientific breakthroughs. Instead, the core principles behind the empowering side of the new paradigm can be found in a short folk song and a parable about kindergarteners.

Those principles start with this chapter's title, which came from Tom Paxton's hit song from the 1970s folk music revival, "Peace Will Come." I have reproduced its lyrics here. The words, of course, are only part of any song, so I encourage you to listen to it in this version, which Paxton recorded shortly after Pete Seeger's death in 2014. If you are reading the printed edition, the link is in this footnote.[5]

Peace
Peace will
Peace will come
And let it begin with me.

---

[5] https://www.youtube.com/watch?v=IsciNPv81KY (Accessed November 3, 2024.)

We
We need
We need peace
And let it begin with me.

Oh, my own life is all I can hope to control
Oh, let my life be lived for the good
Good of my soul.

Let it bring
Peace
Sweet peace
Peace will come
Let it begin with me.

Note how the words build off each other and (if you were able to listen) follow a simple and repetitive chord progression and guitar style which keeps cycling back to the refrain "we need peace, and let it begin with me." And although he only mentions it once, he makes a point that Niebuhr would have loved—my own life is all I can hope to control.

Peace always begins with our own thoughts and actions.

In that order.

At about the same time that my students and George Lopez pulled me up short, a single, simple parable turned the pastor and writer Robert Fulgham into a pop icon. *All I Needed to Know I Learned in Kindergarten* offers a more concrete description of what it means to let peace "begin with me," although I might have left out the cookies or flushing.[6]

Share everything.
Play fair.
Don't hit people.

---

6. Robert Flugham, *All I Really Need to Know I Learned in Kindergarten: Uncommon Thoughts on Common Things.* (New York: Ballantine Books, 1989).

PEACEBUILDING STARTS AT HOME

Put things back where you found them.
Clean up your own mess.
Don't take things that aren't yours.
Say you're sorry when you hurt somebody.
Wash your hands before you eat.
Flush.
Warm cookies and cold milk are good for you.
Live a balanced life -
Learn some and think some
And draw and paint and sing and dance
And play and work everyday some.
Take a nap every afternoon.
When you go out into the world,
Watch out for traffic,
Hold hands and stick together.
Be aware of wonder.

EXERCISE 3.1: AMERICA REMADE

There is no need to return to your kindergarten days or learn to play the guitar to do the first exercise in this chapter.

All you have to do is update the vision of American reMADE that you developed in chapter 2 in two ways.

Start with Fulgham. What difference would it make if you cleaned up your own mess, said you were sorry if you hurt someone, held hands and stuck together, and lived a balanced life? Then turn to Paxton. If it is true that your own life is all you can hope to control, think about how your actions can help turn you into your best kindergarten self and the United States into a better society.

ACTIVELY SEEING WITH NEW EYES

I am greeted with lots of skeptical looks whenever I play Paxton's song or read Fulgham's lines in front of audiences who have never heard of either of these "experts". At that point, I tell them that I will be using their words to help bring their new Proustean eyes into focus. However, I then warn them that I'm going to ask them to bear with me while I get even weirder, because I ask them—and you—to do an unusual exercise that will allow them—and you—to pivot away from just worrying about the world and its problems to doing something about them.

It does so by giving participants a first glimpse into alternatives to business as usual that are based on systems theory and complexity science which they can begin experimenting with right away. It does not offer the answer. Time and time again, however, it has helped participants see that they do have a choice. They can continue to live their lives using a paradigm they are used to but which is also largely responsible for the mess we find ourselves in today. Or, they can choose to begin using a different mindset that is in keeping with what the new realities are telling all of us to do and can help them address the part of the world's wicked problems that they can control.

It also tells them that they still have a lot to learn. While the exercise does show them that they normally have alternatives to choose from, it also helps participants understand they will spend the rest of their lives learning how best to put what reality is telling them to do into practice.[7]

In a classroom or workshop, I start by splitting everyone up into small groups of three to five participants. You obviously can't do that unless you are somehow reading *Peacebuilding Starts at Home* in a study group that is meeting in real time. Still, even if you are limited to a "small group of one," you should be able to see where the exercise would take you if you had a few of your friends by your side in a meeting room at your local library.

I first tell each group to spend no more than five minutes discussing why some global dispute had turned violent. When I wrote this paragraph in August 2025, I would have chosen the war between

---

7. The literature on emotional intelligence is immense. You can start with anything written by Daniel Goleman or recent books by *New York Times* columnist and PBS commentator, David Brooks. Perhaps the easiest entry point to this work is the wet site, Six Seconds.

Israel and Hamas that had recently spread to Iran and now included the United States.

I tell them that I'm not looking for definitive answers, just a list of what they think are the most important reasons why the two sides went to war. In your one-person at-home version of the exercise, get out some sticky notes and write the first words that come to mind. You won't even need five minutes.

I next have someone from each group tell everyone what they came up with. Without fail, they talk about causes which fall into two clusters. I put the objective differences that gave rise to the conflict on the left side of a whiteboard. Israelis and Palestinians both have strong claims to the same land that date back at least to the arrival of the first Zionist settlers more than a century ago. Add to that a history of tension and violence since Israel's independence, which Palestinians refer to as *al-nakba*, the catastrophe. Relatively sophisticated groups will raise some of the other incidents in the three quarters of a century since then—the Six Day War, the Yom Kippur War, the Intifadas, and so on. On the right side, I put the more subjective factors they raise, such as alleged Palestinian anti-semitism, Israeli disdain for Palestinians, or the lived trauma endured by average citizens on both sides. In your at-home version of the exercise you can arrange your sticky notes into the same two clusters on a nearby wall, desktop, or whiteboard.

Then they discuss an intractable domestic political issue, like America's racial divide. After a few minutes, the groups report out again and I put the key points up on the board. On the left side go historical and contemporary trends like the legacy of 250 years of slavery or the recent wave of police shootings. I use the right-hand column for more subjective factors like prejudice, fear of the other side, stereotyping, the perceived cost of losing, and miscommunication. The more perceptive participants have already noticed that the two rounds of questioning produced similar entries in that list of more subjective causes.

Next, they discuss an interpersonal conflict of their own choosing that turned out badly. More often than not, they focus on a failed romantic relationship. When they report out, the group hears tales of different tastes and, sometimes, even the way historically defined gender roles get in the way of twenty-first century relationships. Most of their time, however, is spent putting things like betrayal, miscommunication, or the fear of losing which, of course, go on the right side of the board.

At that point, I switch into professor mode and spend a few minutes on the two conclusions that always emerge. The left hand column drives home the point that intense conflict has deep historical roots that will be hard to overcome—even in interpersonal relationships. These are living examples of Niebuhr's "things I cannot change" or could only change with lots of effort and lots of time.

I then ask the group to focus on the right side of the board. However and wherever I've done the exercise, the participants identified a few common themes which I've summarized in the table below. As I discuss them, the students and/or workshop participants quickly realize that these values shape the way that just about all of us approach just about all of the tough issues they face in just about every aspect of their lives.

Value
Thinking in terms of "us v. them"
Focus on short term self interest
Expect a zero-sum or win-lose outcome in which I would like to win but definitely do not want to lose
Assume that one side will have to use power over the other
Understand that conflict is bad for everyone involved

Table 3.1: Our Current Paradigm

These values are also a version of the paradigm we rely on—consciously or unconsciously—whenever we find ourselves in what

Guy and Heidi Burgess call intractable conflict.[8] We think of ourselves as being in competition with other individuals, groups, or countries, all of which are seeking something we assume is in short supply.

In what some neuroscientists believe is a natural reaction, we split ourselves into camps that pit an "us" against a "them." As economists tell us, we pursue our self-interest, whether that is our personal self-interest or that of any of the "usses" that we are a part of, such as our class or race or religion or ethnicity or nation.

All too often, we magnify those differences, turning disagreements into antagonistic relationships. We start using what psychologists call the "image of the enemy" and demonize the "other," turning them into little more than a cardboard cutout caricature of the real person, group, or country.[9]

Typically, we also assume that any serious conflict will end in a win-lose or zero-sum outcome. In everyday English, that means that I can only win at your expense or, worse yet, your victory has to come at mine. We also assume that intractable conflicts can only be resolved through the use of power. "I" have to make "you" do what I want. That power may not involve physical force or violence, but this kind of "power over" always involves at least the threat of coercion.

That includes me. Remember the threat to take points off when students handed their assignments in late which I used to end chapter 1?

Once we have gotten to this point in the exercise, many participants find themselves depressed. Even worse, they worry that I've lost sight of Niebuhr's distinction between the things we can change and the things that are beyond our control. After all, the values in table 3.1 feel like an integral part of every society they have ever heard of (especially if they had taken my comparative politics courses).

So, I tell them that it is time to take a break and that, after we come back, things will be more uplifting. Nonetheless, when the participants file back into the room, they have their doubts.

---

8. www.beyondintractability.org (Accessed December 13, 2023.)
9. This article from the Beyond Intractability site covers a lot of related material. https://www.beyondintractability.org/CCG/section4A (Accessed February 15, 2025.)

I start by asking the small groups to discuss an interpersonal conflict that had turned out at least reasonably well. Normally, they pick an example in which the stakes were high—a couple deals with the aftermath of an affair or a sexist incident at work.

Still, their discussions are far more upbeat and rarely include anything table 3.1 would lead you to expect. A couple decides to get help so they can put their relationship back on firmer footing for themselves and their children. A supervisor or someone from HR sits down with the co-workers and helps them see that giving women workers the same respect that men get can both improve morale and boost sales and, with it, the company's bottom line.

I almost never have to add anything on the left side of the white board. However, I start making a new list on the right side that includes things like help from a third party, good communication and listening skills, acknowledging one's own role in the problem, and expressing a desire to find a solution that works for everyone concerned.

Then, I have them consider a national issue on which we've made noticeable progress. Here, there are fewer examples for them to choose from, but once the group settles on something like the growing support for marriage equality, they discuss how their own core values and assumptions changed as more and more people realized that there were members of the LGBTQ+ community in their families, workplaces, and neighborhoods—and that they liked them. Some mention effective training programs that help people overcome the homophobic and other prejudices they may have held since childhood.

Many of the themes that came up in the discussion of an interpersonal issue end up in the new list on the right. Learning about people different from yourself. Overcoming prejudice. Wanting what's best for people you care about.

I rarely have to get to a global issue, because the group has begun to see that the values and assumptions in table 3.1 and reproduced as the first column of table 3.2 are not an inescapable part of human nature—a point I will come back to in ending this book. To be sure, some things may be hardwired, including the fight or flight mechanism or the tendency to identify with people who are like us more than those who aren't.

Yet, they can also see that we can choose to base our actions on the constructive values and assumptions that come out in the second half of the exercise. I've summarized them in the right-hand column of this table so that you can see how different they are from the ones that participants stress when they talk about conflicts that don't get resolved well.

Current Value	New Value
Thinking in terms of "us v. them"	Thinking in terms of "us with them"
Focus on short-term self interest	Focus on shared interests in the medium- to long- term
Expect a zero-sum or win-lose outcome in which I would like to win but definitely do not want to lose	Work toward a win-win outcome that benefits everyone
Assume that one side will have to use power over the other	Redefine power as something we exercise with others
Understand that conflict is bad for everyone involved	Understand that conflict can be an opportunity for growth for everyone involved

Table 3.2: Adding the New Paradigm

Whether we get to a global issue or not, I go back into professor mode because I want the people in the room to see one more thing before we explore the second column of table 3.2 in the rest of the workshop, course, or, in this case, the book. The arrival of the first Zionists in Palestine, the centuries of racial inequality in the United States, or the fact that one partner in a relationship "strayed" are a given. They can't be undone. They are the things we can't control.

In my days as a political science professor, I typically limited myself to the top two layers of the chart on the next page. Thus, the students who wrote those insightful exams spent the semester studying the impact of imperialism, the Cold War, constitutional provisions, and the behavior of individual leaders.

Once I started teaching about peacebuilding, I started encouraging the people I worked with to dig deeper and explore the third level—the modes of thinking or paradigms that we use in deciding how to deal with problems at everything from the international to the interpersonal level.

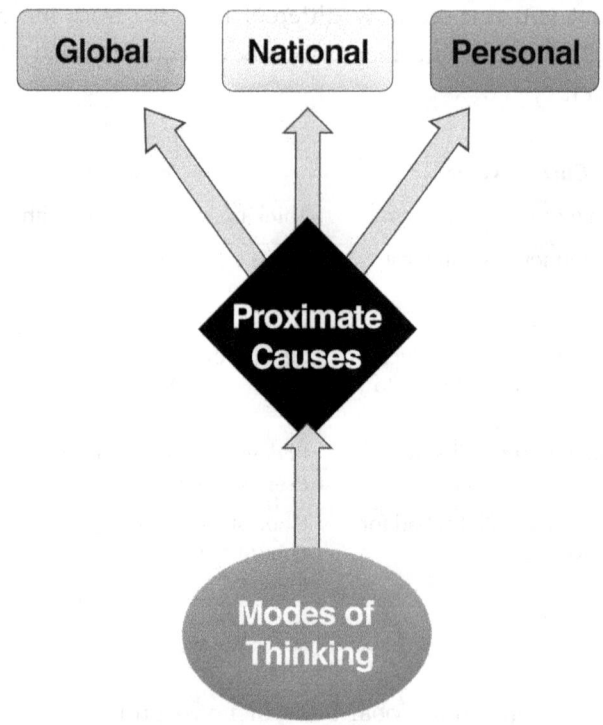

Figure 3.3: Modes of Thinking: The Big Picture

I then suggest that, in Niebuhr's terms, I have just identified the kinds of things we can control. Even when they are faced with the most intractable of conflicts, people almost always have options. They can choose to go down the tried but not so true path of using the values in column one, or they can decide to use the ones they have just brought to the surface in doing the exercise because they have identified the core values of the new paradigm in their discussions after the break. And to use a phrase that wasn't in Niebuhr's vocabulary, it's not rocket science.

Needless to say, most of them are excited—if still skeptical—and want to know more. So, I end the class or workshop as I will end this chapter, by quickly showing how those values in the second column can lead to action, knowing that I will have more time to dig into those issues in more depth, just as I do here in the five and a half chapters to come.

Before doing so, I should note one more thing. I have been doing versions of this exercise for almost forty years. During that time, social psychologists and cognitive neuroscientists have published hundreds of studies that lend empirical support for what I've discovered in my classrooms and workshops.[10]

MY AI REALLY WAS RIGHT: YOU CAN BECOME A PEACEBUILDER

Given the fact that this is a book about peacebuilding at home, I will focus on how the new paradigm helps us deal with the wicked problems in our daily lives. But do note, however, that what follows applies to everything we do.[11]

Each individual I work with is unique and has to deal with a unique cluster of problems under a unique set of circumstances. As a result, I am never able to offer more than general strategic guidelines at this point even when I'm working with a small class or workshop and we are sitting in the same room. A student has to come to office hours or I have to share a meal with a workshop participant to get into the details of what they could or should do. However, because you have responded to my RSVP (and there is still time if you haven't), you can come to the equivalent of office hours with the Peacebuilding Starts at

---

10. The most useful books along these lines that I've read recently are Jamil Zaki, *Hope for Cynics: The Surprising Science of Human Goodness*. (New York: Hachette/Grand Central Publishing, 2024). Amy Gallo, *Getting Along: How to Work with Anyone (Even Difficult People)*. (Boston: Harvard Business School Press, 2022). and Emily Falk. *What We Value: The Neuroscience of Choice and Change*. (New York: W. W. Norton, 2025).
11. There are literally hundreds of references I could cite here. Just as I was finishing this chapter, I read the extremely useful new book by Robert Bordone and Joel Salinas. *Conflict Resilience: Negotiating Disagreement Without Give Up or Giving In*. (New York: Harper Business, 2025).

Home team, which will be glad to help you figure out how you might respond to the issues in your life and go to scale inward.

In the meantime, think of the ideas that follow as more sliders for your mental dashboard that you can consider moving "up" or "down" in ways that make the most sense for you.

Decide. The first step is to "simply" make the decision to base your life on the values listed in the right-hand column of that table. I put the word simply in quotes because I know that making and sticking to a decision of this magnitude is easier said than done as anyone who has been in a twelve-step program and recited the Serenity Prayer can attest.

Alcoholics Anonymous and other recovery programs ask us to acknowledge the problems we face while also understanding that we can choose to break away from the habits that have gotten us into and kept us in trouble. For the purposes of this book, I'm not talking about breaking habits that leave people addicted to dangerous substances. Instead, I am asking you to stop what amounts to an addiction to the values in the left-hand column of the table and begin relying on the second list as often and as fully as you can.[12]

The word decision itself is telling. Its roots lie in the Latin verb *caedere* which meant to cut. Thus, an incision is a cut into an organism's body. By that same logic, a decision is a mental cut that takes you away from something. Decisions are conscious acts. Thus, we make decisions to start exercising or stop drinking. Or to become a peacebuilder.

Because everyone has at least a tiny impact on everything and everyone else, everything you do matters. That includes a decision *not* to act. It doesn't matter why you choose to stay on the sidelines. The bottom line is the same. You are counted among those who either support the status quo or don't care enough to do anything about it.

In my Beyond War days, we thought about decisions in stark, either/or terms You either were a smoker or you weren't—I had easily quit puffing away at my pipe a few years earlier. You either drink or

---

12. Charles Duhigg, *The Power of Habit: Why We Do What We Do in Life and Business.* (New York: Random House 2012) and James Clear, *Atomic Habits: An Easy and Proven Way to Build Good Habits and Break Bad Ones.* (New York: Avery, 2018).

you don't. It was another thirty years before I gave up alcohol, and the difficulties I faced doing so drove home the fact that important decisions are rarely cut and dried.

Nonetheless, deciding how you want to act and practicing how to act that way are definitely things you can control.

As you do so, you will see that my AI that was right. You can be a peace-builder.

Toward win-win. In the 1980s, most peacebuilders made reaching win-win outcomes their highest priority. That made sense since mediation had become a hot topic after Roger Fisher and William Ury's *Getting to Yes* surprisingly turned into a global best seller.[13] As we have added complexity, wicked problems, and the like to the mix, we have learned that peacebuilders have to do more than reach short term deals that satisfy everyone. That said, win-win or positive-sum agreements remain an important component of any successful peacebuilding initiative.

At a face-to-face event, I typically make that point by using an extramarital affair as an example both because the group has already discussed one and because they rarely lend themselves to cooperative solutions!

When, as is often the case today, the parents deal with the situation using the values in the left hand column of the table, they may well separate. If they do stay together, their relationship will remain tense and will probably keep deteriorating. And what about the kids?

What if, however, the couple turns to a family therapist? The ones I know all treat families as a whole and help clients see the value of conflict resolution, systems theory, and other tools that reflect the values in the right-hand column.

Every therapist I've ever met would encourage the family members to talk about everything in ways that hold them all accountable for what happened. More importantly, they help family members find the best outcome for all concerned. In this case, there may not be a single or simple win-win result in which everyone is equally happy. For

---

13. Roger Fisher and William Ury. *Getting to Yes: Negotiating Agreement Without Giving In.* (New York: Houghton-Mifflin 1981).

instance, the best outcome might be a divorce, but even if that does happen, the relationship between former partners, their children, and, often, other friends and relatives will continue.

At that point, the aggrieved partner's power lies less in getting revenge over their "other half" than in finding ways of making the relationships work as well as possible for everyone. This, of course, is what blended families are all about. It is something that I see first-hand whenever I co-grandparent with Gretchen's first husband and his relatives, including his other ex-wife and her adopted child who, of course, is my stepdaughter's non-biological stepsister. Figure out that relationship if you can without getting out some sticky notes and mapping this convoluted set of relationships!

If you will, systems theory and related scientific breakthroughs provide real world support for the Judeo-Christian Golden Rule, a version of which can be found in all of the world's major religions. Put negatively, if I don't do unto you as I would have you do unto me, you will almost certainly resent whatever it is I did and try to get revenge. By contrast, if I treat you well, the odds are much higher that you will appreciate what I did and try to repay the favor.

It is hard to find win-win outcomes, build good relationships, or follow anything resembling the Golden Rule in a troubled family. It is even harder to do so in a community or country that has been divided by racism for centuries or has to figure out how to make the transition away from its reliance on fossil fuels. Nonetheless, one key principle that emerges from systems theory does apply across the board—what goes around comes around.

Making things work beyond the interpersonal level takes a lot of time and goes beyond seeking win-win outcomes. But remember, we still have a few guidelines and a few chapters to go.

Seeking win-win outcomes is another thing you can do to show that my AI was right. You can be a peacebuilder.

Understand that you are probably part of the problem. Because few of today's problems lend themselves to simple solutions, one of the first steps in coming to grips with intractable conflicts is to acknowledge their complexity. In what is undoubtedly the best book on peacebuilding written since *Getting to Yes*, Amanda Ripley encourages her readers to "complicate the narrative."[14] She acknowledges that we all have a tendency to see human conflict—and perhaps all of life—in simple either-or and us-versus-them terms.

The real world, however, is rarely that simple.

More importantly, we don't have to act as if it is.

We do, however, have to come to grips with an uncomfortable fact. Our own actions often make the situation we face even more complicated and harder to solve.

Like it or not, we all contribute to the conflicts we find ourselves in. There is bound to be something that you have said or done that deepened the anger, frustration, and other less than positive emotions your adversary brings to the table. That doesn't mean that you are wrong or did anything out of line. But more often than not, you added to the dispute in part because of something(s) you said or did. For that matter, your attitudes and behavior shape every relationship you are part of, whether it involves conflict or not.

Indeed, the more time you spend developing the self-awareness that going to scale inwardly involves, the more you will come to see the importance of this statement by the lawyer Robert Bordone and neurologist Joel Salinas:

> *It's not hyperbole to say that the biggest hidden barrier to being conflict resilient stems from the inability or unwillingness to face and sit with our own internal conflicts—the negotiations between our divided and sometimes contradictory "selves." Even more surprising is that although there are dozens of self-help books on negotiation and conflict resolution, almost none of them spend any meaningful time on this critical interpersonal barrier to handling conflict.*[15]

Understanding your role in any relationship once again shows that you can be a peacebuilder.

---

14. Amanda Ripley, *High Conflict: Why We Get Trapped and How We Get Out*. (New York: Simon and Schuster, 2021).
15. Robert Bordone and Joel Salias. *Conflict Resilience: Negotiating Disagreement Without Giving Up or Giving In*. (New York: Harper Business, 2025), 95.

Rotary's Four-Way Test. Win-win outcomes and complicating the narrative will not take us very far toward building a healthy society unless they also help forge strong working relationships among everyone who is affected by the conflict. These days, I include Rotary's Four-Way Test in any discussion of cooperative problem solving.

To be honest, I didn't listen when the Richesons and others in Beyond War suggested that we reach out to our local Rotary club. It was just too conventional for someone with roots in the new left and the counter culture. Over the years, however, I came to appreciate Rotary's work more and more until the Richeson's message finally sank in. In 2021, Gretchen and I joined. Now, four years later, only our work for AfP takes up more of our time.

For the purposes of this chapter, Rotary matters because you can use its guidelines when you have to decide how to put these ideas into practice. That starts with its motto—Service Over Self.

Rotary turns that abstract principle into concrete action through its Four-Way Test, which has served as its ethical compass since the 1940s. Its thirty-two words are read aloud at most meetings and many members include them in their email sig files because the test really does lie at the heart of everything Rotary stands for by committing its members to routinely ask these questions before they do anything.

Of all the things we say and do:

- Is it the truth?
- Is it fair to all concerned?
- Will it build goodwill and better friendships?
- Will it be beneficial to all concerned?

Even though the test was devised almost a century before disinformation and fake news became everyday concerns, it commits Rotarians to seeking the truth, which, as we now know all too well, is never easy. After that, it tracks other core values that are at least implicit in my table, especially the need to be fair and to do things that are beneficial to everyone who is even indirectly affected by a dispute.

Last but by no means least is a point that I will come back to in chapter 5. Rotarians themselves are just beginning to explore how peacebuilding can be combined with its other areas of focus. Clubs also work on projects to eradicate polio and other diseases, provide clean water, help mothers and children, support education, expand local economies, and protect the environment. Now, I am part of a growing group of Rotarians who are helping our colleagues see that that this other work can also contribute to peacebuilding if and when they realize that these issues are all interconnected. As I like to put it, they already are peacebuilders; they just don't know it yet.

Using the Four-Way Test will show once more that my AI was right. You can be a peacebuilder.

Call people in and turn toward them. I am also drawn to the Four-Way Test because it steers us away from one of the biggest obstacles that social change advocates have trouble overcoming when they rely on the old paradigm and its values. Social psychologists have known for decades that using our all too common reliance on the image of the enemy gets us in trouble. We stereotype, demonize, and otherwise point the mental (and sometimes literal) finger at people we disagree with. The ongoing "game" of naming, blaming, and shaming makes solving disputes difficult, especially when both sides do it.[16]

But what if we base our thoughts and actions on the other column? In that case, it makes more sense to "call in" the people we disagree with.[17] The term was popularized by the veteran civil rights leader, Loretta Ross, whom you met briefly in chapter 2. Here, I'd like you to consider going even farther and taking the advice of Chad Ford who makes the case that we peacebuilders have an obligation to "turn toward" the people we disagree with and take the first step toward forging a solution that satisfies everyone.[18]

The easiest way to see the importance of what Ross and Ford (and

---

16. The best recent work along these lines was written by the remarkable john a. powell. john a. powell and Stephen Menendian, *Belonging Without Othering: How We Save Ourselves and the World*. (Palo Alto: Stanford University Press, 2024) and powell, *The Power of Bridging: How to Build a World in Which We All Belong*. (Boulder CO: Sounds True, 2024). For what it's worth, powell always writes his name using lower case letters.
17. Loretta Ross, *Calling In: How to Start Making Change with Those You'd Rather Cancel*. (New York: Simon and Schuster, 2025).
18. Chad Ford, *Dangerous Love: Transforming Fear and Conflict at Home, at Work, and in the World*. (Oakland CA: Berrett-Koehler, 2020).

plenty of others) have to say is to recall a time when you were called out. Think about the pain, resentment, and even fear it led to. Then, think about other times when someone approached you with a genuine sense of curiosity and treated you with dignity and respect. Or better yet, when you took that first step yourself....

Turning toward your adversaries alone is never enough to solve a problem, but it can create more mental "space" in which you two can explore options together. It is also the first step toward building trust which, as you will also see, doesn't require agreement.

Calling in and turning toward your "other" both show that my AI was right. You can be a peacebuilder.

Stop. Think. Build peace. The next step has a rather silly origin story, but that doesn't mean it isn't important. A few of my friends, including Gretchen and AfP's executive director, Liz Hume, were talking over lunch at a recent National Association for Community Mediation (NAFCM) conference. I was facilitating the discussion at another table which turned out to be a lot less interesting. Instead of the topic the organizers suggested, Liz and Gretchen's table kicked around ideas for short videos that they could make using TikTok, YouTube, and other platforms that could help people begin making the decision to work for peace in their everyday lives and maybe even have some fun while doing it.

For reasons none of them remembers, Liz recalled a public service announcement from her childhood. In those days, children's pajamas were still made of flammable material. If, in the unlikely event that their pajamas did catch fire, kids were advised to "stop, drop, and roll." Then, someone else remembered Daniel Tiger who sings, "take a deep breath, and count to four" in an ad promoting PBS that I've seen so many times that I sometimes dream about it. After a bit of giggling and brainstorming, the table came up with a line of their own—"stop, think, and build peace."

I don't know how Daniel Tiger learned his version of the lesson. However, research by Daniel Kahneman and others has shown that our "automatic pilot" may lead us to react instinctively, but we all also have the ability to reflect on whatever is taking place around us.[19] If we do the equivalent of taking a few deep breaths or counting to four, it is easier to free ourselves from what cognitive behavioral therapists refer to as automatic thoughts and others call self-chatter. Taking those few seconds and using more powerful mindfulness tools allow us to create the psychological space through which we can at least begin considering alternatives to those gut reactions that reflect the values in the left-hand column of the table. That holds whether we are tempted to lash out at our children or coworkers or, as a society, we are considering lashing out at our geopolitical enemies.

I know from painful, first-hand experience that it often isn't easy to take Daniel Tiger's advice. In my case, I totally lost it on a Zoom call with one of my closest colleagues a few days after I first drafted this paragraph. I still think the point I was making made sense and that she was not doing "her job" on the task we were working on. Still, I failed to learn my own lesson and erupted. Luckily, my friend has a tough skin and no real damage was done. Nonetheless, we have all been in situations in which that wasn't the case and shown that my AI that it was right. You can be a peacebuilder.

Active Listening. Stopping to think makes it easier to do something that is always at or near the top of peacebuilders' list of priorities—active listening.[20] My lapse occurred because I fell into an all too common trap. When we are in the middle of a heated, tension-filled conversation, we typically begin preparing our response long before our partners have finished what they have to say. We haven't really listened. Everyone I know struggles with this, but it's important to fully hear the other person out so that you are at least able to understand where they are coming from, which is literally what empathy is all about.

Amanda Ripley drew my attention to one active listening tool that I

---

19. Amos Tversky would have shared the honor, but he died in 1996, and only living people are eligible to win any of the Nobel prizes. That's also why Kahneman alone wrote the book summarizing their research. *Thinking Fast and Slow.* (New York: Farrar, Straus, and Giroux, 2011).
20. Emily Kasriel. *Deep Listening: Transform Your Relationships with Family, Friends, and Foes.* (New York: William Morrow, 2025).

now use a lot—looping. When you loop, your first response is to restate what you think you just heard your discussion partner say. Although it can be awkward and make a discussion seem stilted, looping matters. If nothing else, your partner will feel heard and be able to "correct" any misunderstandings on your part which, in turn, can help convert animosity into curiosity.

Despite my occasional—and mortifying—lapses, I have been working on looping and active listening for decades. Even in my student activist days in the 1960s, I often found myself in discussions with people whose views were sharply at odds with mine but I still liked and wanted to work with them. They included most of my professors, some of whom became close friends, at least half of the other students in my political science and history classes, and, most instructively of all, my first serious girl friend whose family was extremely conservative.

I got far better at it when I became a professor. Given what I taught and wrote about, I could not hide my opinions about controversial issues. I also did not want to foist them on my students. So, I developed ways of making students feel comfortable disagreeing with me. I learned to get better at helping them strengthen their own arguments, especially when they contradicted mine. They knew I didn't agree with what they were saying, but they appreciated the fact that I took them seriously. Sometimes, it could be as simple as smiling and using other body language that conveyed the impression that what they believe mattered to me. In the language of the 2020s, they felt heard.

Now, I use those skills everywhere I go. Over the years, I've found myself as the atypical secular Jew working with evangelical Christians or the rare peace activist meeting with senior military officers at the Pentagon or just talking to Trump supporters whose children play on the same soccer teams as my grandchildren.

It's not just the tone of my conversations that has changed. So has the way people respond to me. People I disagree with about the Trump presidency, DEI, or a woman's right to choose seem to enjoy working with me. And the feeling is mutual. Along the way, I've learned that the kinds of skills discussed in this entire section and active listening in particular are contagious.

When you listen well, you will prove that my AI was right. You can become a peacebuilder.

Don't try to convince the other person. The next skill might seem counterintuitive. Obviously, when I get into a discussion with someone I disagree with on an issue that I care deeply about, I want them to agree with me.

However, if I have learned anything from all those years I spent teaching inside and outside of the classroom, it is that I almost never convinced anyone of anything. My students had to convince themselves.

I don't keep my own views secret. I also don't try to win the argument. I don't think of these discussions as debates, but as dialogues which the pollster and philosopher Daniel Yankelovich describe as "a discussion that is so intense that it leaves neither party unchanged."[21]

I try to present the material in a way that the person I am talking with is most likely to hear what I am saying and not reject my ideas out of hand. I try to anticipate how they will respond by flexing my empathy muscles. I get creative. I propose ideas that we think might appeal to both of us. I show that I'm ready to listen to and learn from them. Far more often than you might think, they take my ideas seriously, and sometimes they end up agreeing with me—and sometimes I end up agreeing with them.

When you don't try to convince the other person, you can prove that my AI was right and become a peacebuilder.

---

21. Daniel Yankelovich. *The Magic of Dialogue: Turning Conflict Into Cooperation.* (New York: Simon and Schuster, 1999).

EXERCISE 3.2: NAILING IT

My AI actually suggested this exercise.

Choose one thing you could do this week that might address a conflict or tension in your daily life. It doesn't have to be one that could result in an interpersonal version of World War III. In fact, it's probably a good idea to start with something relatively minor—as long as it nags away at you because you harbor some resentment toward the other people involved.

Then, use your imagination to come up with one or more possible outcomes that would satisfy everyone involved in the medium to long term, if not immediately. Approach it using some or all of the values in the right-hand column of the table and/or apply the skills developed in the second half of this chapter (you may want to wait and do this and exercise 3.3 together).

Take note of the times when values like those in the left-hand column shape what you do and consciously use those in the other list instead. Once the conflict has come to even a temporary end however you choose to define it, do your personal equivalent of what the military calls an after action review and assess why things did (or didn't) work.

Be a leader. It is time for peacebuilders to embrace the fact that they are leaders. And that they have to be.

You might have a hard time accepting that, given what most of us think about the institutions and individuals who are running our country in both the private and public sectors. The fact of the matter is that by practicing these and other techniques that my team and I would be delighted to share, you will become a new kind of leader almost by default. As you will see in far more detail starting in chapter 5, cutting edge thinkers in top MBA programs and C-suite executives in hundreds of companies have shown that successful leaders whom you would want to emulate base their work on systems theory and the kinds of ideas I've discussed in this section.

Here, I can point to a single author, Peter Senge, and a single book, *The Fifth Discipline* that revolutionized the way leading corporate executives went about their jobs.[22] As he sees it, leaders need to adopt practices or disciplines that lead them to think of firms as living systems that can become learning organizations for the kinds of reasons I discussed in chapter 2.

New leadership styles show that my AI was right and that you can be a peacebuilder.

Be patient. Finally, understand that our country's problems will not be solved over night. Nor will the ones you face close to home.

Even if you have had experience using these or similar principles before, it will take some time and practice before you can use them effectively, especially as stepping stones for peacebuilding at the national level. If nothing else, you will be a pioneer, since relatively few of the people you deal with will be using a similar "playbook," at least at first. You probably won't need the ten thousand hours of practice that the meme calls for, but it will take time before you begin to see results beyond your immediate circle of family members, friends, neighbors, and co-workers.

So, be patient.

But do keep experimenting. Keep reflecting on whether or not these guidelines—or others that you choose to substitute for them—work for you. Keep adjusting how you use them. It might also help to find a coach or a group of people you try these principles with so that you can reflect on your experiences together.

Here, consider the words of Father Gregory Boyle in describing his half century's worth of work with gang members returning from prison in Los Angeles.

---

22. Peter Senge, *The Fifth Discipline: The Art and Practice of the Learning Organization*. (New York: Currency, 1991).

> *We choose love as our practice. Practice doesn't ever make perfect; it makes permanent, then increasingly habitual. Second nature.*[23]

I don't want to go too far here. To some degree, the values in the left-hand column are hardwired into us. Even if they are not part of our human nature, they are at least deeply ingrained habits and cultural norms that are hard to break. Still, you can choose to anchor your life in the values implicit in the other column, learn how to apply them in your daily life, and begin to see the world change.

All I want you to understand at this point is that we each can make meaningful choices that can help us get closer to what I repeatedly call the three "mosts"—solving most of our problems most of the time mostly without the use of force, coercion, or violence.

And now do this chapter's third exercise. It is my invitation to learn that practice doesn't make perfect but can lead to life-long habits nonetheless. Not just of love but in living as if reality is telling you what to do.

Being patient will show that you that my AI was right. You can become a peacebuilder.

EXERCISE 3.3: THE LUNCH PAIL F***ING JOB

Because I don't know anything about you, this chapter's final exercise was hard to devise. But give it a try any way.

What do you think it would take to keep you engaged for the long haul, especially when you face the setbacks that you are bound to encounter at home, at work, in your community, and in your country?

---

23. Gregory Boyle. *Cherished Belonging: The Healing Power of Love in Divided Times.* (New York: Simon and Schuster, 2024), 142.

THE GHOST OF EMILY POST

I started this chapter with a statement about addiction which is never easy to talk about, let alone deal with. Overcoming it is a Lunch Pail F***ing Job if there ever was one.

So, it might make sense to end the chapter on a lighter note that makes the point that the basics of doing peace in our daily lives is not rocket science from a different angle. One day as I was finishing this chapter, I met with Dr. Whohasnoname for my weekly therapy session. I mentioned that my mother always sent me letters addressed to Dr. Hauss. I didn't like it. Dr. Hauss was my father who was a dentist. My parents had been through one of the most spectacular divorces I have ever heard of, and my mother definitely did not like being reminded of my father.

I told my prim and proper (and very hard to deal with) mother that Emily Post recommended that only medical professionals like my father and Dr. Whohasnoname should be called doctor.

Dr. Whohasnoname responded by asking me if I had read the one hundredth anniversary edition of Emily Post's original book which was written by two of her great grandchildren. I asked her why she even thought that I might have, and she replied that it was all about peacebuilding (she had read the first draft of this book by then).

As soon as I got home, I ordered the book. Emily Post herself would not have been considered a peacebuilder even by her own generation's standards. Her great grandchildren are a different story. To be sure, the book has a lot about when you need to send thank you notes and setting the table properly.

But Lizzy Post and Daniel Post Senning go farther and claim that good etiquette rests on an ethical core that their great grandmother tapped into. So, they decided to update her principles before turning to defining the best ways of behaving in a host of social settings that their great grandmother would have recognized.

Emily Post wrote for what she called Best Society or the highly privileged world that she herself lived in. Her great grandchildren point out that any definition of Best Society in the twenty-first century has to include all of us. Manners still matter, but only in a context that reflects the newfound need for us all to be peacebuilders in a way that makes for a fitting end to this chapter—thanks again to Dr. Whohasnoname.

> *Today we recognize Best Society as being made up of people who are kind, compassionate, and aware. These people speak and act in ways that are inclusive—recognizing that many different lives are lived within each community—and create safe spaces for everyone to be heard and to be themselves. People of Best Society are tenderhearted and fearless all at once. They are aware of their impact beyond the present moment, knowing that the actions they take and the words they say can ripple outward. They see the value and necessities of follow-up action, whether that means self-reflection or outreach. They are equipped with smiles and laughter, bringing a hopeful and positive attitude (when appropriate) wherever they go and they know how to deliver a good apology—one that is sincere, reflective, and focused, while still exhibiting self-respect in our fast-paced world. Members of Best Society recognize the virtue of patience and that slowing down to think first about a problem can be just as useful as solving it quickly.*[24]

---

24. Lizzie Post and Daniel Post-Senning. *Emily Post's Etiquette: The Centential Edition.* (New York: Ten Speed Press/Random House, 2022), 5.

CHAPTER 4
PEACE IS A VERB

If you want peace, you don't talk to your friends. You talk to your enemies.

DESMOND TUTU

I can be a hardliner when it comes to going to scale internally.

I have seen the Serenity Prayer, Emily Post's updated advice, and everything else that I covered in chapter 3 change people's lives. I have seen those same people serve as role models, often without even being aware of the impact they are having on their family members, friends, co-workers, and more. I know this, too, because I have seen it in myself.

I have also seen what happens when peacebuilders don't take chapter 3's lessons to heart. Plenty of my colleagues have demonized President Trump in ways that came back to haunt them. I've heard Rotarians recite the Four-Way Test at the beginning of a meeting and then seemingly forget all about it when they disagree with other club members just a few minutes later. I also have to admit that I do not always live up to my own standards—almost always to my detriment.

In the end, however, I'm only a hardliner up to a point.

Going to scale inward may be a necessary precondition for building peace, but it is not a sufficient one. That's why there are five more steps on the Peacebuilding Starts at Home Loop.

The first of them adds explicit peacebuilding work to your arsenal (pun, again, intended) and your RSVP. Knowing that it, too, won't be enough.

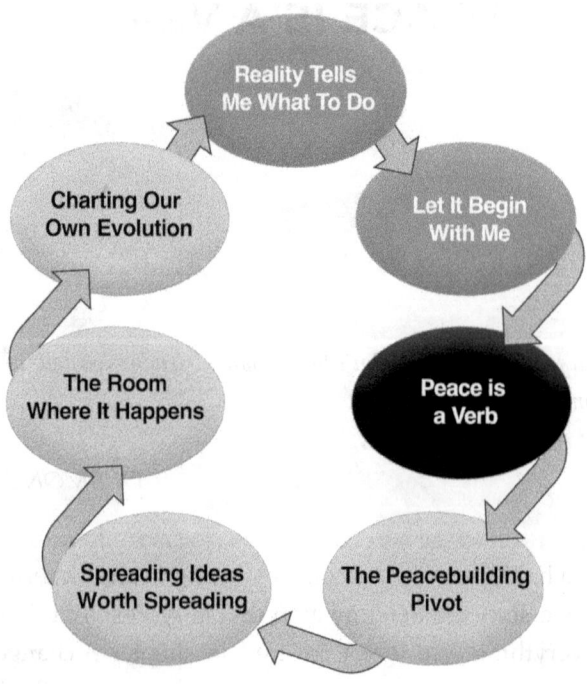

Figure 4.1: *The Peacebuilding Starts at Home Loop*

PEACE *IS* A VERB

For the reasons I mentioned in chapter 1, I had no trouble abandoning Peace Is a Verb as this book's title. I am also delighted that I can use it here, because you are about to see that treating peace as an active verb is the key for turning going to scale inwardly into concrete action steps that could lead to the sweeping social change of a paradigm shift. None of the organizations that you are about to meet have any hope of producing peace on their own. But they can keep getting us closer to a more peaceful society in which most of the people solve most of their problems without the use of force or violence most of the time.

And, once again, practice makes (almost) perfect.

Because I had been doing this kind of work since I was in high school, I assumed that this chapter would be easy to write.

I was wrong.

Not because I didn't "know my stuff."

Rather, it's because "the stuff" that could easily allow you to find your peacebuilding niche doesn't exist.

Although I hate to admit it, there is nothing resembling a one-size-fits-all group for you to join. None of the organizations that I will be highlighting comes close to dealing with all of the issues that reality is telling us to work on. Even more importantly, Rotary is the only one that has anything resembling a nation-wide presence. And as much as I love Rotary, I know that there are people who would never be comfortable joining it.

Add to that the fact that I know nothing about you, including something as basic as where you live. If you are in the Washington DC area as I am, I would have dozens of organizations to suggest. But if you live in Waterville ME (where I used to live) or Waterville OH (where my sister lives), that wouldn't be the case.

Under those circumstances, the best I can do is to lay out criteria that you could use in determining which of the available options are best for you by asking these questions which track the chart below.

What part of peacebuilding do you care about the most?

What options are available to you where you live, including online activism?

What skills and other resources do you have?

Where do you think that you can have the greatest impact?

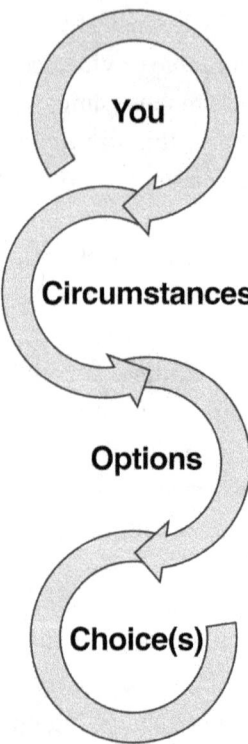

Figure 4.2: Making Your Choice

With that in mind, let the sample of promising initiatives that follow whet your appetite. They reflect the breadth of the American peacebuilding community, recruit average citizens with little or no peacebuilding experience, and could easily be taken to scale before this decade is out. What's more, you can use the three exercises in this chapter to develop a list on your own.

If you still come up short—as my sister did— the Peace building Starts at Home team can help you find your niche. Just fill in the contact form on our website—www.peacebuildingstartsathome.us.

LEARNING FROM DESMOND TUTU

But there is some good news. The groups I am about to introduce you to are doing important work that is anchored in the first two steps along the loop as well the logic underlying the statement by Archbishop Demond Tutu that begins this chapter.

Plenty of people remain convinced that if you want to express moral outrage, your best and perhaps only option is to oppose "the other side."

To some, the second Trump presidency represents a "threat to democracy." We have to do something about it. Right now.

If, on the other hand, you like the Trump administration, you want to give it all the support you can so that it can undo the damage done over the last few decades. Right now.

Tutu suggests otherwise.

His career was based on the assumption that there are times when you do have to say a resounding "no" to what those in power are doing. But we remember him today because he also understood that we have other options.

Tutu, Nelson Mandela, and reformers in South Africa's white leadership came to the conclusion that you can be a powerful advocate for "your side" but make your case in a way that builds support, precisely because you reach out and broaden your coalition. Whatever your political views.

They and other staunch opponents of apartheid were willing to "talk with their enemies" even when the South African government was at its most repressive. To be sure, it took a century of organization and active protest before members of the elite were willing to talk with them. Nonetheless, by the 1980s, front line leaders like Mandela and Tutu along with thousands of grassroots activists had reached out to white leaders—some at the highest levels—who were willing to question whether they could and should continue to rule.

As most readers of this book will already know, Tutu was the first Black head of the Anglican church in South Africa. He literally used his bully pulpit to become one of the leading critics of his country's all white government and its apartheid policies for which he won the Nobel Peace Prize in 1984. After the country's transition to a multi-racial democracy in the first half of the 1990s, Tutu became a global political rock star because of his skillful leadership of his country's Truth and Reconciliation Commission (TRC) which went a long way toward overcoming centuries of racism.[1]

Tutu shook up a lot of preconceptions about peacebuilding. He and others understood that the new South Africa had to do more than just dismantle the apartheid laws and get rid of the institutions that sustained white supremacy.

There were other "realities" that he and his allies had to take into account, including the fact that very few South African whites would want to or be able to leave the country after the transition.[2] Whether they liked it or not, Tutu and his colleagues—Black and white alike—realized that all South Africans had to learn how to get along with each other while, at the same time, they addressed the divisions that led to the transition in the first place. That and his Christian faith led him to reconciliation.[3]

To make a long story short, President Mandela named Tutu as head of the TRC in 1995. Among other things, it held hearings and issued reports in which activists and leaders on all sides would be granted amnesty if they took responsibility for their actions under apartheid as a first step toward racial healing. Without going into the details that would take us far beyond the scope of this book, progress was made in large part because Tutu and his colleagues made it possible for enemies to talk to and learn from each other.

Extremists on both sides resisted. Despite their objections, the commission made remarkable progress. No one would claim that South Africa today has achieved racial or economic equality, but the TRC went a long way toward helping Black and white South Africans figure out how to live more comfortably with each other. It did that by speaking truth to power *and* by bringing strange social and political bedfellows together.

The second reason I chose Tutu's statement is his emphasis on the

---

1. Desmond Tutu, *No Future Without Forgiveness*. (New York: Doubleday, 1999).
2. I should note that I sent this chapter to the publisher during the same week that the Trump administration allowed a group of white South Africans to move to the United States alleging (without any real evidence) that the current regime was racist. The best estimate is that about eighty percent of the white population opted to remain in South Africa after the end of apartheid thirty years ago.
3. I've written on this at some length at https://www.beyondintractability.org/essay/reconciliation. I would also write that essay somewhat differently today.

pronoun that serves as the subject of both of his sentences—you. Tutu, Mandela, and other leaders on both sides of the struggle against apartheid deserve their places in history. However, when we venerate them, we also run the risk of underestimating the importance of the "you" Tutu had in mind—everyday citizens like ourselves.

National leaders do have to make the final "deal." However, the evidence is clear. Those agreements can only work if they rest on grassroots networks whose existence makes it possible for elites to act in new, decisive, and often risky ways.

In the United States today, that means building a network of organizations that can help people adopt new cultural norms and lay the foundation for a movement or movements that can make our equivalent of the South African transition to a multi-racial democracy possible.

American peacebuilders cannot simply copy what happened in a country whose initials once were also USA—for the Union of South Africa. There is no peacebuilding version of the "cut and paste" function I used so many times in moving words around while writing *Peacebuilding Starts at Home*. Nonetheless, there are enough parallels between South Africa in the 1990s and the U.S. today to suggest that we should take Tutu's words seriously, in this case by turning peace into a verb—and an active one at that.

To begin with, the events of the last decade or so make it abundantly clear that our national leaders are reluctant (at best) to start peacebuilding at home themselves. In their absence, organizations like those you are about to meet have no choice but to shift public opinion, build support for social change, and otherwise create an environment in which those leaders have to accede to our demands. For good or ill, that can't be done if all we do is take peacebuilding to scale inwardly.

Tutu's message is also relevant here because the United States is going through a transition which all but requires us to talk across our lines of division. Sometime in the early 2040s, the United States will become a majority-minority country. Whites will make up less than half of the population. Given the "othering" and the tensions that already exist, it is hard to see how we can find a way to deal with the fact that many white Americans fear losing a lot of the power, status, and wealth that they have enjoyed since 1776. And that's just the part of the wicked problem iceberg that sits above the surface.

For reasons I will get to in the next few chapters, we may not end up using terms like reconciliation or talking with the enemy. Still, we are not going to be able to make much progress until we create movements that simultaneously seek to bring adversaries together and solve the underlying challenges that gave rise to our endemic problems in the first place.

A NOT SO REPRESENTATIVE SAMPLE

In fact, there are so many promising groups that I could have devoted this entire book to them. What follows is a far from random sample of organizations that approach peacebuilding from different perspectives and could themselves grow quickly if people like you find a way to work with them.

Common Ground USA. Search for Common Ground is the world's oldest and largest stand-alone peacebuilding NGO. Formed in 1982, it was also the first organization to creatively use the mass media and is best known for television soap operas that dealt with conflict resolution themes in Macedonia, Israel/Palestine, Nigeria, Indonesia, Cyprus, and South Africa.[4]

It is also AfP's only founding member that has always worked on American domestic issues, which is why I joined its staff in 2000. Our team had projects on specific issues including prisoner reentry (in today's terms, welcoming returning citizens home), health care, abortion, and racism. It also came close to creating a United States Consensus Council. Members of the team later founded Convergence Policy, which you will meet in chapter 7.

In the early 2020s, Search (as it is known) resurrected its then dormant American program, repurposed it to deal with ideological polarization, and hired one of the country's most talented young peacebuilders, Nealin Parker, to manage it.

---

4. John Marks, *From Vision to Action: Remaking the World Through Social Entrepreneurship.* (New York: Columbia University Press, 2024).

In the run up to the 2024 election, her team decided to focus on the corrosive effects of polarization. They did some work at the national level, most notably developing some basic principles for dealing with deep ideological communities.

But they also had to overcome a problem that faces all national organizations. Organizations like AfP or Search that are based in Washington have a hard time running grass roots projects on their own, as a Search team discovered in the early 2000s when it tried to "parachute" in to Philadelphia and Cincinnati and create programs without developing much community support first.

Nealin's team applied two of the lessons about locally-led peacebuilding which had not yet surfaced when I was at Search. First, they decided to begin with communities that were at the heart of the dispute and where local partners already knew that they could make a difference. Second, those local partners called the shots. In the jargon we peacebuilders now use, Search decided to "accompany" on-the-ground leaders who will always know more about the needs and capacities of their communities than outsiders like Nealin or I ever would.[5]

Search started working with teams in Texas and Pennsylvania, which are among the most divided states in the country. I will focus on Texas where Search's team was invited in by a group of evangelical pastors—not exactly the kind of group typically associated with peacebuilders based in Washington DC!

The Texas project does more than address the symptoms of deep polarization and the threat of political violence. The team started by doing a poll of what Texans actually thought, feared, and wanted, discovering that almost ninety percent of them hoped to keep their disagreements from getting in the way of what they held in common. So, the Search team gathered a diverse group of leaders from the business, veterans, faith, and education communities who agreed on a charter for what they called a resilient state.

---

5. I borrowed the term accompaniment from John Paul Lederach who is the unquestioned rock star in our generation of global peacebuilders. Learn more about his work in general at his website www.johnpaulledearch.com.

Since then, they have been building support for the charter primarily among evangelicals by issuing their version of my invitation to pastors and their congregations through what they call a peacemakers starter pack. Among other things, it provides church members with basic information on what peacebuilders call the drivers of conflict and introduces them to tools that they could use whenever they see signs that their community might erupt. In essence, it makes a version of the case I made in the second half of chapter 3, urging pastors and their congregants to take conflict seriously, reach out to people they disagree with, and seek cooperative solutions to their problems. While it is hard to tell how effective any of the bridge building programs around the country have been, Stanford University's award winning Politics and Social Change Lab rates the Texas pastors effort as one of the most effective in the country.

The project also plans to go far beyond the text in the manual. Together with the Dallas-based Project Unity, it has launched Together We Dine in an attempt to get Texans of different political stripes to share a meal with each other as the first step in building the kind of relationships that could provide the political equivalent of preventive medicine.

Could you imagine working on a project like this in your community?

The National Association for Community Mediation/TRUST Network. The National Association for Community Mediation (NAFCM) likes to refer to itself as the best kept secret in peacebuilding, because so few Americans know about the great work it has done for the last thirty years. Its origins lie in Part X of the Civil Rights Act of 1964, which created the Community Relations Service within the Department of Justice. The act also spawned about 400 community mediation centers whose mission was to create or hold space in which citizens could solve their problems together—not just those that involve civil rights.

In 1994, their leaders realized they were not getting as much traction as they wanted and decided to form NAFCM to promote community mediation around the country. At the end of that decade, most mediation and dispute resolution professionals combined forces to form the Association for Conflict Resolution (ACR). NAFCM decided not to join the new network because its founders did not want to lose their emphasis on simultaneously co-creating social justice and peace.

Since then, each member center has set its own agenda as long as its actions are consistent with NAFCM's nine hallmark principles. Many of them handle legal cases which are sent to them by judges who understand that mediating a dispute can be cheaper and lead to better outcomes than taking it to trial. Thus, some work with young offenders or handle family-related legal issues, especially for clients who can't afford traditional legal services.

The hallmarks commit centers to hiring staff and training volunteers who can meet the needs of all clients whether they can pay or not. Everyone from judges to individual citizens can refer cases to the centers. Because of its origins, NAFCM members try to address conflict as early as possible and seek systemic change rather than the "simple" transactional win-win outcomes that are the output of most successful court-based mediations. Most NAFCM centers either provide mediation training themselves or hire outsiders (often provided by other NAFCM centers) to provide those services. Its most dynamic centers focus on racial equality by supporting projects that offer people from all identity groups a place to air and settle their grievances. Because many of them have a relationship with the judicial system and they all are anchored in community organizations, NAFCM centers are my first "living" example of what an inside-out strategy that prioritizes social change could look like.

I got my first hands-on exposure to its work when I visited the Warrenton VA center for a racial healing event it co-hosted in that small town on the outer fringes of the Washington, DC metropolitan area. As was the case in all of its work above and beyond mediating individual cases, it brought together a broad cross-section of community members ranging from police officers to teenagers, some of whom had had run-ins with the law.

At about the same time, NAFCM, Mediators Beyond Borders, and the Public Policy program at the University of Massachusetts-Boston created the TRUST Network to provide an early warning and early response system to prevent electoral and other forms of political violence ahead of the 2024 election. TRUST created a national network of observers who could detect signs of trouble and then turn to organizations like NAFCM and other locally-based networks to prevent an actual outbreak of violence. Like NAFCM, the TRUST Network actively seeks volunteers, including people with no prior experience in anything like peacebuilding.

The two years I spent on its board helped convince me to write this book. To my surprise and delight, I saw dozens of NAFCM centers take a leading role in addressing the racial flareups following George Floyd's murder. Additionally, they addressed the rash of evictions that were a byproduct of the COVID pandemic's economic dislocation, the special needs of rural America, police-community relations, and more.

But don't get too excited. NAFCM centers are the best kept secret in American peacebuilding for a reason. Most of them are bare-boned organizations. The average center has a budget of less than $300,000 a year, while only two or three have incomes that reach seven figures.

Is there a community mediation center where you live? If so, could you join it or work with it? If not, what would it take for you and the people you know to create one?

Mary Hoch Center for Reconciliation/Think Peace Learning and Support Hub. The Mary Hoch Center for Reconciliation and the related Think Peace Learning and Support Hub are worth your attention for a different reason. Of all the groups covered in this section, it draws the most explicitly on work done around the world, including by Archbishop Tutu and his colleagues in South Africa.

I met its founder, Antti Pentikainen, by accident. One day in 2019, I attended the weekly potluck lunch at the Jimmy and Rosalynn Carter School for Peace and Conflict Resolution at George Mason University. Antti was about to launch the center and was in town for a few days to set up his office and find a place to live.

Antti had spent the first two decades of his career supporting reconciliation projects in many of the world's hot spots, ranging from his native Finland to the Horn of Africa. He had spent the previous three years promoting similar work with indigenous peoples through the United Nations.

Because of my long-standing interest in reconciliation, I asked him if the Center planned to do any work here. It turns out that the Hoch family wanted them to add an American practice to the center's to-do list. I signed up on the spot.

I was even more excited when Pentikainen talked about how the role insider reconcilers can play in peace processes would be at the heart of the center's work. He developed the idea when he noticed that a certain kind of person often played a pivotal role in moving a divided community beyond conflict, even when its root causes were deeply ingrained and centuries old.

Insider reconcilers weren't traditional mediators whose neutrality helps them bridge divides. Like Bishop Tutu, they couldn't be. They lived in the midst of a dispute in which they found themselves on one side rather than the other. They also understood that reconciliation requires making progress toward solving those problems that had gotten their countries or communities into trouble in the first place. That includes acknowledging the role their own side played in producing and perpetuating problems.

A few weeks after Pentikainen's visa finally came through and his family moved to Virginia, George Floyd was murdered. It became obvious to all of us who were helping set up the center that the United States desperately needed tens of thousands of insider reconcilers, if not its own version of South Africa's TRC.

The Center was well placed to make that happen. Its leaders had already begun synthesizing the lessons that could be gleaned from the roughly 40 truth and reconciliation commissions in countries around the world. They started by defining what reconciliation could look like in the United States. Many activists worried that reconciliation amounted to a sellout. In particular, the skeptics mistakenly believed that reconciling parties produce lasting peace because they are able to restore some sort of harmony that had supposedly existed earlier in their history. Even though no such period ever existed in South Africa (or the United States), some activists were afraid that seeking reconciliation through the widespread issuing of apologies and granting forgiveness rather than, say, demanding reparations, would make achieving social justice impossible.

Like Archbishop Tutu (whose daughter, Mpho, is one of Antti's closest colleagues), MHCR placed itself squarely on the "right side of history," while training more insider reconcilers who could advocate for the demands of people of color and other marginalized communities while also reaching out in a spirit of good will to the millions of Americans who had qualms about phrases like Black Lives Matter or what supporters of the Trump administration today call "woke ideology."

The Center decided to prioritize two things. First, it joined the broad coalition that supported an initiative launched by the former head of the Kellogg Foundation to create a racial healing commission, which they hoped (in vain) that the Biden administration would support. Second, the Center brought its own expertise working for truth and reconciliation around the world to bear on the attempts to do the same in cities and states around the U.S.

It was obvious early on that it could not simply copy the South African model and use it here. If nothing else, too few powerful whites were as willing as the leaders of the Afrikaner community had been to submit evidence to and abide by the findings of any American TRC. Meanwhile, the political turmoil since 2020 doomed efforts to create anything like the national effort proposed by Kamela Harris while she was in the United States Senate.

In keeping with its commitment to locally led peacebuilding efforts, the center has focused on supporting existing truth and reconciliation initiatives in North Carolina, Iowa, Maine, and Oregon. I will return to the Oregon example in chapter 5 when we consider the role that Rotary has played there. Here, it is enough to see that MHCR and Think Peace have offered support for insider reconcilers, which has allowed leaders in those communities to get beyond the slogans of 2020 and begin developing community-based solutions to the host of problems that centuries of systemic racism have left in their wake.

Can you identify issues that could use the help of insider reconcilers in your community? If so, why not reach out to Antti Pentikainen to see if MHCR can help you out?

Rotary. If NAFCM gets the best kept secret in peacebuilding award, Rotary gets its equivalent for the greatest untapped potential. That might seem like a damning statement about an organization I commit a lot of time to.

So, let me explain.

Rotary is the largest peacebuilding network in the world.

Not just by a little.

By orders of magnitude.

Rotary International has 1.4 million members of whom 800,000 live in the United States. Unlike the Lions, Moose, Elks, or Odd Fellows, it has made peacebuilding and conflict resolution one of its areas of focus, along with the environment, children and youth, polio eradication, women's issues, and the like. Its commitment to peacebuilding work dates to World War One, a mere decade after the organization was formed.

It is best known for its Peace Fellows program that has funded 1,800 students who can not themselves already be Rotarians. Its first students were sent to established Masters degree programs at universities in Australia, Japan, the United Kingdom, Sweden, and the United States. About twenty years ago, it began offering shorter certificate programs in Thailand and Uganda for mid-career professionals who did not need an academic degree or could not be away for the year or two that the original programs required. An eighth opened in Istanbul as I was finishing this book.

Rotary members are also involved in peacebuilding projects around the world in part because there are Rotarians everywhere. It has strong working relationships with the United Nations and the Peace Corps and dozens of private sector organizations including the Gates Foundation and, as you will see in the next chapter, the Institute for Economics and Peace (IEP). Perhaps most importantly for our purposes, Rotary anchors its work in the Four-Way Test.

I used the term untapped potential because those 800,000 American Rotarians have largely been missing in action when it comes to peacebuilding efforts in their own country. That's the case despite the fact that there are more than 250 certified Rotary peacebuilding clubs in North America. For good or ill, most of them want to support peacebuilding efforts in places like Ukraine or Gaza, while working on issues troubling the United States often seem "too political" for members of a service club that prides itself on its impartiality.

That helps explain why it took me a long time to get to Rotary. Also, I have to admit that I did not find the idea of going to weekly meetings at what it calls brick and mortar clubs appealing. Besides, I was fixated on peacebuilding. Sure, its other areas of focus were important, but there were only so many hours in my day.

Then, in 2022, I learned that Rotary was experimenting with cause-based clubs that focused on a single issue, including peace. Some of them only met online and did so outside of normal business hours. So, Gretchen and I joined one that is based in California whose meetings started at 10.00 PM on the east coast. We quickly realized that this didn't fit our early-to-bed-early-to-rise lifestyle. We then learned about the E-Club of Global Peacebuilders, which is based in our time zone and met at the far more convenient 7:00 PM.

So, we joined and began doing what we could to tap that untapped potential. To begin with, our club's members do not live up to anyone's stereotype of a peace activist—other than me. It includes three former military officers, a retired as well as a serving foreign service officer, a veterinarian, a few retired teachers, and even a former intelligence analyst (Gretchen).

Because cause-based and online clubs are both new, we couldn't just copy what other Rotary clubs did. We had to define what an online peace club would do.

Even before we joined, the founding members had decided to focus on the Institute for Economics and Peace and its work on positive peace. I will discuss the IEP's contributions in the next chapter on the peacebuilding pivot and concentrate here on how our club has used it to expand our own influence.

My first observation might strike you as obvious, but came as a delightful surprise to someone who has been a peacebuilding professional and educator for decades. From the beginning, club members realized they had to learn more about peacebuilding. Rotary itself provides self-paced courses on a wide variety of relevant topics, which club members worked through. The club also started a book club, which has discussed Amanda Ripley's *High Conflict* among others.

Because she is a friend of ours, Ripley herself attended the last session at which we talked about how Rotarians could use her ideas in their peacebuilding projects and beyond.

Shortly after Ripley's visit, the members pointed out that they have busy lives and couldn't carve out the time to read more than a chapter a month. So, we substituted hour-long podcasts that the Next Big Idea Club has done with authors of new nonfiction books (including Ripley). We also have been able to invite well-known peace-builders like Ripley; AfP's Liz Hume; the former U.S. ambassador to the Vatican, Miguel Diaz; and the head of IEP's American office, Michael Collins, to speak to the club at its regular meetings.

Because our club is located in northern Virginia where we also happen to live, it was assigned to the Rotary District which covers half of the state, including the Washington DC suburbs, most of its exurbs, and some rural areas that still feel like they are part of the old south. As we got involved in District peacebuilding work, we were delighted to discover that the organization now has plenty of women and people of color despite the fact that it resisted racial integration for decades and only admitted women members in 1987. We also realized that our club could help our fellow Rotarians more explicitly connect their other service projects to peacebuilding, a point I will also return to in the next chapter.

The club also organizes annual peacebuilding conferences for our district. The conferences typically draw about seventy Rotarians who have even less exposure to formal peacebuilding than our club's members did when they started it in 2021. We have done enough of them now that attendees come with the expectation that we will help them incorporate peacebuilding themes into their existing service projects, which generally fit more squarely into one of Rotary's other areas of focus.

In the last year, we have also been asked to help area clubs deal with broader divisions facing our country. Thus, a colleague and I facilitated a district-wide training in September 2024 that gave the seventy or so attendees tools to use when they found themselves in the middle of difficult conversations during that year's presidential election campaign. The following spring, the same friend and I met with a local club that was trying to find ways of reconciling differences among its own members. Needless to say, I drew on what I had learned from the Mary Hoch Center and would have dragged Antti along had he been available that evening.

As I write, we have begun making plans to bring these initiatives together into a package that other clubs (in person or virtual) could use in ramping up their own peacebuilding initiatives. We are also talking with the organization's international leadership about ways of publicizing what our club has done to the broader Rotary community so that the untapped potential becomes at least a bit more tapped.

Could you get in touch with your local Rotary club? Then, see if it has any peacebuilding projects and develop your own if it doesn't.

Youth and Peace in Action. Patricia Shafer is a force of nature who has taken the American peacebuilding community by storm. After a couple of MBAs and a career in the business world, she spent three months in Thailand as a Rotary Peace Fellow in the early 2010s, which changed her life.

Patricia returned home raring to go on a project that had little to do with her previous life in corporate America—turning high school and college students on to peacebuilding. She started by creating New Gen Peacebuilders, which works with teenagers in South Sudan, Lebanon, and the Philippines as well as the United States and usually has Rotary as a key partner.

Patricia was already laying the groundwork for Youth and Peace in Action (YPA) as a separate organization when the two of us met at a workshop on peacebuilding in the United States which I organized in 2019. In fact, she stole the show when she outlined the proposal to the group. Unlike New Gen, it would focus on the United States and be sponsored and partially funded by Rotary Zones 33 and 34, which serve the Middle Atlantic and southern states, Washington DC, and parts of the Caribbean. After some pandemic related delays, she launched YPA at the start of the school year in 2021. [6]

---

6. Hers are by no means the only projects involving K-12 students. For another, quirkier example, check out John Hunter. *World Peace and Other 4th-Grade Achievements*. (New York: Houghton Mifflin Harcourt, 2013). I will return to his work in chapter 8.

Perhaps because she came to peacebuilding after twenty years in the corporate world and studied it in a setting as far removed from home as you could possibly imagine, she understood the importance of blending classroom and "real world" experience from the beginning. That included making certain that students understood the importance of the root causes of any dispute, which led her to focus on the structural or long-term causes of conflict.

In the last four years, her team has developed curricula for students, teachers, and parents that reflect what peacebuilders have learned from their work around the world. The student version starts with a core curriculum that introduces basic concepts in peace and conflict studies. Students, for example, create conflict "maps" like those I discussed in chapter 2 for problems facing their own communities.

YPA also deserves your attention because it goes beyond the classroom. Students who complete the educational component of the program do receive a certificate/certification to put on their resumés and college applications.

YPA stands out, however, because the students are also expected to put what they've learned into practice by creating local peacebuilding projects that put anything that looks like a conventional internship to shame. Some of them do revolve around peacebuilding, per se. However, Patricia and her colleagues learned early on that young people are most likely to remain engaged if they work on a specific issue that touches their own lives. More often than not, they have chosen to take on a local problem such as homelessness, poverty, immigration, or intolerance and then address it using a peacebuilding lens—much as my Rotary club is trying to do with other clubs in our district.

To help students choose a project, YPA coined the acronym SMART:

- **S**pecific and focused on a single pressing need
- **M**easurable in much the same way that a Rotarian's business activities are monitored and assessed
- **A**ctionable or specific enough to be carried out

- **Realistic** rather than a holistic "moon shot" project that the teens could never pull off
- **Time bound** so that it can be done in the weeks or at most months the students have left before graduating, although YPA hopes that many of the projects will last more than a year and become a permanent part of the school and community's landscape

Meanwhile, teachers, Rotary members, and other mentors go through an "adult" version of the curriculum. Because almost no American high school teachers have training in peacebuilding, the YPA team has created toolkits for them to use in creating their lesson plans and grading rubrics that can be used where the courses are offered for academic credit.

In its first year, YPA enrolled 8,000 students, teachers, and community supporters; delivered over 70,000 hours of peace education and mentoring; initiated almost 100 student-led peace projects; certified 2,250 young peacebuilders; and distributed over 1,000 peace education toolkits to teachers. By the end of the 2024-2025 school year, it had reached 20,000 students. All of the high schools in Birmingham AL now have peacebuilding integrated into their ninth-grade curriculum.

As is the case with Rotary's work in general, YPA prepares students for a lifelong journey. After all, YPA is preparing them for a future of building peace in much the same way that Junior Achievement does for business or Junior ROTC does for the military.

Could a project like YPA work at high schools in your community? What would it take to make one happen?

EXERCISE 4.1: AMERICA REMADE

Youth and Peace in Action had reached 20,000 high school students by the time I wrote these words in early 2025.

Pick another group that you either already work with or could see yourself joining. Develop at least the outline of a project that could reach even one tenth the number of people that Youth and Peace in Action worked with in its first three years.

Unify America. I learned about Unify America after I had finished the first draft of *Peacebuilding Starts at Home* which meant that I didn't have room to add (m)any new organizations. After hesitating for a while, I realized that I had to to make space for Unify America because it offers two promising pathways (the second appears in chapter 7) and does so with a lightheartedness that is rare in a field whose champions understandably take their work extremely seriously.

Unify America is also unusual because its founder, Harry Gottlieb, is even more of a newcomer to peacebuilding than Shafer was when she left for Thailand. As an undergraduate, he created his own major in individualism and community and the possibilities for balance—whatever that means.[7] After graduating, he started a business career that led him to create Jellyworks Lab which helps companies "take boring, complex subjects and make them interesting, simple and delightful" in humdrum parts of business life like benefits management. He then started Jackbox which creates online party games that also take boring, complex subjects and make them interesting, simple and delightful. The website had 240 million players in 2020, including my grandson, but not me.

In the early 2020s, Gottlieb returned to his old desire to find balance

---

7. I had no idea what that meant until I asked and learned that he had taken courses that launched him on a career path that led him to the use of new media in education, corporate management, and then cooperative problem solving.

between individualism and communities by creating Unify America. His decision came at a time when polarization had reached an all-time high and he began worrying about what life would be like for his teen-aged children. Among other things, that led the quirky Gottlieb to have his then thirteen-year-old son interview him and use a transcript of their discussion instead of a mission statement on the organization's website. As he told Moshe:

> *I founded Unify America so that by the time you children are adults, our country has stopped making civic decisions based on power and influence. Instead, our country will make decisions based on reason and empathy.*

And I would add, it does so in ways that take boring, complex subjects and make them interesting, simple and delightful.

Its projects draw on his Jackbox experience to reduce tensions on polarized college campuses, starting with a variant of the radio and television College Bowl franchise which was a big hit when I was in college. The original—and its 2020s revival—pit teams from competing colleges against each other. But instead of scoring touchdowns, field goals, or safeties, they gain (admittedly less) glory for their schools by answering tough questions on obscure topics.

Unify America redesigned the game to the point that anyone who grew up watching the show would have a hard time recognizing this version of the game. It doesn't even have teams. Instead, participants are paired with students they disagree with. Over the course of about an hour, they meet in pairs for what amounts to political speed dating by holding lightning-fast discussions on up to eighteen hot button issues.

By the end of 2024, over 20,000 students from 219 campuses had taken part in this twenty-first century version of what was, frankly, a pretty boring vintage television program. Almost ninety percent of them loved the experience. Eight in ten felt more confident in their dealings with people they disagreed with, and fully three quarters of them expressed more hope for America after their time together. No one knows if the speed dating led to any real dates....

Gottlieb and his team realized that their version of the College Bowl could never be more than a first step. In 2023, they introduced what they think of as a deeper dive into disagreement in which they work with professors who are willing to integrate enjoyable learning exercises that cross ideological lines into their courses. Unify America has adapted the tools Gottlieb's companies developed into modules that faculty members can assign in much the same way that they have their students read books or write papers. It helps them develop the critical thinking, listening, and cooperative problem-solving skills that College Bowl like experiences can't get at.

What's happening at colleges and universities near where you live? My experience as both a student and a professor has shown me that input from "townies" is almost always welcome. Many universities and community colleges offer courses explicitly designed for geezers and other community members.

EXERCISE 4.2: NAILING IT

This chapter has introduced you to organizations that are far from satisfied by the fact that they amount to a bunch of small islands in what is for the moment a politically insignificant archipelago. If, in Kelly Corrigan's terms, we want to nail it, we will have to greatly expand those efforts. That starts by exploring what it would even mean to reach anything resembling that level of success.

So, take the organizations or type of organization you identified in this chapter's first exercise and do something that startup companies often do. Write a press release that you would issue on the day that your initiative has found success and reached one of its major goals.

Living Room Conversations and the Bridging Movement. Until the beginning of the 2010s, Joan Blades fit a lot of conventional stereotypes about northern Californians. She was a liberal who had begun her professional career as an attorney and mediator and then became a tech entrepreneur whose company introduced the wildly popular "flying toaster" screen saver in the 1990s—and, as I learned when I showed her the first draft of this book—helped Harry Gottlieb market his first games.

During the impeachment trial of President Clinton in 1998, she and her husband started a one-sentence petition drive asking Congress to "censure and Move On to pressing issues facing the country." To their surprise and delight, Move On became a large, progressive, grass roots organization. Disturbed by the political divisions that only heightened after the dawn of the new century, Blades co-founded Moms Rising, an organization that mobilizes mothers and people who have mothers to fight bias against mothers and support policies that are good for families.

By the time Barack Obama was elected, Blades decided it was time to come to grips with the fact that the United States was becoming even more polarized, given the rise of the Tea Party, the Birther movement, and more. Unlike most of her progressive colleagues, she had an ideologically diverse set of friends and had always appreciated the more nuanced understanding of the issues that she got from talking with people she disagreed with.

So, she and a conservative friend decided to reproduce the kinds of discussions they had when they met for a meal or went for a hike or played soccer.[8] By 2011, they had created a template for hosting conversations that would literally take place in living rooms. Two people with different political viewpoints would each invite two or three of their friends for a structured discussion using questions and ground rules that Blades and her team developed. It offered plug and play dialogues that people who knew nothing about peacebuilding could organize. They are even planning to host them about the themes in this book as soon as it is published.

Today, Living Room Conversations is one of the best known of the

---

8. I only know about her soccer-playing efforts because Blades plays in a weekly intergenerational game that includes my college roommate who is in his late seventies and is not the oldest player.

roughly four hundred organizations that are trying to "bridge" ideological divisions of all sorts. It has written 165 discussion guides, some of which deal with hot political topics such as Guns and Responsibility, Immigration, and Abortion. All are designed to help people begin to see some shared values and interests that could rebuild trust or expand everyone's sense of belonging. Most have now been packaged in an "off the shelf" format so that you can simply download the material and host a conversation on your own.

Discussions now take place in all sorts of places—libraries, schools, places of worship, clubs, and online. Indeed, executive director, Becca Kearl, started its 2022 annual report by joking that she had actually held a living room conversation in her own living room for the first time since the pandemic shut down almost all in-person gatherings.

Living Room Conversations is also working with other organizations. In 2023, it formed a partnership with NAFCM to start a pilot project on conflicts that have disrupted local school systems. The two organizations together developed the curriculum. However, unlike its earlier projects, these conversations are part of a multifaceted program being organized by trained professionals from NAFCM's community mediation centers.

As is the case with all of the dialogue and discussion-based groups I could have included here, Living Room Conversations does not pretend that it can fix all of America's problems. I chose it because it offers an easy way to begin practicing the skills I have been discussing for the last chapter and a half. Indeed, because you can now do them online, you don't even have to leave your own living room to participate.

Who could you invite for a living room (or patio) conversation? What would you talk about? What's keeping you from hosting one?

The Peace on Earth Game. The Peace on Earth by 2030 game isn't for everyone. However, it is the only example I could find that both stands for a lot of what Peacebuilding Starts at Home embraces and is available to everyone reading this book.

And I almost missed it.

I had already drafted most of this chapter when I got an email from David Sloan Wilson who gave me the islands-in-an-archipelago metaphor. He thought that I might be interested in attending an introductory meeting that the Peace on Earth Game leaders had called for the next day. I went, and immediately realized that I needed to find room for it, too.

The game is the brainchild of long-time social entrepreneurs David Gershon and Gail Straub who met decades ago when Gershon organized a torch-passing project to celebrate the American bicentennial. In the nearly half century since then, they have put together similar events involving other runners who carried other torches for other causes, including one for global peace at the height of the Cold War in 1986.

They later established the Empowerment Institute which pioneered ways of using behavioral change techniques for reaching environmental and other social goals. The through line in their work is a desire to produce what Gershon calls second order change in which something happens that alters the underlying order of things, which is another way of saying that a paradigm shift takes place.[9]

Theirs is not a traditional game. No one keeps score. There are no winners or losers. Rather, it is an attempt to gamify behavioral change that promotes peace.[10]

Gershon and Straub began developing the game in the late 2010s and rolled out the current, scalable version in 2024. For the moment, it is easiest to play online. You and a team of two or three others meet weekly over two months. In each session, players experiment with ways of building unity, social health, cooperation, and the like while identifying at least seven action steps they can take in real life to promote empowerment, oneness, unity, cooperation, abundance, love, and faith. At each week's session, they share what happened with their teammates and record their results into a global data base that Gershon, Straub, and their team maintain.

As of January 2024, 6,000 people had played the game in 567 cities

---

9. David Gershon, *Social Change 2.0: A Blueprint for Reinventing Our World.* (New York: High Point, 2013).
10. It is what economists and others refer to as an infinite game. For a non-technical introduction to a topic that many of the organizations you will meet in the second half of this book think is important, see Simon Sinek. *Infinite Games.* (New York: Portfolio, 2019).

in 59 countries and engaged in 67,000 actions. My cohort alone added 143 participants who reported engaging in 7,888 Peace Actions; or an average of 55 per player. Many of them reported profound increases in their self-confidence when it comes to taking initiatives for peace that involve interacting with other people.

If they meet their goal of 40,000,000 players by 2030, they will have reached 0.5 percent of the world's population. According to their understanding of social change, reaching this target will ensure their vision of peace will be embedded (a point I will return to in chapter 6), and as it continues to grow, its impact will become unstoppable on either cultural or policy levels.

Along the way, it also plans to create at least 10,000 peace zones which will give it a beachhead in each of the planet's population centers. That work is progressing more slowly than Gershon and Straub would like in part because most people have to play the game online. Once local networks are established, players will be able to join larger teams that meet in their own communities, physically do some of those actions together and build those peace zones through which participants can help produce cultural and policy change.

The first zones have been created in the Pacific Northwest, Louisville, and, most surprisingly and intriguingly, in Afghanistan where a network of teenage girls are playing the game because they can no longer attend school. Each is based on at least three three-person teams that have completed the basic version of the game and who have agreed to adapt it to whatever conditions they face which means that the ones in Kentucky and Kabul are quite different.

The realist in me doubts that Gershon and Straub will be able to meet their ambitious goals for 2030. However, it may not matter because the Peace Game is the kind of initiative that can attract newcomers to the peacebuilding world, give them tools that they can use without disrupting their daily lives all that much, and help us all build the kind of movement I will be discussing in the rest of this book.

Why not give the Peace on Earth Game a try? Gretchen and I were skeptical when we signed up, but, in the end, we had a good bit of fun, met some interesting people, and took the world a tiny step closer to peace.

PEACEBUILDING DOES START AT HOME

These organizations and others I didn't have room to include here have accomplished a lot. When I joined the Beyond War movement in 1982, next to no one knew what the phrase win-win meant. Today, it is deeply embedded in everyday conversation to the point that I have heard it used to describe everything from business deals to baseball trades. The same is true of mediation, meditation, mindfulness, and more.

At the same time, I am not ready to take a self-congratulatory victory lap.

How could I, given the problems facing our country and the planet as a whole?

Or given the likelihood that many—maybe most—readers will have a hard time finding a peacebuilding group in their community to work with?

Or given the fact that none of the organizations I included or could have included in this chapter are even close to having a national impact?

At best, there are gaping holes in what they have accomplished or could reasonably hope to accomplish in the foreseeable future because next to no one who could be a highly effective peacebuilder even thinks of themselves as one. To see how and why that is the case, return for a moment to my sister in Waterville OH. I have always known that Leslie is a much better "natural" peacebuilder than I am. She is far more patient than I will ever be, as reflected in her career choice—teaching learning disabled children. Add to that the fact that she and her husband almost have to be bridge builders. They live in a community that is far more diverse in socioeconomic or political terms than Falls Church VA where I am based. Now that they have retired, they spend half of each year camping and attending folk music festivals where they meet an even more diverse sample of Americans.

I had always known this about Leslie, but it really got driven home during the final two decades of our mother's life. Neither of us ever got along with Amy whose values and personality were as far from being a "good peacebuilder" as you could possibly get.

Things only deteriorated as she entered her nineties until she died at age 102 as I was finishing the first draft of this book. Leslie almost never lost her temper with our mother. I got mad at her almost every time we spoke, including just a few weeks before she died—yet more proof that living up to the values laid out in chapter 3 is easier said than done!

But that's not why I sing my sister's praises. Or want to use her as an intellectual bridge to AfP's plans for Peacebuilding Starts at Home.

Despite having been a freshman at Oberlin when I was a senior and one of the most visible activists on campus and despite sharing most of my social and political views, she has never been tempted to follow me into the peacebuilding trenches. That reflects both her personality and the fact that she lives where she does.

Yet, if we are going to succeed, we have to reach people like Leslie, her family members, her neighbors, and the people she runs into at those folk music festivals and campgrounds. We also have to reach people like Dr. Whohasnoname who introduced me to Emily Post's great grandchildren. Or the realtors who helped us sell our house and buy a condo in the same month that I sent this book to the publishers. Or to the Moose and Elks and Lions who see the need to provide service over self, but just not through peacebuilding.

That world contains lots of dissatisfied voters of all persuasions as well as everyday Americans who understand that we need to do things differently but don't see peacebuilding as a viable option. Indeed, they are the target audience for this book, not my fellow peacebuilders.

As you saw in chapter one when I explained why I changed this book's title, AfP decided to step up its domestic peacebuilding game, largely by creating the scaffolding for an ecosystem of domestic peacebuilders. The work on the ground will still largely be carried out by AfP's member organizations and other partners that have the resources that can build and sustain grass roots networks to reach every corner of our country—sooner rather than later. Our role will largely be to focus on taking that work to scale, which will range from helping you find your on-ramp into peacebuilding to building the much broader movement that I will be describing in the second half of this book.

For now, it is enough to see how the Peacebuilding Starts at Home network has taken its first steps in filling in these gaps in three broad ways, as stated on its website on the day this book went to press. I will add more to its agenda in the chapters to come and our team will continue to do so after this book is published. So, check the website for updates: www.peacebuildingstartsathome.us.

Raise awareness about the drivers of instability and conflict in the United States, while restoring trust and building support for evidenced-based constructive solutions from the local to the national level. The first task is educational. Just about everyone I meet is unhappy with the state of our country and the world. At the same time, just about everyone I meet in the course of my work knows little or nothing about the analytical tools in chapter 2 or the self-awareness techniques in chapter 3. We plan to change that.

Develop and disseminate ways of showing how anyone can learn to build peace and prevent conflict (that doesn't take hours of classes) so you can spark change in your home, community, online, and beyond. This is what I have in mind when I talk about on-ramps to the peacebuilding starts at home loop. Through the projects I've just discussed, others we know about, and yet others we hope to incubate, we plan to recruit tens or even hundreds of thousands of new activists. For the moment, all we can say with any certainty is that next to none of them will be professional peacebuilders. That almost certainly includes you. And my sister and her family. We can also offer some basic coaching to help those new peacebuilders decide how best to use their limited time and resources. That led us to create what amounts to a help desk for the peacebuilding starts at home community at AfP. In fact, I briefly introduced this idea in chapter 1 when I offered to help you wherever you are on your personal peacebuilding journey.

Connect people to organizations that are working to build peace and prevent conflict in their communities and beyond, as well as developing activities where nothing exists. As will become easier to see in the next two chapters, we can take advantage of the fact that AfP is a national (and international) organization to help spread successful local initiatives. Given my penchant for oceanic metaphors, we expect to:

- Help speed the growth of existing islands by working with individuals and organizations who already have projects underway
- Create new islands by incubating projects both in new communities and in those that cross issue-based or ideological lines
- "Fill" in the "water" between the archipelagos by connecting the dots that could tie them together intellectually and/or politically, a point that will also structure the second half of this book.

EXERCISE 4.3: THE LUNCH PAIL F***ING JOB

We will have made some progress and modified our project by the time you started reading this book. In other words, we know that Peacebuilding Starts at Home will still be a work in progress.

So, return to the press release you wrote in this chapter's second exercise. Now, develop a short strategic plan outlining how you might get to that point in the next five years.

We also know that AfP can't do it all. It is a small organization based in Washington DC. Add to that the fact that even if we could create a large peacebuilding network, it would not be able to address all of the wicked problems that divide our country – which is why there are four more steps on the peacebuilding starts at home journey waiting for you.

CHAPTER 5
THE PEACEBUILDING PIVOT

The same factors that create peace also create many other outcomes to which societies aspire, such as thriving economies, higher levels of happiness and well-being, stronger social inclusion, and increased resilience and adaptability.

THE INSTITUTE FOR ECONOMICS AND PEACE

Before I invite you to take the next step along the Peacebuilding Begins at Home Loop, take a moment and consider the following scenario.

Peacebuilding Starts at Home succeeded beyond my wildest expectations. My sister, Dr. Whohasnoname, my realtors, most Rotarians, and, of course, you all decided to do peace as a verb. Somehow, we managed to stop the fighting in Ukraine, Gaza/Israel/Iran, and Sudan and reduced tensions here at home.

Like me, I assume that you would be delighted and (I expect) surprised. After all, we would have created the most broadly based and successful peace movement in American history.

Like me, I assume that you would also realize that even our dream-team like movement would not be able to pull off my beloved paradigm shift.

Don't get me wrong. Getting that far would be amazing and unprecedented. Given the news from Ukraine, the Middle East, and Sudan when I clicked save for the last time while writing this book, achieving what scholars call a negative peace in which leaders agreed to stop the fighting would be one hell of an accomplishment. The same holds true when I looked at the situation here in the United States. To be sure, not many literal bullets were flying across our political divides. Still, it was not hard to imagine how we could get to a point when real as well as metaphorical ones were ripping away at our country's civic well-being.

But let me add one more reason to be dissatisfied with the status quo that emerged from our work around the world.[1] Our colleagues have helped forge dozens of those so-called negative peace agreements over the last half century. Only about half of them lasted for as long as five years. Yes, the fighting did stop. Social stress levels may well have been reduced, too. However, once something happens to heighten those tensions again, even a seemingly minor event can trigger a new round of fighting.

Scholars and practitioners alike have spent a lot of time exploring why that is the case. At first, they studied why so many of those agreements broke down. In the last twenty years, they have begun paying more attention to a different question. Why did a few of them succeed beyond anyone's wildest expectations?

We are far from having a definitive answer. Nonetheless, researchers have found a powerful common denominator in every example of stable or positive peace.

Their leaders understood that negative peace would never be enough. As you can see if you watch videos of Nelson Mandela's presi-

---

1. The allusion to former Vice President Al Gore's game changing book and movie on climate change is intentional. *An Inconvenient Truth: The Planetary Emergency of Climate Change and What We Can Do About It.* (Emmaus PA: Rodale Books, 2006). The film is available on most streaming services, including Apple, Google, Amazon, Netflix, and YouTube.

dential inauguration, peacebuilders definitely celebrated their victories. However, they also knew that they had to do more than just celebrate. They also had to address whatever it was that gave rise to the conflict in the first place. In so doing, they made enduring peace possible.

In South Africa, the African National Congress, Archbishop Tutu, and other leaders assumed from the beginning that a post-apartheid South Africa would also have to address the economic inequality that centuries of imperialism and racism had spawned. So, too, did the leaders who brokered the Good Friday Agreement in Northern Ireland or helped lead Brazil back to democracy after decades of military rule.

They may not have used terms like interdependence, complexity, or wicked problems or drawn on a table like the one I introduced in chapter 3, but they took it for granted that their reality was telling them to come up with holistic solutions. To use the term I used as this chapter's title, they made their peacebuilding pivot to take on the wide variety of problems their country faced.

When AfP first started working on what became peacebuilding starts at home, we were surprised by how little attention our colleagues paid to other issues like climate change or racial injustice. Of course, they knew that those problems existed and that they could not ignore them. Yet, few of them found ways of integrating those other wicked problems in their peacebuilding work. While we knew that no one organization could tackle everything, we were surprised by how rarely our colleagues took their work beyond what you might think of as the traditional peacebuilding silo.

Our need to pivot was driven home for me at a workshop I helped organize with a diverse group of American peacebuilders in 2019. By that time, we had been working with the Institute for Economics and Peace whose statement begins this chapter for more than a decade. We knew from our own first-hand experience as well as their research that lasting peace had to rest on a bedrock of social well being, including a flourishing economy, high levels of happiness, social inclusion, increased resilience and adaptability, and all of the other issues they allude to in that statement and in all of their research.

At that point, I realized that the American peacebuilding movement would have to do something that our colleagues in South Africa or Northern Ireland understood from day one. We would have to be intentional when it came to pivoting.

Since then, things have begun to change. First, peacebuilders themselves have begun to include those other issues in their own work. Second—and frankly somewhat to my surprise—a growing number of organizations who focus on those other issues have come to realize that they need to work with us. Both should make the "party" I've asked you to come to more interesting—but also more demanding.

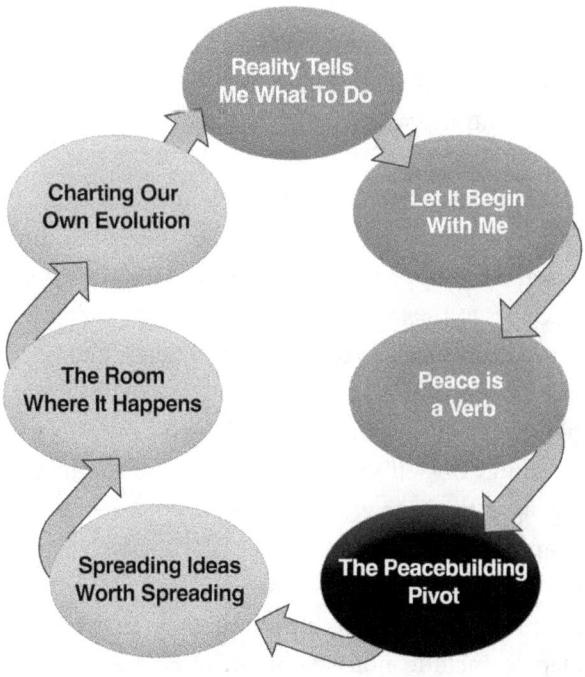

Figure 5.1: *The Peace as a Verb Loop*

ON PIVOTING

Basketball players pivot when they place one foot firmly on the court and then take a bold step toward the hoop so that they can set themselves up for a slam dunk or a sky hook. Companies pivot once they realize that their current strategy is not going to be profitable (enough).

At that point, they plant their metaphorical foot on the metaphorical floor and change direction by, say, developing new and more marketable products.

You can get a glimpse of why pivoting needs a whole chapter in a book on peacebuilding by thinking about what happened when two iconic companies failed to take decisive action.

Kodak scientists invented most of the technologies that made digital photography possible. However, the company was so wedded to its film-based products that it never seriously considered selling digital cameras.

Until it was too late.

Blockbuster was the darling of the video rental world in the 1980s and 1990s. However, its store-based model could not compete once Netflix started sending subscribers cassettes and DVDs through the mail.[2]

Until it was too late.

If I'm right, it isn't too late for the peacebuilding community...

... if we seize the opportunities I will be presenting in the rest of *Peacebuilding Starts at Home*.

Nothing is guaranteed. Still, I'm convinced that we can avoid Kodak's and Blockbuster's fate if we and our colleagues in related fields execute what will amount to a double pivot.

Luckily, I found myself in a position to see both the need to pivot and the early signs that one was underway because of two unexpected things that happened years ago.

The first occurred before my career officially got started. While I did begin my professional life as a peace activist in the 1960s, my interests expanded to include nonviolent social change in general by the time I got to graduate school. My PhD advisor, Roy Pierce, suggested that I do my dissertation and first book on the new left in France on the assumption that it would help me become a more effective radical leader here at home.

---

2. Not to mention the pivot toward streaming which Netflix initially got right but then almost got wrong. Although it would take us beyond the scope of this book, Netflix itself might need to do some pivoting of its own today.

Although I didn't realize it at the time, Roy's suggestion that I spend a year with the Unified Socialist Party (PSU) — which was a full-fledged political party rather than a peace movement — prepared me for everything that I have done since then. Before heading off into the field to do my research, he also wanted me to study with the likes of Bob Putnam (whom you already briefly met in chapter 1), Charles Tilly, and Everett Rogers (both of whom will be featured in the next chapter). Together, they sparked my interest in broader movements for social change. Although none of them had this in mind, their mentorship set the stage for my enthusiastic embrace of Beyond War rather than a more conventional peace movement a decade later. In short, by the early 1980s, I was ready for the peacebuilding side of the peacebuilding pivot even if took another forty years for it to begin to materialize.

The other was an unintended byproduct of attending my thirty-fiftth high school reunion in 2000. I had had next to no contact with my New London High School classmates after we graduated and only went because I could use the trip to see my mother who was about to turn eighty.

I was already nervous when I walked into the banquet hall that my classmates had rented. Who would I talk to? About what? My anxieties neared panic level when I realized that there weren't going to be any nametags with or without pictures of what we looked like in the (good) old days. I stumbled through some stilted conversations during the cocktail hour and made my way to a dinner table where, as my nametag-less luck would have it, I found myself sitting next to someone who was a realtor in suburban Maryland and I had actually known and liked back in the day.

Nancy and I talked over dinner and rekindled a friendship that had been interrupted when she went to prep school after the eighth grade. At some point in the course of the evening, she suggested that I get in touch with her childhood next door neighbor Dick O'Neill—to whose memory this book is dedicated—because he did the same kinds of work that I did.

I was perplexed.

As she knew, Dick and I had been close friends from the time we met in nursery school until we headed off for college. In elementary school, he and I were in the world's worst-ever boy band whose career mercifully ended when we broke up after two performances.[3] As high school freshmen, we attended a Pete Seeger and Joan Baez concert together, which kindled a mutual life-long interest in folk music and the arts in general.

What little I knew about his career had come from my mother who sent me the occasional clippings from the local newspaper, one of which informed me that he had recently retired after thirty years as an officer in the Navy. Nancy didn't know much more, but her rumor mill had told her things that suggested that I might be interested in since I had just started working at Search for Common Ground.

Her instincts were on target. Dick's final tour of duty had been as a senior U. S. Navy officer on the staff of the then Secretary of Defense William Perry. Perry was an unusual leader who came to the Pentagon after a long career in the Engineering School at Stanford where he had worked with some of my Beyond War friends.

To make a long story short, Perry and others were not happy with the fact that few of his senior advisors knew much about complexity science and other ideas that were already taking hold in Silicon Valley. So, knowing that Dick would soon be retiring, Perry and his team asked him to take off his uniform and go meet everyone who could help the Pentagon think outside the clichéd box. Then, he would turn those contacts into a network of advisors whom future Pentagon leaders could learn from which Dick would run as a consulting firm after he officially took off his uniform.

We got together a few weeks after the reunion and hit it off immediately. Nancy was right. We really did have a lot of interests in common, including almost all of the scientific topics that found their way into chapter 2 because his travels for Secretary Perry had taken him to Xerox's famous PARC research center in Palo Alto which the Beyond War team also knew well. He had also spent time at the USC

---

3. To give you a sense of how bad The Emeralds were, at our first and only rehearsal before our first performance, we realized that we had two clarinetists. So, the (alleged) band leader turned Dick into a drummer. Need I say more?

Film School and at the Santa Fe Institute where modern complexity science was being developed which had also been on my radar screen since my Beyond War days. Although we had both left our Pete Seeger and Joan Baez fan days behind, we each still had a deep interest in the impact the arts and creativity in general could have on social change.

I did a few things with his Highlands Forum in the rest of 2000 and the first half of 2001.

Then, 9/11 happened.

On 9/13, he came to a launch party for a book I had just published that was held at Search for Common Ground which was uncommon ground for someone who had spent thirty years in uniform. We ended up doing the Q and A session together. On the basis of our answers, no one in the audience could have told which of us was the career peacenik and which the career intelligence officer.

In the chaotic weeks that followed, he asked me to bring peacebuilding ideas into the Pentagon as part of its internal discussions about how to respond to the attacks in New York and Washington and to terrorism in general. This was quite a stretch for me since I had been a conscientious objector and never imagined that I would find myself in constructive discussions with senior military leaders, let alone search for common ground with them. As a result, I still keep the guest pass from my first visit to the Pentagon on my desk to remind myself of how far I have come.

We were asked in because Dick and other Pentagon leaders realized that the military could not defeat terrorism on its own. That led to more discussions with serving officers and civilian national security intellectuals that included the visit to SOCOM where I first saw the Spaghetti Map.

Once we discovered that Dick had worked with the husband of AfP's then CEO when Melanie and Lawrence Greenberg were in graduate school, we started including him in our projects and realized that he could do more for us than just get us into the Pentagon—although that was amazing in and of itself. So, in the early 2010s, we asked him to join the AfP board, on which he served until the first of several debilitating illnesses forced him to retire.

In the end, his contacts with and curiosity about science, technology, and the arts had a huge impact on all of us at AfP. For the purposes of this chapter, one of the first and most important things we did was to explore the idea of creating an edge lab for the peacebuilding community.

When Dick told us about it, we had no idea what he was talking about. It turns out that the first ones had been developed by management consultant John Hagel and physicist turned entrepreneur John Seely Brown. They had recently landed at Deloitte where they created an office that would help clients look beyond their own industry's frontiers for ideas that they could adapt and use to spark innovation in their home company.[4]

In the end, we decided not to seek funding to create a formal edge lab at AfP, but everyone agreed that I should turn myself into something like one in my role as its senior fellow for innovation. That put me in a position from which I could meet individuals and organizations whose groundbreaking ideas might not otherwise find their way into the peacebuilding community. That also made it easy for me to see it once other organizations started pivoting toward us earlier in this decade.

So, for reasons that had a lot of dumb luck built into them, I found myself in a doubly good position by the end of the 2010s. I had the personal experience that helped me make the case to my fellow peacebuilders that we had to pivot and a long-standing interest in social change, entrepreneurship, technology, and the arts that brought me into contact with social entrepreneurs in those other fields who were open to pivoting toward us.

PIVOTING PEACEBUILDERS

I don't want to go too far here. The most I can claim is that the peacebuilding pivot has begun and that the following four examples give you a sense of how my colleagues have begun to shift their metaphor-

---

4. John Hagel III and John Seely Brown, *The Only Sustainable Edge: Why Business Strategy Depends On Productive Friction And Dynamic Specialization*. (Boston: Harvard Business Review Press, 2005).

ical feet. It is worth noting, too, that all of them began as global peacebuilders whose experiences elsewhere may have made it easier for them to see the importance of working holistically than it was for our colleagues who worked exclusively in the United States. As I learned from my career as a comparative political scientist, it is easier to see the "big picture" when you can take a step back and put whatever it is you are interested in into a larger context.

Rotary and the Pillars of Positive Peace. The Institute for Economics and Peace (IEP) is an Australian-based think tank which made a splash in peacebuilding circles when it published its first Global Peace Index in 2007. Every year since then, it has ranked the world's 162 largest countries on more than twenty indicators of peacefulness, most of which measure aspects of what I earlier called negative peace. The first index caused more than its share of controversy because the United States did not fare well, ranking ninety-sixth. It has since fallen to one-hundred-thirty-first place meaning that only thirty countries in the world are less peaceful than we are.

In some ways, America's score was misleading. Given our global role, it would be hard for us to do as well as a country like Iceland or New Zealand which routinely appear at or near the top of the rankings.

While the IEP researchers knew that "the data don't lie," they were perplexed by some of their findings which led them, in my terminology, to pivot in the early 2010s. They realized that most of their indicators—the use force at home and abroad, spending lots of money on defense, or incarcerating a large proportion of a country's own citizens—tapped what I have called negative peace. So, they set out to gather data on the forces that allowed countries to sustain peace for an extended period of time which led them to create a second, Positive Peace Index.

They have since found that the most peaceful societies do the best job of strengthening the eight "pillars" of positive peace depicted below.[5] The causal links between the pillars and lasting peace are still murky. The data that IEP uses do not show how or why any of those

---

5. Steve Killelea, *Peace in an Age of Chaos: The Only Solution for the Future.* (Sydney:

eight factors make such a difference. Still, it isn't hard to see how having an effective and corruption-free government, a reasonably equitable distribution of resources, good community relations, an effective communications system buttressed by an open media ecosystem, a healthy business environment, and widespread support for human rights would contribute to a society where few people would even think of using force or violence to settle their disputes.

It also helps explain why the United States does better on the positive peace index than it does on the original one, although our score is declining on it, too. Still, the fact that we continue to do fairly well on each of those pillars helps people see what some of those often ill-defined guardrails sustaining our democracy include.

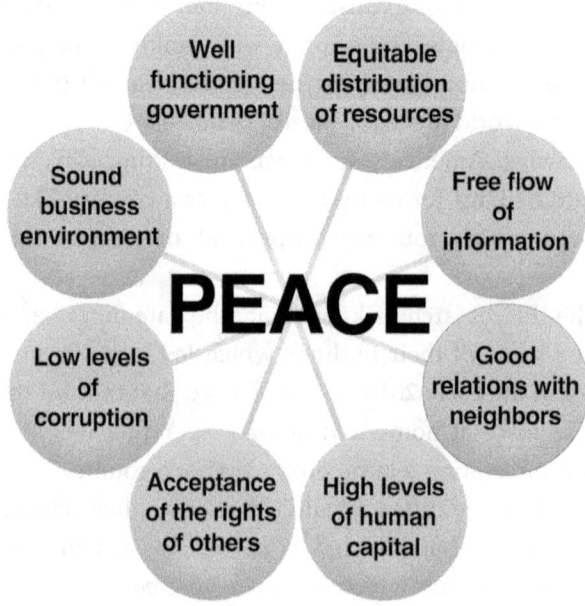

Figure 5.2: *The Pillars of Positive Peace*

Because IEP is a think tank, the index would not have found its

---

Hardie Grant, 2020). The most recent data can be found at https://www.visionofhumanity.org/maps/positive-peace-index/#/ (Accessed December 4, 2024).

way into this book if Rotary International hadn't decided to bring its statistics to life. Its leadership had known for some time that few local clubs made peacebuilding at home a top priority, choosing to emphasize one or more of its other areas of focus instead.

When they learned about the Positive Peace Index, they realized that it could breathe new life into one of Rotary's oldest and most cherished traditions by showing how the service projects that most clubs focus on also contribute to peace. That led its peacebuilding team to forge an alliance with IEP to support its work all over the world, including the United States.

Few American clubs have found ways of including peacebuilding at home in their service work for reasons I mentioned in discussing my own club in chapter 4. That led us and other Rotarians scattered across the country to begin using the pillars to show Rotarians that their existing service work at home should also be seen as contributing to peace once they explicitly draw the connection between their work and one or more of those five pillars.

That is particularly important for the rest of this book because few Rotarians (Gretchen and I are exceptions even in our own club) join because of its peacebuilding work. Rather, Rotary is as strong as it is because it attracts successful professionals who all seek ways of "giving back" to their communities. If they join out of an interest in a specific issue, it usually was one of its other areas of focus.

As a result, as I also noted in chapter 4, my own club has decided to use the pillars to help deepen our fellow Rotarians understanding of peacebuilding. And, as I have hinted at throughout this book so far, if we don't attract the kinds of people who join service clubs like Rotary, we will not be able to build the kind of movement that could spark a paradigm shift in ways I will begin describing in the next chapter.

Maybe Rotary isn't for you. Nonetheless, you can still think about how you could use its Four-Way Test (see chapter 3) and the pillars of positive peace in sparking a broadly based peacebuilding pivot in your community.

EXERCISE 5.1: AMERICA REMADE

Put yourself through a version of the same exercise we used at our most recent Rotary District Conference. Make a rough estimate of how successful your community has been at "constructing" any one of the eight pillars (define what you mean by community and success in any way that makes sense for you). Then, ask yourself how a change in any one of them would affect all of the others. Even if your answers are tentative and vague, the exercise should deepen your understanding of how complicated wicked problems are. It should also help you see why peacebuilders realized that we had to pivot and consider all those other issues that amount to what we refer to in our internal jargon as the drivers of conflict.

Youth and Peace in Action. Return, too, to Youth and Peace in Action. Recall that each group of high school students chooses its own peacebuilding project. Very few of them decide to work on anything like ideological division, political violence, or any of the other kinds of issues associated with negative peace.

Instead, almost all of their projects deal with issues that can be found in one or more of the eight pillars. While it is true that they had been exposed to them in YPA's coursework, they probably would have gravitated in those directions anyway because these are the issues that young people tend to be interested in these days.

Thus, a school in Boca Raton FL worked on the environment, a military academy's group developed programs to welcome immigrants to their rural Virginia community, and a charter school in Americus, Georgia spent the academic year 2022-2023 setting up a mentoring program to help students from less than privileged backgrounds prepare for college.

The Birmingham AL team has pivoted in two ways each of which has gained the attention of city leaders. The students have taken the lead in addressing gun violence which took 152 lives in a city of

200,000 residents in 2023. Meanwhile, YPA teachers and students have made huge progress in adding peacebuilding themes to the general curriculum. During the 2024-2025 academic year, all ninth grade English teachers began integrating elements of its peacebuilding fundamentals course into their analysis of the novels that they assign during the course of the year. By the time they graduate, just about every high school student in the city will have had some peacebuilding training, something that cannot be said of any other student population anywhere else in the country.

Maybe working with high school students isn't for you. Nonetheless, you can still think about how people in your community could execute a peacebuilding pivot by using the school system as a leverage point.

Urban Rural Action. I met Joe Bubman at a conference in Cyprus in 2016. While on the long flight back to Washington, he laid out his early plans for what turned into Urban Rural Action three years later.

Joe was then a member of Mercy Corps' peacebuilding and conflict resolution team and spent most of his time managing projects in Africa. He loved his work. But, he also realized that the United States had its own problems that he could help address. Besides, he was tired of living out of a suitcase and was ready to settle down.

During his time at Mercy Corps, Joe had noticed two things. First, wherever he worked, he saw a growing disconnect between people who had moved to cities and those who chose to stay in the countryside. Second, he also noticed that people only stayed involved in Mercy Corp's projects for the long haul if they had a good time while doing the hard work.

In the aftermath of the 2016 presidential election, Joe decided to leave Mercy Corps and start his own American-based NGO. He quickly realized that the original ideas he floated past me on the flight back from Cyprus put too much of an emphasis on the fun side of the equation. That plan would have brought urban and rural residents together to simply spend a day or two playing games and hanging out with each other. As the project evolved, however, the game playing slipped into the background, although it did not disappear.

By 2019, he had launched Urban Rural Action and moved to Los

Angeles where his new family was establishing its own urban roots. Since then, Urban Rural Action has drawn on Joe's experience with Mercy Corps but adapted it to the realities of life here in the United States. It has focused on incubating projects that bring together volunteers in regions that contain both a medium-sized city and rural areas. The first projects brought liberals and conservatives together in south central Pennsylvania for a discussion of gun safety—not gun control.

Joe and his team start by meeting with local leaders, often including the staff of the community mediation center. Together, they hone in on a single problem facing the entire region. The one in Adams and Franklin counties chose the threat of electoral violence. Others picked less overtly political issues such as the provision of physical and mental health services or the status of returned citizens who had been released from prison.

Then, Urban Rural Action and its local partners put out a call for volunteers who are willing to spend between eighteen months and two years working together on whatever problem(s) the team selected. Because there are always more applicants than available slots, the team is able to select a group that reflects the diversity of the region's population, however you choose to define it.

Urban Rural Action is also in expansion mode. As I was finishing this chapter, it launched the United Safe and Strong Communities project which it launched in four south-central Pennsylvania counties which are home to Hershey, Gettysburg, York, and the state capital, Harrisburg. Any citizen could apply. In April 2025, Urban Rural Action chose a steering committee of about 20 who, together, who broadly represent the region's demographic.

Participants spent a month getting to know each other. Then they devoted a few more weeks developing their collaboration skills while learning how to minimize our human tendency to "other" the people we disagree with. At the same time, they designed a project that meets a glaring need of their own choosing which they can implement over the course of a few months. The program will end when the team communicates what it has done, takes stock of their successes and failures, and plans for the next phase of Urban Rural Action's work in a (presumably) even larger portion of Pennsylvania's heartland.

Maybe working on the urban/rural divide isn't for you. Nonetheless, think about how you could focus on one burning issue given your community's demographic divides and do a peacebuilding pivot based on them.

Resetting the Table. Other groups have found it easy to pivot and move beyond peacebuilding because they always had an eye on other issues, too. Here, the best example is Resetting the Table that started out working with Jewish congregrations and now is a key player in the broader interfaith community.

As is the case with many of those organizations, the key to understanding Resetting the Table's history lies with its innovative founders. In the mid 2000s, Melissa Weintraub and Eyal Rabinovitch each made a professional pivot. Melissa had recently been ordained as a conservative rabbi, while Eyal had started his career as a sociologist teaching at Wesleyan University and Baruch College. Then, they both realized that they had another calling—getting American Jews to support peacebuilding between Israelis and Palestinians. That led Melissa to found Encounter which has taken more than 3,000 Jewish leaders to visit the Holy Land where they learn about the conflict from thought leaders who represent all of the viewpoints along the ideological spectrum—which is saying a lot given the region's many divisions.

As Encounter grew, Melissa and Eyal decided that they had to pivot again. Members of the congregations they worked with disagreed with each other on a lot more than policy toward Israel, including marriage in all of its forms, who should be ordained as rabbis and cantors, and the role that their synagogue should play in the broader community.

So, they created Resetting the Table to bridge all of these divides. They started working with synagogues, Hillel clubs on college campuses, Jewish federations, and more. They don't just do the kind of superficial one-off events that DEI trainers today are often and justly criticized for. Instead, like Urban Rural Action, they realize that they have to dig deeply into the material so that as many of the people they work with as possible could themselves facilitate difficult conversations when Resetting the Table trainers could not be in the room.

In *High Conflict*, Amanda Ripley featured their work with New

York's B'nai Jeshurun (BJ for short) which is one of America's oldest, largest, and most influential Conservative synagogues.[6] Unfortunately, as it was nearing its two hundredth birthday, the congregation was on the brink of collapse because its members were deeply divided over the situation in Israel which is near and dear to almost every practicing Jew's heart. In particular, the left-leaning rabbis publicly supported forging closer relationships with Palestinians, which many in the congregation opposed. Some prominent members quit.

In an attempt to stop the exodus, the embattled chief rabbi took a congregant's advice and called in Resetting the Table. Its team began by surveying the members and holding in-depth discussions with fifty of them. They started by using a phrase that Ripley would put at the heart of her own work a few years later. They helped the members complicate the narrative. People learned to listen to each other with curiosity and to loop or verify that they had heard things right by repeating back what their interlocutor had said. Then they began to understand—if not agree with—what the others were saying. Gradually, the members noticed that they had a lot in common, whatever their differences about the peace process. They found it easier to disagree with but also learn from and even enjoy spending time with other members of the congregation.

Their conflict didn't disappear. But they had learned to disagree better.

In time, the community took on other divisive issues, including interfaith marriage which had long been a taboo in the Conservative Jewish community. It also prepared them for perhaps their most remarkable accomplishment of all, an exchange trip to meet with Trump-supporting, gun-toting members of a corrections officers' union in Michigan who themselves then came to New York. Although Resetting the Table was not involved in this project, the work it had done made these visits possible.

Meanwhile, Resetting the Table itself realized that its tools could

---

6. Amanda Ripley, *High Conflict: Why We Get Trapped and How We Can Get Out*. (New York: Simon and Schuster, 2021) p. 240-250, but that whole chapter on complicating the narrative helps.

help all Americans deal with the differences facing our country that did not center on the Jewish community. So, after Donald Trump's first election, they began exploring tensions in communities that had supported President Obama in 2008 and 2012 but had swung to Trump in 2016. They did the same kind of training they did with BJ in a mostly rural four county region where Illinois, Iowa, Minnesota, and Wisconsin meet—and there are not a lot of Jews.

After a few weeks of community-wide work based on the model they had developed for BJ, they brought a diverse group of leaders together for a day in 2019, the highlights of which are captured in a video, Purple, which has now had hundreds of showings and related discussions in civic associations around the country.[7]

At the time, they planned to do more of these intensive local projects, but the pandemic ruled that out. Nonetheless, it convinced Weintraub, Rabinovitch, and their growing team to work on bridging America's broader divides that affect the ninety-seven percent of the population that does not identify as Jewish. The organization became involved in the broader efforts of the so-called Bridging Community which I will get to in the next chapter.

More importantly for our purposes here, Resetting the Table decided to build on its strengths and work with locally based faith communities that wanted to do something about polarization where they lived—and worshiped. That work started by seeking common projects with conservative Christian congregations, especially in the South. And as I was finishing this book, they started putting out some feelers in Hollywood.

Maybe working with the Jewish community isn't for you. Nonetheless, you can still think about ways of doing a peacebuilding pivot with faith based organizations in your community.

OTHERS ARE PIVOTING, TOO

I did not expect to include anything resembling the rest of this chapter when I started writing *Peacebuilding Starts at Home*. Then, much to my

---

7. https://www.resettingthetable.org/purple (Accessed December 4, 2024).

surprise—and delight—I discovered that a handful of individuals and organizations that focused on the kinds of issues included in the pillars of positive peace were beginning to pivot toward us. None define themselves as peacebuilders, but they all are beginning to see ways in which our community could add value to their work and vice versa.

If nothing else, I want to introduce you to a sample of what I jokingly refer as our first cousins. None of them is more than another one of those tiny islets in the archipelago of social change activists that David Sloan Wilson described. Some may not even survive. Nonetheless, as was the case with the peacebuilding organizations you have already met, each has had its share of success and could get significantly larger and more influential in the not so distant future.

Stranger's Guide. As was the case with most of the organizations covered in the rest of this chapter, I discovered *Stranger's Guide* by accident. I was at my fiftieth college reunion in 2019 when Ron Rapoport handed me a copy of a new travel magazine that his daughter Abby had co-founded. I took it back to my room and immediately realized that it was a peacebuilding publication—in addition to whatever Abby and her colleagues thought it was. The next morning, I reminded Ron that Abby and I had met when she was in junior high school, which prompted him to ask if I would be willing to meet with her and help her figure out how to expand the magazine's audience. I agreed immediately. We have been meeting weekly ever since.

Stranger's Guide can best be described as an unconventional magazine for people with global interests and a social conscience. It normally publishes four issues a year, three of which cover a country or community somewhere else in the world while the fourth is on some place in the United States. Unlike a conventional travel magazine, it has had issues on Tehran, Ukraine (which was planned and published in the six months after the Russian invasion), and other global hotspots.

Abby and her team want to turn readers into mental "travelers" by offering them new insights into other parts of the world through nonfiction reporting, short stories, poetry, and photography. At least eighty percent of the material in each issue is produced by locally based authors and photographers. Each issue, too, includes articles on sports, youth, and the LGBTQ+ community as well as cute factoids (who knew, for example, that Ukraine is home to the world's largest toilet bowl museum). The tiny team brings the material together in a visually stunning product that has won four National Magazine Awards which typically go to publications with national reputations, several of which sit on my coffee table.

I also saw its peacebuilding potential the minute I opened the first issue. Ron is no fool. He made a point of giving me the issue on Vietnam since he knew that I jokingly refer to myself as having majored in ending the war there back in the day. The next steps followed quickly and easily. Abby is now a regular participant at AfP's PeaceCon. It has featured AfP members and the issues it focused on in many of its issues. With AfP, it has begun exploring how we can incorporate story-telling and place-based journalism into peacebuilding initiatives in the United States. More generally, Rapoport and her team have helped AfP find ways of pivoting beyond its own silos of peacebuilders.

Last but by no means least, Abby co-founded N/A Books, which published *Peacebuilding Starts at Home*.

Maybe travel journalism isn't for you. Nonetheless, you can still think about how journalists could be part of a peacebuilding pivot in your community.

The Super Crowd. I met Devin Thorpe because he was the first person to subscribe to my Dot Connecters Substack. Having nothing better to do when the notification arrived, I decided to check him out, which was the beginning of a remarkable friendship.

After getting an MBA, he began his career as a conventional investment banker who gradually developed a powerful social conscience. By the time we met in 2021, he had run for Congress as a liberal Democrat in his native Utah—and lost badly.

His electoral ambitions quashed once and for all, Devin then shifted his attention to projects that grew out of a podcast he had been hosting twice a week for nearly a decade, Superpowers for Good. Over the years, he has interviewed over 1,000 change makers, some of which he has pulled together into a book of the same name which is an utter delight to read because their personal stories are so inspiring.[8]

When we met, he had pivoted again, having decided to focus on a new way for startups to raise investment capital—equity crowd funding.[9] Many Americans had already given money for specific causes through crowdfunding platforms like GoFundMe. On the day I drafted these words, its home page promoted fund raising efforts to support victims of the war in Gaza, tornado relief, and a holiday gift giving campaign. No one should scoff at those efforts which raised over $100 million in disaster relief in 2023 alone.

Devin, however, has something different and more lasting in mind. Before the passage of the JOBS Act in 2012, only so-called accredited investors with assets of at least two million dollars could put money into startups. That meant that only conventional bankers (like Devin in his first professional incarnation) and venture capitalists could get involved. Not surprisingly, they tended to fund companies that seemed likely to make a big profit, most of which did not make social justice a high priority—if they cared about it at all.

The JOBS Act carved out a niche for small investors. Companies can seek backers who commit as little as $100 and therefore get their seed capital from a large number of individuals who can't come up with the seven and eight figure investments that have made the venture capitalists based on Sand Hill Road in Palo Alto (in)famous. As Devin and others see it, the act makes it easier for community members to invest in local projects, including those that help underserved communities of all sorts and, in the process, could make the so-called American dream accessible to the millions of people who have been "left behind" as American capitalism has evolved.

To be eligible, a company has to be listed on one of the eighty-four (as of 2024) online platforms through which all such trades have to be made. While no two platforms are alike, companies seeking investment funds typically include a product description, the amount of

---

8. Devin Thorpe, *Superpowers for Good: The Skills You Can Master to Leave Your Mark on the World*. (Salt Lake City: Devin Thorpe, 2021).
9. Devin Thorpe, *How to Make Money with Impact Crowdfunding: Your Guide to Investing Profitably to Support Diverse Founders, Social Entrepreneurs and Community Builders*. (Stockton, CA: Devin Thorpe, 2024).

money sought, investment terms, and a descriptive video. The offerings usually are available for a period of a few weeks to a few months as is also the case on sites like GoFundMe or Kickstarter.

If you decide to invest, all you have to do is fill out a simple form that is only a bit more complicated than the one you might have filled out if you bought a copy of this book from an online bookstore. When and if the company reaches its target, it gets the funds minus the small fee the platform charges for its services. But without the symbolic ringing of the bells that accompanies a splashy IPO at the New York Stock Exchange.

Being an entrepreneur at heart, Devin also created the Impact Cherub Investment Club to build support for equity crowd funding in general and help fund the best startups in particular. He chose the name because (mythological) cherubim are small and good-natured angels—whether or not they are investors. In its first year and a half, the club has grown to about seventy members, roughly ten of whom make it to each month's meeting.

The group considers two companies seeking equity funding on one of those platforms. Most of the members (especially me) are rank amateurs when it comes to investing. Despite our limited experience, one or two of us volunteers to do something like due diligence on one of the companies we are considering that month, and we then decide if we want to make an investment.

Typical was Block Energy which I reviewed. It provides no-money-down funding for solar panels and other renewable energy services for property owners in underserved communities, especially in inner cities. It was one of the larger groups we decided to support even though it had raised some of its funds from more traditional venture capitalists. We also decided to fund Garden for Wildlife which is a for-profit subsidiary of the National Wildlife Federation that sells native plants directly to customers who are interested in revitalizing their local habitat.

Most of the companies we consider are far smaller and based in a single community which means that they are more in line with my idea that peacebuilding which starts at home literally has to start as close to home as possible. To that end, we have decided to make our hundred dollar investments in companies that build 3D printed homes or support BIPOC owned startups in cities all over the country.

Just as promising is Devin's newest enterprise, the SuperCrowd, Inc which he created to build support for crowd equity funding in the general public, something we Cherubs could not do using our monthly meetings as a platform. In keeping with its mission, Devin has crowd funded SuperCrowd on one of the platforms to give himself the working capital to spread the word about equity crowdfunding. So far, it has run four large virtual conferences on crowdfunding. He is also beginning to hold in-person events in cities like his native Salt Lake, Baltimore (where I first learned about Garden for Wildlife), and Chicago that already have substantial equity crowd funding communities.

The events themselves resemble conventional trade shows with a dose of SharkTank thrown in. Speakers discuss the benefits of crowd funding writ large. Devin even invited me to lay out the rationale behind Peacebuilding Starts at Home at the first SuperCrowd online conference in 2022. Breakout sessions allow attendees to do a deeper dive into aspects of crowd funding. Finally, companies make pitches to all of the attendees who then are free to invest in all, some, or none of them.

I am particularly drawn to Devin's initiatives because of the centrality of local peacebuilding in our own work. Whether it's in Burundi or Baltimore, the evidence overwhelmingly suggests that initiatives that are locally created and managed are most likely to succeed, especially if success involves working across either ideological or issue-based lines.

Maybe equity crowd funding isn't for you. Nonetheless, you can still think about how locally based startups could be part of a peacebuilding pivot in your community.

Nursha is by far the edgiest organization you will meet in this entire book. That starts with its self-description.

> *Together we co-create experiences and opportunities for True Do-Gooders to deliver their offerings with flavor.*

Created in 2003 by yet another force of nature, Shalonda Ingram, Nursha is also one of the oldest groups covered in this book. Nursha and Shalonda's many other ventures reflect her wide-ranging interests and the fact that she describes herself as a personal and professional nomad who resists efforts to pin herself down to a single idea or even a single place to live.

Like all of Shalonda's projects, Nursha defies simple description. On one level, it can look like a non-conventional branding and event planning organization. Indeed, that is how I first met them because Shalonda and her team helped facilitate a conference that I attended. A few weeks later, she was on the West Coast doing grand rounds on intergenerational trauma at the Stanford and University of California-San Francisco medical schools that led to a co-authored article in the *American Journal of Public Health*.

For the purposes of this book, Nursha's most promising initiative is its New Stained Glass Project. Although she does not identify with any single religious tradition, there is a strong spiritual dimension to many of the projects that Shalonda takes on. That led her to think about how her team could help breathe new life into underused churches and their congregations.

Nursha's project draws on two uses of stained glass that can be traced back to its origins in the eighth century CE. It provided images of what Christianity stood for at a time when most believers were illiterate. At the same time, making stained glass provided an income for artists and artisans who might otherwise have gone hungry.

The new stained glass project seeks to shed new metaphoric light on what it means to believe and the role that a church (or other religious building) can play in a community. In many cities, once prominent, mainline Protestant churches have seen the size of their congregations plummet as members moved to the suburbs. Their buildings—many of which have sizable endowments—are at best underutilized. In some cases, the buildings as well as their congregations are falling apart, as literally happened in January 2024 when the First Congregational Church in New London CT—my home town—collapsed.

Nursha has projects to repurpose church buildings in a number of eastern cities, two of which are within walking distance of the AfP office and the White House. The Church of the Holy City (Swedenborgian) and the Universalist National Memorial Church sit two blocks apart on 16th Street in Washington and as recently as the 1960s, they served largely white and upper middle class congregations. With Nursha's help, they have become home to job training and English as a Second Language centers. At the Church of the Holy City, it has redesigned some of the building's internal spaces and rented them out, netting the congregation about $500,000 in income a year. At the Unitarian National Memorial Church it has installed solar panels and new audio-visual equipment in an attempt to rebuild the congregation.

Maybe working with underutilized houses of worship isn't for you. Nonetheless, you can still think about how the interfaith community could be part of a peacebuilding pivot in your community.

Build IRL. Just as I was finishing the next-to-last draft of this book, a friend introduced me to Colton Hewerd-Mills and Saumya Gupta, the co-founders of Build IRL. At first glance, they are unlikely candidates to include in a book on peacebuilding. Colton is a first generation Ghanaian-American who somehow made it to Exeter, Princeton, and Stanford Business School. Saumya graduated from the selective and prestigious Indian Institute of Technology before getting her MBA at Harvard.

After they finished their graduate degrees, the two of them and their respective families moved to San Francisco. They soon discovered that they and the people they knew had a hard time building meaningful personal networks given everything from the isolation imposed by the pandemic to the fact that so many of their contemporaries worked long hours and spent a lot of their free time looking at screens which contributes to what some call an epidemic of loneliness.

So, they joined a social club that was designed to attract young professionals like themselves. They loved it. They were disappointed, however, to learn that the club's founders were not interested in expanding beyond its single location. At that point, Colt and Saum decided to pivot away from their budding tech careers, use the entrepreneurial skills they had learned in grad school, and start their own business to help people create, sustain, and grow social clubs in the Bay Area.

By the summer of 2024, they had scraped together enough early stage investors to enroll a cohort of twenty-four new clubs into what amounts to a Silicon Valley-style incubator. Only one is a traditional place-based club that serves the delightfully named Cow Hollow neighborhood. The others bring together people from around the metropolitan area with other shared interests that include swing dancing, a group that deals with neurodiverse friends and family members, a cooperative pet walking service, and more.

Maybe joining a hip, cool social club is not for you. Nonetheless, you can still think about how adding to the social capital in your community can be part of the peacebuilding pivot wherever you live.

Daryl Davis and the ProHuman Foundation. Eighty years ago, Gunnar and Alva Myrdahl called race relations the American dilemma.[10] No one reading this book needs to be reminded that racism is still the one wicked problem that looms over just about everything else that divides our country. Thus, George Floyd's murder, Black Lives Matter, the opposition to DEI and "Wokism," and the like are but the most recent "symptoms" of a "disease" that won't go away no matter how much progress we have made—and we have made a lot of it over the course of my life time.

Hundreds of organizations are trying to come to grips with the legacy of racism that literally stretches back to the day that Columbus "discovered" the Americas. For reasons that should be obvious by now, I am drawn to those that emphasize calling in all Americans rather than the ones that explicitly or even implicitly name, blame, and shame people that are not perceived as anti-racist enough.

I decided to include the two that have reached out to us at AfP, starting with the ProHuman Foundation. I actually met its cofounder, Daryl Davis, at Gretchen's first husband's seventieth birthday party which was a swing dance. Ed attends at least one dance a week which

---

10. Gunnar and Alva Myrdal. *An American Dilemma: The Negro Problem and Modern Democracy*. (New. York: Harper Brothers, 1944). Note that Alva's name did not appear on the cover of the original book. Now, she is universally given equal credit for writing it.

is how he met Daryl who plays keyboards at many of them. When he introduced us, Ed said something about his civil rights work, but it didn't really register until Daryl ended up as the speaker at Zoom meetings I attended in the weeks after George Floyd's murder. At that point, I realized that I had missed a golden opportunity at that birthday party when Daryl talked about his work leading more than two hundred people out of the Ku Klux Klan.[11] In almost every case, Daryl was the first Black person with whom the Klansmen had ever had a civil conversation. Relationships that started over a shared love of honky-tonk and rockabilly music turned into friendships and then to the KKK members questioning their racist values.

We physically met for the first time at a workshop on pluralism organized by the Mercatus Center, a libertarian-leaning think tank at George Mason University.[12] We got a few minutes together before his talk when we mostly talked about Ed and the party. I then asked a question during the Q and A period at the end of his presentation about how people who weren't Black and weren't high end musicians could use his work. My question must have grabbed the attention of the ProHuman staff members in the audience because we spent a lot of time talking during the rest of the workshop and afterward which led to their decision to ask me to join their board of advisors.

In fact, the ProHuman Foundation is in many ways the answer to the question I posed to Daryl that evening. His work is the inspiration for everything it does. Like me, the rest of its staff can't do the kind of work that made him famous. But, they can use his efforts as a springboard for addressing the social-psychological drivers of ideological division in our country that have also been at the heart of my own work for the last decade or so. As they see it, American history is filled with huge steps forward and equally huge periods of stagnation and

---

11. https://youtu.be/ORp3q1Oaezw?si=BwXB4KKwWWv2nSo8 (Accessed December 10, 2024).
12. Oddly enough but also as a sign of why a book like this one was needed, GMU's Jimmy and Rosalynn Carter School of Peace and Conflict Resolution is located one floor above Mercatus in Vernon Smith Hall. Until I started hanging out with colleagues at Mercatus, faculty and staff at the two centers rarely even nodded to each other in the elevator.

even regression culminating in the situation we find ourselves in today when so many of us feel that the country is heading in the wrong direction—no matter who they voted for. Thus, as they put it:

> *The defining question of our time is: How do we break through the demonization and division, and find the courage to move forward together?*
>
> *We believe that embracing the foundational truth,*
> *that every person is a unique individual united by our shared humanity, is what will allow us to continue to advance.*

They bring a lot of recent research from social psychology and neuroscience together in defining an organization whose mission revolves around promoting social harmony, building positive connections, and adopting a growth mindset.[13]

As a new organization, the foundation is still defining its role. Still, it has begun developing three separate initiatives each of which seems promising. They are actively seeking volunteers to serve as ProHuman ambassadors who will work directly with Daryl and staff members, developing curricula beginning with elementary school students, and providing grants for educators.

Maybe talking people out of the Klan isn't for you. Nonetheless, you can still think about how the ideas Daryl brought to the ProHuman Foundation could be part of a peacebuilding pivot using education in your community.

One Million Truths. At about the same time that I met Daryl Davis, yet another friend introduced me to Mark Eckhardt, the founder of One Million Truths. Mark had spent the previous fifteen years as CEO of Common, which he still leads, despite launching his new organization.

Over the years, Common has become a leading partner for businesses that wanted to change the world. It drew on its team's collective

---

13. Carol Dweck, *Mindset: The New Psychology of Success*. (New York: Random House, 2006).

experience in social entrepreneurship and pivoted toward becoming an innovation enterprise dedicated to conflict transformation worldwide. As such, it serves as an execution partner for peacebuilding organizations, other nonprofits, corporations, and solo practitioners that can leverage its experience working with government agencies and Fortune 1000 corporations. In the late 2010s, its own research revealed shortcomings that were preventing peacebuilding organizations and their potential partners from measuring up to many of the new realities of the digital age.

Common and now One Million Truths have done this kind of work in dealing with conflicts in Ukraine, the Middle East, and Africa. For the purposes of this book, it makes sense to focus on the work it has done on racial healing in the United States.

Formed at the height of the 2020 protests, the organization seeks to gather personal stories about racism in the United States and then use them to help heal our country's divisions. As Eckhardt put it in a guest column in *Time*:

> In June 2020, I founded One Million Truths, a media platform dedicated to truth and reconciliation, a centralized place for Black Americans to go to feel safe, be seen, heard and validated and a place for non-Black Americans to listen, respond and amplify truth. What if we could really see each other and feel each other's experiences? What if all Americans understood racism and how it shows up in everyday life from the insidious to the overt? By sharing first-person testimonies from Black Americans, One Million Truths pierces through today's sense of separation and shines a light on the humanity and struggle of racism. We should be connected, not fragmented, and instead of being afraid to act, we should be emboldened to. From this place of restoring dialogue, we move powerfully forward.[14]

The friend who introduced us did not realize how far One Million

---

14. https://time.com/5958495/one-million-truths-mark-eckhardt/ (Accessed December 10, 2024).

Truths had already pivoted toward peacebuilding. To begin with, Eckhardt has served as an advisor to the head of Search for Common Ground and helped design some of the Common Ground USA projects I discussed earlier. Moreover, as the statement I just quoted suggests, Eckhardt understood that white Americans as well as people of color had to be part of any effort to address systematic and institutional racism in the United States and that efforts that focus on calling people out rather than calling them in is likely to be counterproductive. Finally, his team is explicitly using Dave Snowden's analytical tools for probing, sensing and responding to complex adaptive systems which I ended chapter 2 with.

On one level, his stories are not surprising. His Black respondents echoed his own experience with racism which, in his case, he experiences as a middle aged, middle class, highly successful professional who had once been a professional musician before becoming an environmental and social change entrepreneur. Once he found how far removed most white people he interviewed were from that experience, he shifted gears and asked his next round of interviewees how race had directly or indirectly shaped their lives without casting blame or demanding that they come to grips with their "white privilege."

Unlike most activists who were mobilized in the aftermath of 2020's tumultuous events, Eckhardt has been patient. In fact, he put the systematic gathering of stories on hold for months before we met as I was putting the finishing touches on *Peacebuilding Starts at Home*.

Now, he is planning a major push in the run up to July 4, 2026 and our country's two hundred fiftieth "birthday." He is currently seeking support from companies that still want to do some kind of DEI work but are reluctant to do anything that seems even vaguely confrontational given the "anti-woke" backlash. For the moment, I am working with him to develop partnerships with a few grassroots organizations through which he can gather a few thousand stories by the time this book is published, do a preliminary analysis using Snowden's Cynefin framework, and begin planning projects that would grow out of the data gathering and partnerships it establishes between now and our semiquincentennial—a term I hope never makes into our everyday language.

Maybe working on the stories Americans tell themselves about racism isn't for you. Nonetheless, you can still think about how our collective experiences with racism and other wicked problems could be woven into our semiquincentennial celebration as part of a peacebuilding pivot in your community.

Optimal Work is the most conventional organization I will be introducing you to. It is another group that I met by happenstance. One of its young staffers, Aviva Lund, had taken a course on using peacebuilding skills in political work shortly after she moved to Washington after graduating from Notre Dame with a BS in neuroscience. My friend who taught the course put the two of us together because he assumed that I would find her work appealing.

Optimal Work is also the first (but not the last) for profit business you will encounter in *Peacebuilding Starts at Home*. Founded in 2018, the organization is based on the work of Dr. Kevin Majeres, a practicing psychiatrist who also teaches at the Harvard Medical School. When his co-founder Sarif Younes discovered Majeres's unusual packaging of psychiatric and neuroscience concepts, he realized that they could help people bring their best selves to work without spending the hundreds of dollars an hour it costs to see a mental health professional. It does so by teaching its clients how to use a combination of mindfulness practices and a version of cognitive behavioral therapy (CBT). CBT is particularly helpful for peacebuilders because its founder, Dr. Aaron Beck, talked about the importance of reframing one's personal problems in much the same way that mediators help their clients do the same with their conflicts as a step toward finding win-win outcomes.

Majeres and Younes never thought of the peacebuilding community as a likely market for their services until I met Aviva. She and I had no trouble seeing how what she did in her day job could help her deal with the tensions that grow out of her own multicultural background and the fact that she had been a conservative student at a predominantly liberal university.

As with Abby Rapoport, we clicked immediately. Within an hour, we were joking about our very different positions on life v. choice issues, the role of Judaism (part of her family is Jewish while I have not been a practicing Jew since my bar mitzvah), and national politics.

I began including her in AfP's peacebuilding starts at home work once it became clear that others were pivoting toward us and that we would need to enhance our ability to work with people who had other areas of focus. In time, I expect that many of the organizations that join the coalition I'll be describing in the next chapter will find a way to use Optimal Work's self-paced and face-to-face trainings.

Maybe working with mental health professionals isn't for you. Nonetheless, you can still think about how bringing our best selves to work could be part of a peacebuilding pivot in your community.

Prosocial World. You have already met the founder of ProSocial World, David Sloan Wilson, who likened existing peacebuilding and other social change movements to tiny islands in an archipelago scattered across an enormous ocean of social change initiatives. As you will see in the rest of this book, David's contribution to peacebuilding starts at home goes far beyond his ability to come up with one liners.

I had been a fan of his research on evolution for years. Then, in 2023, friends from the national security community whom I met through Dick O'Neill told me that Wilson had done a twenty-four part series of video interviews on the noosphere.[15] On the assumption that the term noosphere is new to you, it was coined by the French Jesuit priest Pierre Teilhard de Chardin to reflect the integration of all human learning. My friends were going to be among the interviewees because of the way Teilhard's ideas had shaped their understanding of how warfare was changing and thought I might find their session interesting. What they didn't realize is that I ended up spending an entire weekend watching what turned out to be forty hours of serious nerd television, because I couldn't tear myself away from my screen as David and his guests explored everything from advanced neuroscience to Australian aboriginal traditions.

Since David frequently mentioned his main initiative, Prosocial World, I decided to check it out. Once again to my surprise, I found an organization that adds a lot to peacebuilding here at home. That's the case because ProSocial World weaves together three distinct intellec-

---

15. https://www.humanenergy.io/science-of-the-noosphere-series/science-of-the-noosphere (Accessed December 10, 2024).

tual threads—psychological flexibility, Elinor Ostrom's core design principles for living in an interdependent world, and social evolution. Because I will get to the commons and evolution in chapters 7 and 8, I will limit myself here to what the term ProSocial itself means and why psychological flexibility is so important to David's work—and now mine.

The word "ProSocial" itself is not widely used in peacebuilding circles even though it describes behavior that is wholly consistent with everything in this book. As Wilson uses it, ProSocial acts themselves benefit the entire community, including the people who engage in them. It's Fulgham's kindergartners or Corrigan's neighbors celebrating essential workers at the height of the pandemic. It does not downplay the importance of individual freedom or accountability but puts them in the context of a world that is inextricably intertwined and filled with wicked problems.

As Wilson and his colleagues see it, their challenge is to help people develop the skills that make them as effective as possible when they decide to act pro-socially. To that end, Wilson and his team launched the ProSocial Action Labs in 2023. I was part of a team and sponsored four others that went through its second and third cohorts in 2024. Each team of three to five members learns about all three of the organization's core tools over the course of a two-month workshop which had a huge impact on all of the peacebuilding teams that took part in the training.

The psychological side of the work is anchored in acceptance and commitment therapy and, to a lesser degree, on the same CBT that Optimal Work uses. Both are popular enough in psychological circles that Dr. Whohasnoname used them with me as I was writing this book. I do not have the room to go into the details here, but both help prepare people to do a few things that build on the conclusions I reached in chapter 3:

- You can't do much of anything about what has already happened (acceptance)
- But you can focus on what you will do in response to whatever it is that bothers you (commitment)

- If you are able to reframe the situation and see that you have more alternatives than you previously thought (cognitive)
- And, in the language I used in chapter 3, you then turned toward the people you disagree with (behavior)

In the six months before this book went to press, David and his colleagues began spending time exploring ways we could work together given our professional, political, and intellectual similarities, more of which you will see in the final two chapters. For now, it's enough to sense that I left the most promising example for last because it also provides an intellectual bridge to the rest of this book.

Maybe working with ProSocial World isn't for you. Nonetheless, you can still think about how psychological flexibility could be part of a peacebuilding pivot in your community.

EXERCISE 5.2: NAILING IT

Take any of the organizations included in the second half of this chapter or another organization that you know about that does not think of itself as a part of the peacebuilding community. Spend no more than ten minutes exploring what it would take for that organization to work more effectively with the peacebuilding community.

PEACEBUILDING DOES START AT HOME

I've barely scratched the surface in this chapter. Shortly before I finished it, I spent three days in Atlanta at the Pluralism in Action summit which, as you will see in the next chapter, opened the door to dozens of new potential partners. Some of them have already begun taking their work to scale, a subject I have largely kept on the back burner so far.

You also won't be surprised by the way AfP's Peacebuilding Starts at Home Team reacted to my "discovery" of these organizations that wanted to work with us. They all started finding potential partners all over the place, including through two members of our board of directors who work in corporate America.

In fact, finding all of these potential partners convinced the AfP team that it had to add a fourth theme to the three that initially structured the campaign. Now, we will be seeking as many of these partnerships as possible and doing so in a way that changes the entire country, not just the people who come into direct contact with these and similar groups.

That is where we are heading next.

EXERCISE 5.3: THE LUNCH PAIL F***ING DEAL

Return to the Nailing It exercise you just completed. Clearly, building even the limited partnership you discussed will take time. So, ask yourself what it would take for the organization(s) you just about to sustain the active engagement of people like yourself. Because we are all in it for the long haul.

CHAPTER 6
SPREADING IDEAS WORTH SPREADING

What do you do when you have a problem and there is no known solution? Think bigger.

SHEENA IYENGAR

You don't waste time with reactionaries; rather you work with active change agents and with the vast middle ground of people who are open-minded.

DONELLA MEADOWS

The very essence of capitalism is a win-win-win philosophy.

JOHN MACKEY

Neither basketball players nor startup founders pivot for pivoting's sake. They take those bold new steps in order to reach a more important goal—scoring a game winning basket or making more money for their company.

The same holds for peacebuilders. And their allies.

To see why, cast another skeptical eye on what you've seen so far.

Yes, peacebuilders have accomplished a lot. Those islands in that archipelago do exist. Some of them are growing despite the depressing news we are bombarded with every day.

But, we haven't come close to reaching our goal. We haven't figured out how to bring those local initiatives together into a unified and powerful whole that would make a paradigm shift possible. We haven't come close to addressing the mismatch between the problems we face and the tools that we use to deal with them which has loomed over this entire book. To echo the words of Diana Chigas and Peter Woodrow, it is hard to see how what we are currently doing could "add up to peace."[1]

If we are going to meet today's unprecedented challenges that call for unprecedented responses, we will have to up our game. We won't be able to do that unless we shift gears, become more creative, find ways to extend my invitation to far more Americans, and bring our country's cultural norms in line with those that are at the heart of *Peacebuilding Starts at Home*. In short, we have to build a movement that can make America great again by turning the United States into a country where most of us solve most of our problems without the use of force or violence most of the time.

The minute I use a word like movement, I have to confront a massive elephant-in-the-room problem—politics. Like it or not, all movements seek political as well as social or economic change which means that we have no choice but to deal with something that Americans increasingly dislike or even despise.

Rest assured. I am not going to try to lure you into the world of partisan politics. Even if I wanted to, I couldn't. The Alliance for Peacebuilding and almost every other initiative mentioned in this book is a non-profit organization and cannot legally take sides in election campaigns.

More importantly, the movements I will be describing in this

---

1. Diana Chigas and Peter Woodrow. *Adding Up to Peace: The Cumulative Impacts of Peace Initiatives*. (Boston: CDA Associates, 2018). This book can be downloaded for free from the CDA website, https://www.cdacollaborative.org/publication/adding-peace-cumulative-impacts-peace-initiatives/ (Accessed December 17, 2024.)

chapter and the two that follow are not designed to succeed in the cutthroat world that is political life today. Instead of pitting some "us" against some "them," they are trying to build the kind of inside out coalitions that I've already alluded to which rally as many Americans as possible around what they are for rather than what they are against.

You could and should have plenty of doubts about how far any such movement can go. Frankly, it is hard to see how average citizens like ourselves could change "the system" given the realities of American life as I write in mid-2025. Yet, because I've spent the academic half of my career studying what I inelegantly call large scale change, I know that paradigm shifts can and do happen in social, economic, and political life as well as in scientific laboratories. There is also evidence that some Americans—including some surprisingly powerful ones—have begun laying the groundwork for making one happen here and now.

The next stage of the loop, therefore, involves reaching out to "mainstream America," changing core cultural norms, and building a new kind of movement. My challenge here is to convince you that it can be done and is, indeed, already being done.

CULTURES AND NORMS

Although I would not have been able to explain things in these terms at the time, I first got interested in cultural values and norms when I spent the summer between my junior and senior years in high school as an exchange student in Italy. I had to adapt to lots of (seemingly weird) new things, ranging from the anti-Americanism of the kids I played basketball with who were members of the Communist Party to the fact that my teenaged brother-for-the-summer drank wine every night with dinner.

My teenage culture shock turned into a life-long fascination with the impact of social norms on a country's political life. If anything, cultural issues became more important once I became a professional peacebuilder. You actually saw some of that in the exercise I discussed in chapter 3 that showed both how our often-unspoken values and assumptions shape what we do and how we can change how we act once we bring them to the surface.

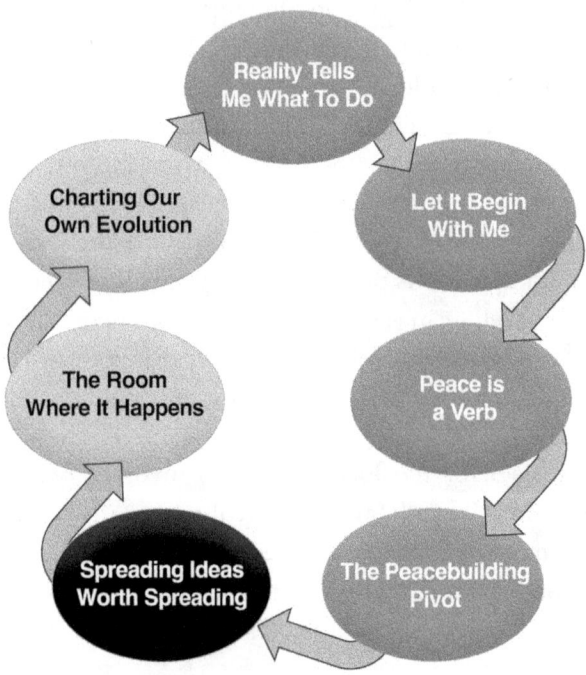

Figure 6.1: The Peace-is-a-Verb Loop

I created that exercise to help students and workshop participants come to grips with what is going on in their own lives. Now, it is time to see how we can change what we do together, too.

Without rehashing decades of not very interesting or fruitful academic debates, it is enough to think of cultural norms as history's lingering impact on the values that most people accept most of the time. For Americans, that includes our commitment to individualism and free speech as well as our understanding that we all support "one nation, under God, indivisible, with liberty and justice for all."

As such, cultural norms run far deeper than our attitudes toward what is happening at the moment. To cite but one obvious example, they reflect our attitudes about the Congress in general, not how we assess what it is doing on a single issue, let alone piece of legislation.

We often take those values for granted to such an extent that we have a hard time putting them into words because they are part of what amounts to our collective second nature. In that sense, cultural norms rarely tell us exactly what to do. Instead, they define the boundaries of what is—and what isn't—acceptable behavior. To anticipate a term that I will keep coming back to in this chapter, they provide clues about what "people like us" could and should do. In that sense, cultures can be particularly important because they rule things out, which is one of the reasons why so many Americans refuse to take socialism seriously.

Cultural norms often seem as if they are set in stone. It is hard, for example, to imagine rugged individualism or patriotism disappearing from the American psyche. That said, cultures can and do change. Since the middle of the nineteenth century, almost all Americans have expanded the statement that "all men are created equal" to include everyone regardless of race or gender. In my own adult lifetime, the same thing has happened on a number of LGBTQ+ issues.

It is high time that we did the same with the cultural norms that shape how Americans deal with conflict and the wicked problems that produce it. If we succeed in doing that, we can also take our work to scale outwardly in addition to doing the personal or inward work I focused on in the first half of this book.

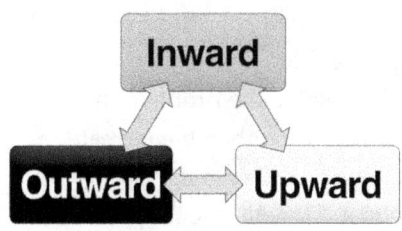

Figure 6.2: Going to Scale Outwardly

To begin seeing why that's the case, start with this chapter's title and epigraphs.

Fans of the TED media empire already know where the title came from. The organization has long done a terrific job of living up to its tag line—identifying and promoting ideas that are worth spreading.

That hasn't always been the case. TED began in 1984 as a conference on Technology, Education, and Design (hence TED). For its first fifteen years, TED lost money and was never anything more than a cult event that was only of interest to the three hundred or so people who made their way to Monterrey CA for its annual gathering.

Chris Anderson bought the struggling company in 2001 and turned it into the juggernaut it is today. TED still puts on the annual conference in Monterrey. It, however, is now best known for TEDx conferences held around the world, the TED media conglomerate with its online archive of lectures, podcasts and radio programs, and TEDed talks and other products for young people. It also names TED fellows, grants the Audacity Prize, and Anderson has written a book on infectious generosity that was published as I was finishing this one.[2]

Unlike Anderson, I am not interested in every idea worth spreading, just those that foster a culture of peacebuilding and could lead to a paradigm shift, which is why this chapter has these epigraphs. None of their authors is a self-identified peacebuilder. Yet, they each suggest ways of spreading my subset of those ideas worth spreading in support of peacebuilding at home.

Sheena Iyengar teaches in the business school at Columbia University. Her courses and her research both revolve around a single key idea. Successful entrepreneurs can do remarkable things when they seek innovative responses to a problem that does not have an obvious solution. The men and women she studies don't play it safe. They start by finding an inspiring idea that has worked in some other field, adapting it to help them solve the problem they face, and then building a market for whatever it is that they have created.[3]

Or, as she put it, they think bigger.

As a young scientist, Donella Meadows and her team did much of the pioneering research on the environmental problems of the 1960s and 1970s. She went on to introduce systems thinking into business

---

2. Chris Anderson, *Infectious Generosity: The Ultimate Idea Worth Spreading*. (New York: Crown, 2024).
3. Sheena Iyengar. *Think Bigger: How to Innovate*. (New York: Columbia Business School Publishing, 2023).

school curricula in ways that I will return to toward the end of this chapter.[4]

As you saw in chapters 2 and 3, systems theory leads us to anchor our thoughts and actions on the fact that what goes around comes around which, in turn, predisposes us to seek win-win or cooperative outcomes in our everyday lives. Meadows and her colleagues made the same case at the societal level, too. If we develop new strategies for working with all "active change agents" in the "vast middle ground" of open-minded people, we stand the best chance of moving an entire system in the direction we want. That also left her more open than I was in the 1960s to adopting inside out strategies because she realized it is possible to convince people in the mainstream rather than those on the ideological extremes to change their ways.

John Mackey was one of the four counterculture (in other words, hippie) entrepreneurs who founded Whole Foods Market in 1978. He went on to serve as its CEO for more than four decades. Under his leadership, it became the world's largest organic food retailer[5] and was at the heart of a much broader cultural transformation that brought mindfulness, yoga, and spirituality as well organic food into the mainstream. And as Mackey's own libertarian leanings suggest, that has happened in ways that can appeal across ideological lines.

Mackey and Whole Foods are by no means unique in that regard. Think of Patagonia, Ben and Jerry's, Salesforce, and other highly successful "companies with a conscience." I chose Mackey's short sentence here because his sense of win-win-win could prove to be a kind of glue that helps connect the metaphoric dots I've raised so far and will add to in this chapter.

Peace activists know that the term win-win is used to describe solutions that benefit all parties to a dispute. By adding the third win, Mackey alludes to a phrase that one hears a lot in his wing of the busi-

---

4. Donella Meadows. *Thinking in Systems*. (New York: Chelsea Green, 2008). This book was actually written in the 1990s and was pulled together and published posthumously by her friends and colleagues.
5. That claim can seem misleading. Costco and Walmart may well sell more organic food products. There is no question that Whole Foods is the largest supermarket chain in the organic market place.

ness world—the triple bottom line. First used by the British environmentalist Jon Elkinton, this idea refers to individuals and organizations that seek outcomes that promote social responsibility (people), environmental sustainability (planet), and economic success (profit). Taking our work to scale geographically will thus add another "win" and more to the list so that it reads win-win-win-win-win-ad infinitum.

TOWARD A CULTURE OF PEACEBUILDING

Those three statements also bring us back to the ideas in the table I first introduced in chapter 3 when I invited you to take your peacebuilding journey to scale inwardly. Here and in the rest of this book, I will be drawing your attention to doing the same thing for our country (and planet) as a whole. As a result, few of the themes in the pages that follow will be entirely new. However, once you add the nine overlapping strategic steps in this section to your mental version of an editing app's sliders, you should be able to see ways of meeting Chigas and Woodrow's desire to see our work add up to peace.

It is also worth reemphasizing another point I made in chapter 3 as your attention shifts from individual to collective action. You can't build that movement on your own, but when my AI turned this chapter into a podcast, it realized something I had missed. Think of each of them as pointing you toward a small step you could take today whose impact could ripple out into your community and other networks you are a part of for days, weeks, months, and years to come. As the sociologist Mark Granovetter pointed out fifty years ago, that impact sometimes is the greatest when you work with people you actually don't know all that well.[6] In this case, that definitely includes working with individuals and organizations that are quite far removed from conventional peacebuilding that would take us beyond those covered in chapter 5.

---

6. Mark Granovetter. "The Strength of Weak Ties." *American Journal of Sociology.* (78) 1973: 1360-1380.

Current Value	New Value
Thinking in terms of "us v. them"	Thinking in terms of "us with them"
Focus on short-term self interest	Focus on shared interests in the medium- to long- term
Expect a zero-sum or win-lose outcome in which I would like to win but definitely do not want to lose	Work toward a win-win outcome that benefits everyone
Assume that one side will have to use power over the other	Redefine power as something we exercise with others
Understand that conflict is bad for everyone involved	Understand that conflict can be an opportunity for growth for everyone involved

Table 6.1: New Cultural Norms

Help people see that we need a paradigm shift. Next to no one took me seriously when I talked about the need for a paradigm shift in my Beyond War days. Times have changed. The term itself has entered everyday conversation. More importantly, public opinion polls suggest that far more people today believe that our institutions are no longer up to the task, including those who have never heard of the term paradigm shift.

Few of them believe that we currently have a viable alternative to business as usual. That's one of the reasons why I have asked you to spend a good bit of time thinking about what an America reMADE would look like. It is also why I keep harping on Daniel Tiger's (and real scientists') suggestion we take a deep breath and count to four so that we can find the mental space to reorient our actions along the lines suggested by the likes of Optimal Work.

People like us. Return, too, to interdependence which is the most important reality that is telling us what to do. Its most powerful cultural implication grows out of research on what academics call narratives which most of us refer to simply as story telling. Among other things, we have learned that we are drawn to stories that we relate to because they involve a real or idealized version of what Will Storr calls people-like-us—replete with the hyphens.[7]

In his most recent book, Storr discusses how businesses use new and engaging stories to convince people-like-us to try something new. Apple did that with its famous Super Bowl ad introducing the Macintosh in 1984 and in the messages it ran in the late 2010s that pitted a hip, cool Mac user against a stodgy PC guy. Iconic campaigns like these succeed in part because they appeal to people-like-us whom they differentiated from people-not-like-us in ways that lead us to change how we think and act not just in the here and now but over the long haul.

Now, as peacebuilders, our challenge is to help our fellow citizens see that, in many ways that matter, we are all people-like-us.

It probably is true that humans are hard wired to think in terms of ingroups and outgroups. Nonetheless, over the roughly 10,000 years of recorded history, our ancestors expanded who they included in their "wes" while reducing the number of "theys."

Now, reality is telling us that the problems we face are increasingly ones that we all share and that we have to treat them as such. If more of us do that more of the time, we will come to see something my high school English teacher would never let me get away with. Everyone is people-like-us.

Even when we disagree. As someone who has never bought a phone, tablet, or computer that wasn't made by Apple, I can still share concerns about technology with my sister who is devoted to Windows and Android.

Can't I do the same with Red Sox fans?

Russians?

Conservatives?

Expanding who we include in our definition of people-like-us will be the first step in making it easier for us to reach the kinds of societal agreements that mirror the interpersonal ones I included in the first half of this book. Can't we do a better job of linking the islets in David

---

7. Will Storr, *A Story is a Deal: How to Use the Science of Storytelling to Lead, Motivate and Persuade*. (London: Platkus/Little Brown, 2025).

Sloan Wilson's archipelago so that it becomes easier to see that we are all people-like-us? That doesn't mean that we agree with Donald Trump or Kamala Harris any more than we agree with that annoying cousin who raises controversial questions at our family's holiday dinner parties? How can we call them in because we are all a part of a single human family and because everything we do affects everyone and everything else? Perhaps most challengingly of all, how do we treat the people who do not seem to be people-like-us?

That applies to each of us. Including you.

And me.

I have mostly kept my own political views off of center stage in *Peacebuilding Starts at Home* because its message should make sense wherever you sit on the ideological spectrum. However, it would only take a click or two to discover that I have been on the left since I was a teenager.

Needless to say, I was less than overjoyed by the results of 2024 election and the first months of the Trump administration which unfolded as I was putting the finishing touches on this book. In other words, I felt like I was in the middle of an experiment of my own design in which I was the "lab rat."

I clearly could not accept a lot of what was done. USAID. DEI. Ukraine. Taxes. The Budget.

Still I kept asking question like these:

Could I disagree with my friends who supported the new administration without deepening our divisions?

Could I learn anything from listening to them?

Could I help others do anything that would make it easier for us to solve our problems together?

What could I do to get others to think and act in a similar way?

Once I began finding affirmative answers to questions like these, I also realized what spreading ideas worth spreading and building a new culture of peacebuilding are all about.

EXERCISE 6.1: AMERICA REMADE

Go back and watch the Australia reMADE video again and reread the answers you came up with when I asked for your ideas about what an American ordinary paradise would be like. If you need or want to, tweak your version of that vision.

Then, ask yourself what values would most Americans have to espouse if we were to make significant progress in that direction. How would our value system have to change? How would you have to change? And the people you interact with on a daily basis?

From the inside out. Return, too, to the idea that a successful twenty-first century movement will not and can not look like the ones I was part of in my youth. In those days, everyone assumed that they had to start on the social and political fringes and work their way "inward" into the mainstream.

The great social movements that reshaped American history did pit one side against another.[8] Abolitionists v. slaveowners. Antiwar protesters v. the government during Vietnam. Prolife v. prochoice activists. Climate change advocates v. the petrochemical industry.

I am not suggesting that those kinds of protests could or should disappear.

Times have changed so much, however, that it is time to flip the assumption that this is the only way to go on its head. In the 2020s, it makes more sense to build movements for social change from the inside out.

In our increasingly interdependent world, almost every issue we face amounts to what psychologists call a superordinate problem that can only be successfully addressed if almost (if not) everyone involved finds a cooperative solution to it. Thus, if Donella Meadows is right, we have the best chance of moving any system in a sustainable and

---

8. Linda Gordon. *Seven Social Movements That Shaped America.* (New York: Liveright, 2025).

constructive direction if as many of us as possible work together to find mutually beneficial solutions. Indeed, given the logic of systems theory which she helped pioneer, no other strategy makes much sense. Whether they start in the middle of the political spectrum or not, we do have to build the broadest possible coalitions.

The challenge is to identify solutions that will benefit us all in the medium to long term. Take climate change. Katherine Hayhoe is both a leading climate scientist and an evangelical Christian who happens to live in west Texas. She makes the news both because of her contribution to the research on the threats we face but also because of her ability to convince her neighbors who raise cattle or work in the oil industry that it is in their best interests to limit our use of fossil fuels.

The fact is that almost every issue area dividing Americans has its equivalents of Dr. Hayhoe who are spreading ideas and strategies that can span ideological and other divisions. The challenge is to build the kind of support for them that could produce lasting change.

Bridging Social Capital. Much of the research that made Robert Putnam famous revolves around two types of social capital. First is the bonding type in which people join associations with people like themselves. Second and far more important for the health of any democracy is bridging social capital in which individuals join forces with people-not-like-us in Storr's terms.

Putnam and his protégés do not define themselves as peacebuilders. Still, they make a convincing case that peaceful societies, like democracies, are most likely to thrive if and when their citizens are actively engaged with groups across lines of division.

Network building. Spreading ideas worth spreading next involves creating a new kind of social network that builds metaphorical bridges across the islands in David Sloan Wilson's archipelago. Organizations like AfP were created to do just that *within* a single field. Now, our challenge is to build those kinds of networks *across* lines of division, whether they be professional (environmentalists with peacebuilders) or ideological (left with right).

My thoughts along those lines were shaped in large part by two other graduate school professors who would not have taken this line of thinking as far as I do. I decided to do my PhD at the University of

Michigan because it had the world's best program in quantitative political science. Even as an undergraduate, I realized that the then path-breaking use of computers and statistics in social science research could be of use to the New Left and assumed that Michigan's faculty members who specialized in American politics and research methods would help me build a career as an activist/scholar.

Because none of them were interested in anything other than pure academic research that focused on elections, I switched to comparative politics after my first semester so that I could focus on the new left and radical change. My new advisor, Roy Pierce, told me about Chuck Tilly, who had just joined the history and sociology departments and studied social movements in Europe.[9] Tilly's own research project focused on the nineteenth century, but given the ability of the French and Italian new left to reach beyond students and other intellectuals, he was eager to have me join his team of graduate students.

Once he realized how little I knew about the nineteenth century, he gave me a copy of Emile Zola's *Germinal*, which was one of twenty novels he wrote between 1871 and 1893 that chronicled life in France as it urbanized and industrialized.[10] In it, Zola tells the story of a strike in a mining town whose impoverished workers had little sense of hope for a better future until a socialist organizer, Etienne Lantier, arrived and starting working in the mines. Because he could put the conditions the miners faced in a broader perspective, he became what Tilly thought of as a movement entrepreneur who could fuse the anger and spontaneity in those local protests and turn them into a powerful force proactively demanding change from the state at the national level.

It wasn't just Lantier, of course. In his dozens of books and articles, Chuck showed how what he called contending groups normally began life as grass roots movements in a single town or mine or factory and then spread until they forced the powers that be to go along—or failed to do so as the case may be. In a way, everything I have done since

---

9. Charles Tilly and Sidney Tarrow, *Contentious Politics*. 2nd ed. (Oxford: Oxford University Press, 2015).
10. Emile Zola (translated by Roger Pearson). *Germinal*. (New York: Penguin, 2004).

then has revolved around understanding and supporting the work of movement entrepreneurs along the lines I learned from his network.

While I was in Ann Arbor, I had to take two years off to perform my alternative service as a conscientious objector. To say that I got off lucky is an understatement. I spent those years as the lead data analyst and computer wizard for Pierce's project on the politics of representation in France.

During my time at the Institute for Social Research, he introduced me to Everett Rogers whose office was down the hall from ours. Rogers never did research on radicals or insurgencies or social capital or even political science. Instead, he started his career as an agronomist, studying how Iowa farmers like his parents decided to plant new varieties of corn seed. I sat in on a research seminar he presented after I returned from doing my field research in France. I was impressed, but seed corn didn't seem all that important to a guy who was trying to plot a political paradigm shift!

It was only after he moved to Stanford and Beyond War's leaders and other Silicon Valley entrepreneurs saw how his models helped them understand how the adoption of any new and innovative idea followed something like the pattern he had first noticed among Iowa farmers, as depicted in this chart.[11]

At first, only a handful of people take the new idea seriously because it is, frankly, too outlandish given prevailing beliefs. If you could, for example, project yourself back to the 1930s or 1940s, you would find that few white Americans would have accepted the idea that the phrase "all men are created equal" could or should be extended to Blacks.

---

11. Everett Rogers. *The Diffusion of Innovations*. 5th ed. (New York: Free Press, 2003).

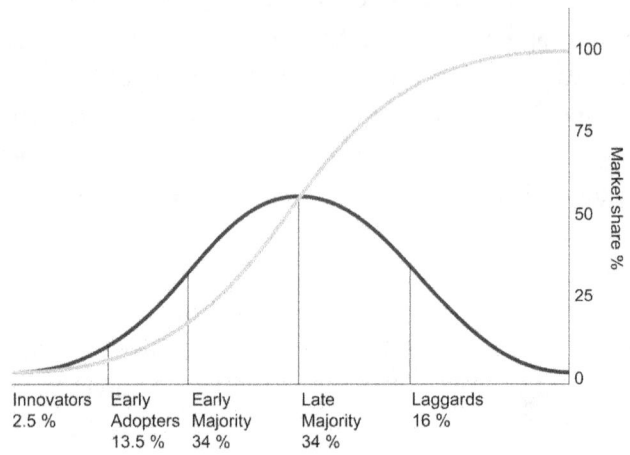

Figure 6.3: The Diffusion of Innovation

Then, a series of seemingly unrelated events laid the groundwork for the movement to spread, including the Great Migration before, during, and after World War II and President Truman's decision to desegregate the military in the late 1940s. Once something like that happens, it becomes easier for respected local opinion leaders to buy into a new idea. At that point, support for a movement can truly take off, often with the same kind of speed with which the COVID pandemic spread in the first half of 2020.

Indeed, much of what follows in the rest of this chapter focuses on creating the preconditions for the inflection point that occurs after you begin reaching enough early adopters who are also community leaders, however you choose to define community. As Malcolm Gladwell popularized it twenty years ago, once an epidemic, support for a movement, or anything else reaches such a tipping point, it enters a period of exponential growth.[12] Once *that* happens, the S-shaped curve in my chart deserves our attention, because by the time you've reached the middle of the bell-shaped one, you already have half of the population on board.

---

12. Malcom Gladwell, *The Tipping Point: How Little Things Can Make a.Big Difference.* (New York: Little Brown, 2000).

Personal efficacy and agency. For reasons that I don't recall, neither Putnam nor Tilly ended up on my PhD committee. That was all for the best, since Roy Pierce turned out to be the best mentor any 1960s radical could have had—even if I didn't realize it at the time. Roy always kept his own political views to himself. So, it was only after his death that I first learned that he had studied at an alternative university based at a ranch in Nevada before he was drafted during World War II. It was his service in post-war revolutionary China that convinced him to take up a conventional academic career after he was discharged. After he died, his wife told me that he had always respected my activism and nudged me toward doing my dissertation and first book on the French Unified Socialist Party (PSU) because he felt I could learn a lot about sustained activism by spending a year with them as a participant observer.[13]

By the time I got to France in 1972, the PSU was in terminal decline. Still, it had tens of thousands of active members, many of whom understood that the party had reached its peak in 1969 when its candidate won five percent of the presidential vote. What I learned from hundreds of interviews and meetings filled with toxic smoke from *Gaulloise* cigarettes is that its *militants* stayed active if and only if they were convinced that the party could turn its fortunes around.

Ron Rapoport (who introduced me to *Stranger's Guide*), another friend, and I reached a similar conclusion when we polled our Oberlin classmates to discover who was still politically engaged five years after we graduated and American involvement in the war had ended. After that, my research interests drifted away from what I then called organizational efficacy and what psychologists today refer to as a sense of agency.

But that same discussion with Winifred Pierce that took place a few months before I joined AfP's Board of Directors led me to revisit what I had learned in France. Now, without the Gaulloises or a scripted research agenda, I found myself watching peacebuilders come and go.

---

13. Charles Hauss. *The New Left in France: The Unified Socialist Party.* (New York: Praeger/Greeenwood, 1978). This is not worth reading unless you think you might enjoy a book on activism that is filled with lots of advanced regression equations.

In the twenty years since then, it has become clear to me that my new colleagues who don't burn out developed something like the sense of organizational efficacy and personal agency I saw in those PSU activists. Thus, just about every organization I met while writing this book understands the need to create mechanisms that enhance the psychological and social well-being of their teams. That need will only grow as more people like you get involved.

Plan for a long journey. The final lesson is one I drew from the "careers" of people like Etienne Lantier. Even before I read *Germinal*, I had learned that convincing people to join something flashy and dramatic like a strike would not be enough. Then, systems theory and my own research on the PSU convinced me that lasting change that builds toward a paradigm shift requires the political equivalent of a distance runner's stamina.

Nothing has happened to change my mind on that score. Paradigm shifts can't happen over night. That might seem like an odd thing to say for someone who was seventy-seven when he wrote these words and realistically can't plan on much of a long-term future for himself. Still, the fact is that it is going to take time to build the kind of movement that will truly change the face of American social, political, economic, and environmental life.

GLIMMERS OF HOPE

I have no desire to pull the clichéd wool over your eyes. We are nowhere near close to having spread those ideas worth spreading. At best, we can find glimmers of hope that we could build a movement that can do so. Not surprisingly given what you've seen so far, three of them come from Rotary.

Youth and Peace in Action. There is no need to describe Youth and Peace in Action's work in any more detail here. Rather, let me simply point out that it is one of the few peacebuilding organizations that has made any progress toward going to scale geographically.

You also don't have to look very far to see why Youth and Peace in Action was able to reach hundreds of schools and thousands of students. Even before she reached out to more than a handful of schools, Patricia Shafer and her team had built a partnership with regional Rotary leaders who helped her convince hundreds of clubs to make YPA one of their service projects which also meant that they partially fund it.

Now, as the organization nears its fifth anniversary, its challenge is to spread its ideas worth spreading throughout the country. And to figure out how to develop other projects on other topics with other long-term partners that can scale geographically as well.

Obviously, I know that she has just scratched the surface here.

So read on.

Rotary Peace Activators. As part of its partnership with the Institute for Economics and Peace, a group of Rotarians (including Patricia) created the Positive Peace Activator program. It recruits senior Rotarians and deepens their understanding of the IEP's pillars of positive peace so that the newly minted Activators can help rank and file members incorporate peacebuilding themes more effectively in their existing service projects that focus on other problems and vice versa.

By the end of 2024, more than 100 senior Rotarians from around the world had completed the twenty-hour training program. The on-line course starts with the pillars of positive peace and then helps participants see that traditional service projects can become even more effective if and when Rotarians stress their peacebuilding implications as well.

As the program expands, Rotary will be able to use the Peace Activators to do two things. First, it can perform its own version of the peacebuilding pivot by helping its members see that everything they do in their communities amounts to peacebuilding whether they think of it in those terms or not. Second, because there are about 800,000 Rotarians in the United States, they can take on leadership roles in almost every community in the country.

I had not personally been involved in this program until I realized that our club had stumbled onto a very similar idea as we planned the next stage of our own growth. So, the minute I finished drafting this paragraph, I signed up for the training.

Obviously, I know that they have just scratched the surface here.

So read on.

The Saturday Racial Justice Group in Portland. One final Rotary story should also help you see what *could* happen once peacebuilders commit to taking their work to scale. Shortly after George Floyd's murder in 2020, an ad hoc group of senior Rotarians in Portland, OR launched a project on racial healing that just oozes with spreading-ideas-worth-spreading potential.

Portland might not seem like an obvious city to use as an example when it comes to racial healing given its reputation as one of the most liberal cities in the country. If you dig into its history just a little bit, it is easy to see why it grabbed my attention.

As recently as 1950, Portland was an almost all white city in an almost all white state. Since then, however, both have diversified to the point that people of color make up just about a third of Portland's and a quarter of the state's population today.

Until 2020, most outside observers thought that Portland had handled all of these transitions fairly well, although people with roots in the region knew better.[14] Despite Portland's liberal reputation, Oregon had been a Ku Klux Klan stronghold in the 1920s and rural areas of the state—including Portland's exurbs—are home to militias, neo-Nazi groups, and other right-wing extremists to this day.

As a result, Portland residents were not all that surprised when their city erupted following George Floyd's murder. Almost daily protests reflected decades-old dissatisfaction with the police department in the Black and Brown communities. At least in part because of the city's reputation and because the federal building was a focus of the violent side of the protests, the Trump administration sent armed marshals to Portland, which heightened tensions even further.

That fall, a friend told me that a group of veteran Rotarians had started the Saturday Racial Justice Group as a creative way of addressing the situation in the city they loved. It turns out that Al Jubitz, whom I had met during my Beyond War days, was one of its

---

14. In one of the weirdest coincidences in journalism, Nicholas Kristoff and James Tankersley grew up in the same small town in Oregon featured in both of their books. Nicholas Kristof and Sheryl WuDunn, *Tightrope: Americans Reaching for Hope.* (New York: Vintage, 2020) and James Tankersley, *The Riches of the Land.* (New York: Public Affairs, 2020).

leaders and also one of the most respected peacebuilding advocates in the global Rotary community. Because it was born during the pandemic, the group had always met on Zoom. So, it was easy for Gretchen and me (along with a few other Rotarians who do not live in Portland) to attend its weekly meetings.

The regular participants live up to most people's stereotypes about what Rotarians are like. They are older and privileged. That holds for the half dozen men and women of color who are part of the group.

But perhaps because they had spent years applying Rotary's principles in all aspects of their lives, they didn't fall into the traps that have limited the impact of many middle class whites who decided to take a stand on racism in the aftermath of Floyd's murder.

Instead, they started by inviting religious leaders, economic reformers, civil society activists, and entrepreneurs trying to build businesses based in the BIPOC community and beyond to speak to the club's weekly meetings. Most were local, but some were visitors to the region, including Daryl Davis whom you met in chapter 5. The Rotarians attended neighborhood festivals, concerts, and youth training sessions. They supported entrepreneurs—many of whom had recently returned from prison—who have created companies and training projects aimed at underserved communities of all sorts. They have connected grass roots activists with leaders in the public and private sectors which was particularly important as the city adopted a new model of local government, itself largely inspired by the shortcomings we all watched on our television screens in 2020. In Rotary's own terms, they have put its Four-Way Test (see chapter 3) into practice and, with it, the importance of changing our own personal paradigms.

After six months, the group started acting and now estimates that its members have devoted upwards of 6,000 people-hours to service projects that grew out of their meetings. Two weeks before I sent this book off to the publishers, it held its fourteenth community gathering with members of Portland's BIPOC community. It sponsors blues concerts. It mentors grass roots organizations and businesses, many of which are run by Portlanders who have recently finished lengthy prison sentences. Typical here is Lionel Irving, founder of Love is Stronger who spent a decade in prison for manslaughter. For the last decade—and now through the Saturday Racial Justice Group—Irving and his team launched programs to help today's young Portlanders avoid making the same mistakes that he did. To be honest, seeing Lionel and his friends hanging out with my Rotary friends is a delight in part because networks like theirs are so rare.

Because its members are part of "the establishment," the group has also worked with city officials, especially in its troubled police bureau as the department is officially known. There, it has helped build ties between the serving officers and the community, especially in campaigns to curb gun violence. Thus, it promotes a program that it did not start itself. Talk a Mile has paired about 350 young police officers and at risk teenagers who literally walk four laps around a track. They start by getting to know each other. Then, on the second and third laps each partners tells their story. In the last quarter mile, they explore whatever came up in the first three laps. Often, the officer and teen stay in touch after they finish their walk. Even if they don't, neither leaves the walk unchanged.

Unfortunately, I emphasized the word could in the first sentence of this section for a reason. As much as I love the work that my friends have done, it has one obvious shortcoming which is why I can only call it a glimmer of hope. They pretty much flunk the spreading side of the spreading-ideas-worth-spreading test. I do not hold that against them. The Portland Rotarians are—and should be—laser-focused on what they can do to improve their own community. They have resisted any suggestion that they should export what they've done to other cities with an active Rotary presence and racial problems of their own. That's up to the rest of us.

Obviously, I know that our friends in Portland have just scratched the surface here.

So read on.

Join or Die. Recall that the very first words in this book were Bob Putnam's impassioned reminder to a group of Georgetown students that the country's future was in their hands. He was in Washington for the local premier of a documentary film about his life and work, *Join or Die*.[15]

In one of the eerie coincidences that seem to happen all the time as I have gotten older, Gretchen and I had met the film's co-producer, Pete Davis, a few months earlier. A mutual friend invited us because he knew that we were both interested in faith-based progressive organizations. We also already knew that Pete lived in the same suburb that we did and knew Liz Hume.

During the course of the lunch, Pete happened to mention that he and his sister were making a documentary about Putnam who had been his mentor at Harvard. He, of course, had no way of knowing that we had taken classes from Bob in his Michigan days and had kept up with him as our interests in democracy and peacebuilding converged.

By that point, they had finished shooting the film, and we helped them edit the rough cut. That night at Georgetown was the first time that we saw the final version and realized that it had tremendous spreading-ideas-worth-spreading potential.

It captures not only the essence of Bob's message but the Energizer-bunny and infectious nature of his personality. Like just about everyone else in the room that evening, we were ready to sign up to do some bridging social capital building of our own.

At a reception between the screening and the discussion at which Bob uttered those words from chapter 1, I suggested that we could help Pete and Rebecca spread the word about the film and then some. We could get Rotary clubs, NAFCM centers, and others to show it, host discussions, and offer attendees on-ramps for getting involved in projects in their own communities.

Patricia Shafer of Youth and Peace in Action organized several such showings through her local Rotary Club in Charlotte NC. Build IRL did the same in San Francisco. I have since learned that a network of urban librarians have used it. Now that the film is available for streaming, anyone could organize a combination screening/discussion/re-

---

15. https://www.joinordiefilm.com/ (Accessed February 24, 2025).

cruitment event. We are planning to host one in the new condo development we moved into while this book was in production.

And, of course, it isn't just *Join or Die*. You could do the same thing with any film or book or podcast. For example, you could use George Mason University's Mercatus Center's equally moving video *Undivide Us*.[16]

My Rotary club has conducted a similar experiment. We started with a conventional book club until we realized that our members didn't have time to read more than a chapter a month. So, we switched to podcasts made by the Next Big Idea Club that feature interviews with authors of the best new nonfiction books. Instead of reading a book or even a chapter, we have great discussions after listening to an hour's discussion in which authors who take on peacebuilding and related questions discuss how people can use their books in their daily lives.

Obviously, I know that the Davises and the Next Big Idea Club authors have just scratched the surface when it comes to using videos.

So, read on.

Weave. In 2018, the New York Times columnist and PBS commentator David Brooks created Weave.[17] I had followed his work for years and found it thought provoking even when I disagreed with what he had to say, which happened frequently when he was one of the country's most articulate neoconservative pundits. But as the 2000s turned into the 2010s and as American conservatism took on a more populist and, then, Trumpian tone, a different, community-focused side of his political persona rose to the surface.

After Trump's first election, Brooks decided that he had to do something to literally reweave the fabric of American society in ways that explicitly drew on research by Putnam and others. He also used reporting and organizing work that his wife, Anne Snyder, had done

---

16. https://undivideusmovie.com/ (Accessed March 1, 2025).
17. The best book on his thinking that led to Weave is David Brooks, *The Second Mountain: The Quest for a Moral Life*. (New York: Random House, 2019).

on things that average citizens were doing to rebuild their own communities.[18]

As Weave took shape, it focused on two things, the second of which has become far more important in the mid-2020s and convinced me to include it in this book.

Then and now, it wants to serve as a clearing house for ideas about rebuilding America's social fabric and for experiments that could connect people who decide to turn those theories into practice. Among other things, it helps train people anywhere to learn how to "weave". More importantly, it has created a national trust map that measures the degree to which people trust each other and join civil society organizations by zip code. It is also building a national network of weavers and will help you connect with potential colleagues in your community much like AfP does with its virtual help desk.

That led to their decision to support local initiatives in specific communities, including major urban areas (Baltimore and Chicago), smaller cities like Danbury CT, and rural areas in western North Carolina.

Obviously, I know that the Weave team has just scratched the surface when it comes partnering with other national networks.

So, read on.

The New Pluralists. The New Pluralists are funders, not activists Their founders came together because they realized that political polarization was tearing our country apart.

You don't need to be the head of a major foundation to reach that conclusion, of course. What is remarkable about the New Pluralists is that the founding funders themselves represent a diverse coalition that spans the political spectrum, including the Lubetsky Family Fund (of Kind Bars fame), the Rockefeller Brothers Foundation, the Templeton Foundation, and Stand for Us (run by the surviving Koch brother).

Despite their differences, the New Pluralists realized that if we began thinking in terms of all Americans as people-like-us, our differences could become a source of strength when and if we learn to

---

18. Anne Snyder. *The Fabric of Character: A Wise Giver's Guide to Supporting Social and Moral Renewal.* (Washington: The Philanthropic Roundtable, 2019).

respect and even cherish each other. They do not want to sweep America's divisions under the rug by, as they put it, "sacrificing deeply held beliefs or compromising to meet in some gray, featureless middle." Rather, they want to (re)create an America in which we heartily disagree with each other but make progress toward shared goals since we respect each other precisely because we don't see eye-to-eye.

From their perspective, pluralism is both an idea and an ideal. It starts with the understanding that any diverse society consists of dozens of different groups all of which vie for and deserve their "piece of the pie." Despite their ideological differences, they share a common concern that the declining respect for the "other" could tear the country apart.

Their own common ground is powerful enough to be worth quoting at length.

> *Since the earliest days of our nation's founding, the seeds of racial and social injustice were sown by slavery, displacement, and genocide. Ever since, the work of living up to our founding ideals has been unfinished, with hopeful steps forward alongside profound failures.*
>
> *America is on a precipice, but this is also a moment of possibility. Most of us are exhausted by the prevailing culture of "us versus them" and long for a better way forward. There are countless examples of people and communities working together across divides to tackle hard issues and to imagine a new future. Will we seize this moment of possibility or will we squander it?*
>
> *To realize the vision of a politically vibrant, multi-racial, multi-faith democracy, we must renew the promise of America by ushering in a new pluralism.*[19]

Therefore, they have chosen to support organizations that foster community, mutual respect, and dignity while confronting our current

---

19. https://newpluralists.org/about/ (Accessed January 4, 2025).

and historical problems and addressing them in a way that heals our communities. There is a lot of overlap between their goals and peacebuilding. A half dozen of its original grants went to AfP members. Another third went to organizations with which we have done some work because they are already pivoting toward peacebuilders on issues such as faith, economic and racial inequality, and mental health.

AfP had not done much with the New Pluralists until 2024 when one of my former students who is an active libertarian and peacebuilder got me invited to a workshop on pluralism at the Mercatus Center. There, I met Lauren Higgins who is the New Pluralists' staff member in charge of ecosystem development.

As we talked, we realized that we had a lot to learn from and offer to each other. AfP brought years of experience working abroad using the kinds of holistic systems-based approaches that the New Pluralists found sorely lacking in the groups they worked with. We continued talking while they made plans for a workshop and hackathon on pluralism in action in Atlanta in early 2025. In the end, they also asked Liz Hume to give a keynote address while I stayed on to participate in the hackathon session on better measuring the impact that pluralists have on society as a whole.

The workshop began ten days after Donald Trump's inauguration. He and his team were beginning to dramatically reshape the American political system. That helped Liz's argument about the need for peacebuilding and social change in general hit home in ways I had never seen happen before. The fact that we had already spent the better part of a decade helping our member organizations measure the impact of their work then made me and the other AfP members stand out in the hackathon. More generally, we met dozens of people we plan to work with in the future, including the YMCA, the Urban Library Association, and lots of local groups, including a number of interfaith networks.

Last but by no means least, Lauren, Liz, and I together came to see that the New Pluralists had a major role to play in putting goals like those I've described in this book into practice. Yes, the New Pluralists could and should focus on the funding side of things. At the same time, it had to step up its role in network or ecosystem building. Liz and I were only too happy to offer our help.

Obviously, I know that the New Pluralists have just scratched the surface when it comes partnering with other national networks.

So, read on.

Civic hubs. I learned about this final pair of examples after my manuscript came back from the copy editor and no traditional publisher would have allowed me to add any new material. Luckily, Abby and her team let me violate one of the cardinal rules that previous editors had ruthlessly enforced over the years.

In July 2025, I met Vinay Orekondy of Better Together America at the International Listening Society's annual conference where we each led a discussion. Before that afternoon, I knew next to nothing about the organization other than the fact that a few people I knew sat on its board of directors.

However, Vinay blew me away when he started talking about the forty or so civic hubs they had helped create around the country. All are organized by local citizens and grass roots leaders who take on one or more of the issues that matter in their community.

My first reaction was that this was *Join or Die* in action. But then, he mentioned the one in Scottsbluff NE which had been started by the head of its local community mediation center with whom I had served on the NAFCM board. That really grabbed my attention because Charles Lieske is one of my favorite colleagues who reflects the fact that he has lived his whole life in one of the reddest states in the country. So, Vinay, Gretchen and I spent the rest of that day talking and discovered that, among other things, that Pete Davis, who made *Join or Die*, was a mutual friend.

At that point, I mentioned Falls Church Forward, which Pete had helped create a few years earlier. Coincidentally, Gretchen and I had just moved to Falls Church City and had plans to attend the group's annual potluck the following weekend.

At it, we discovered a network of new neighbors who had developed a vibrant organization that included the mayor and two other city councilors. Together, they had created the kind of civic hub that Vinay and his colleagues had in mind. Even as new residents, Gretchen and I could see that everything from the traffic flow to commercial development patterns were different from what we had experienced in Fairfax County. And we had moved less than half a mile.

Just before I wrote these words, Gretchen and I agreed to represent Falls Church Forward in the new neighborhood of one hundred condos and four hundred rental apartments that we have moved into. I also introduced Vinay to my new friends in my new town.

EXERCISE 6.2: NAILING IT

> Pick one of these organizations or another one that I did not include but you know something about. Ask yourself what it would take for that organization to become a household name that people turned to when they wanted to deal with divisive issues. What could you do to help it get there? How could you help it spread its ideas worth spreading in the communities you live and work in?

CLEARER BUT MORE DISTANT GLIMMERS OF HOPE– CONSCIOUS CAPITALISM

What follows is also the only section in this book that is not based on my own first-hand experience. It's not for a lack of trying. I have been obsessed with startups and entrepreneurship since I joined Beyond War. I have learned a lot from what I have read and otherwise learned about social entrepreneurship as you saw in the section on the Super-Crowd in chapter 6.

That said, I've had almost no direct contact with the movers and shakers behind conscious capitalism. At the same time, I could not leave them out of this chapter, because the companies and individuals that you are about to meet have made huge progress in shifting American cultural norms and could become partners in future peacebuilding starts at home initiatives.

Emphasis very much on could.

As always, I do not want you to read too much into what follows. It would be absurd for me to claim that a paradigm shift has taken place in American business at a time when tech giants and their "bro" leaders dominate the news because of their (alleged) greed and thirst for power.

Still, lurking just below the headlines are other companies whose corporate cultures reflect "macro" level versions of the themes I introduced in chapter 2 and 3. In particular, they have realized that corporate leaders can prioritize what reality is telling us to do.

Firms of endearment. This book is not the place to go into the details of why what Raj Sisodia calls "firms of endearment" are doing so well. It is enough to see that they are already helping spread new cultural norms (this chapter) as well as new ways of making the decisions about how our society is governed (the next one). As he put it in his most recent book:

> *You can do good all along the journey, enrich people's lives, and help the planet—while making more money.*[20]

The entrepreneurs he has studied over the years have explicitly built their companies on the basis of values that track those in the right hand column of my table. They know that they have to make money. If not, their company will go bankrupt. At the same time, they also understand that they cannot pursue short term profits or shareholder value if doing so comes at the expense of what some refer to as their triple bottom line or the three "p's" I mentioned earlier—seeking to benefit people and the planet as a whole while also making a profit.

You can see this in the history of two very different companies.

Formed in 1885 by members of its namesake families, Barry-Wehmiller made equipment used in the beverage industry, like beer barrels. By the 1950s, the last Wehmiller realized that the company had to shift gears and brought in William Chapman as President and CEO.

After his sudden death in 1975, Chapman's then thirty year old son

---

20. Raj Sisodia and Michael J. Gelb. *The Healing Organization: Awakening the Conscience of Business to Help Save the World*. (New York: Harper Collins Leadership, 2019), 12.

Bob took over. The company enjoyed some growth spurts over the next decade but it was still not out of the woods until the late 1980s when the younger Chapman started buying small, often troubled industrial firms.

When it subsequently spun off some of them, their sale brought in a lot more cash than anyone had expected. That led the younger Chapman to use those funds to pivot the company toward what it is today. At the time, there were no conscious capitalism role models for him to emulate. So, he cherry picked ideas from the few businesses that inspired him, lessons he could draw from his faith, and his experience as a parent to gradually put together a company that in his words, successfully "touch[es] the lives of all of our people."

And succeed it did. When it began its pivot, Barry-Wehmiller had a net income of about $20 million a year. By 2024, it had acquired (or as Chapman prefers to put it, adopted) more than 120 companies that generated $3.6 billion in revenue. Most were small, failing industrial firms that produced industrial tools and packaging equipment that no one outside of the relevant industries (including me) had heard of.

The key to the story for our purposes is what the new owners did with those struggling companies. The Barry-Wehmiller team turned them around using what they now call B-W's Guiding Principles of Leadership in order to create a workplace based on trust that also frees its employees and the teams they form to do their best while performing meaningful work.

As Chapman put it:

> *I had come to understand that my responsibility as CEO transcends business performance and begins with a deep commitment to the lives of those in our care—the very people whose time and talent make the business possible.*[21]

He had never read any of the books and articles that lay out the concepts underlying conscious capitalism let alone this book. None-

---

21. Bob Chapman and Raj Sisodia. *Everybody Matters: The Extraordinary Power of Caring for Your People like Family.* (New York: Portfolio/Penguin, 2015), 11.

theless, Chapman understood that the best leaders empower their workers by treating them well, including them in all decision making, and giving them a stake in the company's future.

The companies it bought were in trouble in large part because their workers felt that they were little more than cogs in a machine that called on them to do boring work in a setting where what they wanted didn't matter. Chapman set out to change each company's culture—a term he explicitly used—by focusing on improving the lives of its employees.

Chapman set out to foster virtuous circles in which each Barry-Wehmiller company constantly improves because of the way it empowers its employees. They started small by gamifying some sales and customer service jobs so that employees would look forward to going to work. Later, they introduced ways for including employees in all decision making that affected their work place. Chapman and his team dramatically increased the company's training programs, creating the Barry-Wehmiller University that offers leadership courses to its employees that are taught by other employees. The commitment to their employees is not limited to the work place but includes helping them meet challenges at home and in their communities.

The second company is a household name—Whole Foods Market.[22] It comes second because it is a more ambiguous case than Barry-Wehmiller in ways that reflect why the transition to a new paradigm will inevitably happen in an uneven series of fits and starts.

With 524 stores in forty-four states at the end of 2024, Whole Foods Market is by far the world's largest organic supermarket chain. Unlike Barry-Wehmiller, Whole Foods was created with something like conscious capitalism in mind. Mackey and his cofounders lived up to many stereotypes about those of us who came of age in the 1960s and early 1970s. Long hair and beard. Lived in a commune. Free thinker. Dabbled in democratic socialism and drugs. Active in local food coops.

---

22. John Mackey and Raj Sisodia, *Conscious Capitalism: Liberating the Heroic Experience of Business*. (Boston: Harvard Business School Press, 2012). Readers who are more interested in the story than the rationale behind conscious capitalism would enjoy Mackey's memoir, *The Whole Story: Adventures in Love, Life, and Capitalism*. (New York: Matt Holt Books, 2024).

PEACEBUILDING STARTS AT HOME

After dropping out of college and spending a few years adrift, Mackey and his then girlfriend opened a vegetarian food store and café in Austin TX in 1978 which they called Safer Way (a play on the name Safeway), renaming it Whole Foods Market when it moved the next year.

The store gradually built a small but loyal clientele until it was nearly destroyed by a flood three years later. Because it didn't have insurance, that could have been the end of the Whole Foods Market story. To everyone's surprise, hundreds of its customers came to help the staff clean up and reopen the store. Their generosity as well as Mackey's newfound interest in market dynamics turned Whole Foods into one of the last half century's most spectacular corporate success stories that had little or nothing to do with Silicon Valley or information technology.

Mackey himself came to adopt libertarian economic values which will also make a cameo appearance in the next chapter because modern market theories helped him see the importance of blending competition and cooperation and opened the intellectual door to new ways of governing which will be the next step on our journey. That and Mackey's personal competitiveness also led to its share of controversy, including Whole Foods' opposition to recognizing trade unions.

Through it all, Mackey wanted his stores to reflect the values in this chart which also reflect those in the values in the right hand column of my table. Somewhat surprisingly, almost all of them survived Amazon's purchase of the company in 2017 and Mackey's retirement five years later when he turned seventy. [23]

---

23. Image source: Adapted from John Mackey and Raj Sisodia, *Conscious Capitalism: Liberating the Heroic Experience of Business*. (Boston: Harvard Business School Press, 2012), 43.

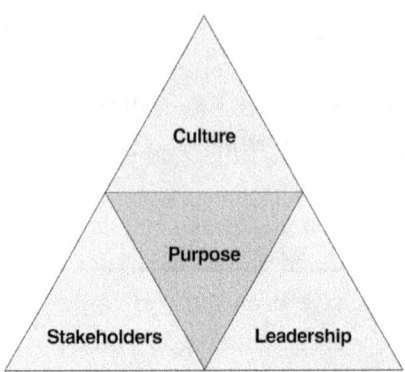

Figure 6.4: *The Whole Foods Triangle(s)*

As suggested in Mackey's statement that begins this chapter, Whole Foods Market was never "just" a conventional business that stressed its bottom line. The same is true of Barry-Wehmiller and dozens of other companies I could have featured here. The new business paradigm starts with the founders' belief that businesses not only *can* combine what Mackey calls profit and purpose but that they increasingly *have to*.

Their vision of capitalism stresses stakeholders rather than shareholders. Despite the fact that those two terms share all but two letters, no two words could be less alike. Many mainstream economists stress that the only thing that matters is the return on investment that the owners make. The conscious capitalism community rejects that idea out of hand and makes the case that companies that see to the needs of their employees, suppliers, communities, and the environment as well as their investors do far better at least in the long run.

Such companies go out of their way to avoid hierarchical or top-down leadership. In Mackey's day, individual Whole Foods stores organized themselves through largely self-managed teams that ran the deli, produce, nutritional aids, and other departments. Senior leaders did make more money than the men and women who stock the shelves or pack grocery bags, but the gap between the highest paid executives and the newest hire in the warehouse still is lower than in most companies in the retail food sector. While Whole Foods was an independent company, all workers with a certain amount of seniority were entitled to stock options. Beginning in 2007, Mackey himself stopped taking a salary and donated all of his personal stock options to the Whole Planet Foundation which was created so that some of the company's profits could be used to help pull people out of poverty in the Global South where many of its employees come from.

Although I can't measure its impact on general cultural norms with any degree of precision, Whole Foods has made a huge contribution to the spreading of ideas worth spreading in ways that go far beyond its direct impact on Americans' growing fascination with healthy dining, mindfulness, and a culture of cooperation.

I don't want to make Whole Foods or Barry-Wehmiller seem idyllic. Both have had to make compromises in order to compete. The economic crisis of the late 2000s forced both to retrench. Both have had to fire staff members—including senior executives—who did not fully endorse the company's commitments. Both "have" to pay those same executives a lot more than they might prefer because they risk losing them to competitors who offer higher salaries and better benefits.

That's the case because we are still in the early stages of the paradigm shift that lies at the heart of this book. The economic center of gravity still lies in the large hierarchical companies that grab most of the headlines.

Obviously, I know that the conscious capitalism community has just scratched the surface when it comes to partnering with other national networks.

So, read on.

Beyond conscious capitalism. Chapman, Mackey, and entrepreneurs like them are outliers. Most business leaders don't think or act the way that they do, including the likes of Jeff Bezos who was directly involved in Amazon's purchase of Whole Foods.

At the same time, it is also true that the values that Chapman and Mackey stress have entered the corporate mainstream because they are now part of the core curriculum of most top business schools. To be sure, MBA students still learn economics and accounting. Most still want to make money and head off to Wall Street or Silicon Valley as either venture capitalists or as founders of the next great tech startup. At the same time, almost all of them take courses that help prospective

C-Suite executives learn how to deal with disputes, alienation, and other workplace problems that reflect the logic of what reality tells us to do, often by explicitly drawing on the kinds of peacebuilding practices in this book.[24]

I only have room to discuss one of those pioneers, Amy Edmondson, whom I met long before she became the Novartis Professor of Leadership and Management at Harvard Business School and one of the leading management experts of her generation. Our paths crossed a few times in the mid-1980s and she continues to have a huge impact on the way I think about leadership even though we haven't seen each other in almost forty years.

At the time we met, she had just formed her own consulting firm after having worked as the chief engineer for the legendary R. Buckminster Fuller until his death in 1983. A few years later, Edmondson went back to graduate school and was one of the first of hundreds of people with a PhD in psychology who ended up teaching in MBA programs where they revolutionized the business education curriculum.

Edmondson is best known for research that connects corporate success with leadership skills that include effective conflict resolution. She got her start with research projects that explored why some surgical teams avoided making mistakes in the operating room. Traditionally, surgeons have called the shots and often ran their teams with something like an iron fist. To her surprise, Edmondson discovered that the most successful surgical units were characterized by what she calls psychological safety. Nurses, anesthesiologists, technicians, and even members of the maintenance crew felt comfortable raising problems when and if they saw them.

As she and her colleagues studied more teams in more professional settings, they discovered that leaders needed expertise beyond traditional things like managing budgets or work flows. Their success depended just as much on their ability to handle the conflicts that

---

24. The most enjoyable entry point into the literature on all this is David Bradford and Carol Robin's book about the Interpersonal Relations Course that they taught at Stanford. *Connect: Building Exceptional Relationships with Family, Friends, and Colleagues.* (New York: Crown Currency, 2021).

inevitably arise when a team takes on a difficult or unprecedented challenge. These problems are so common that I almost don't need to mention them here—inflated egos, selfishness, poor communication, hidden agendas, passive aggressive behavior, and, of course, denial that any problem exists.

Her research also suggests that our failure to take cooperation at work seriously is particularly problematic today because we face unprecedentedly complex problems that don't have obvious solutions. The best leaders don't impose solutions. Instead, like good peacebuilders, they help their employees find common ground through what she calls extreme team-building. What's more, they understand that building teams is a never-ending process that modern corporations can't ignore. It is hard to think of any meaningful work project—including writing this book—that can be done by any individuals working on their own. If you don't believe me, read the acknowledgements section at the end of this book.

Edmundson doesn't use the term wicked problems. She doesn't have to. Corporate leaders have to deal with them all the time. That is especially true in hospitals or technology workspaces where most employees are well-educated and want to find meaning in their work.

Obviously, the likes of Amy Edmondson have just scratched the surface when it comes partnering with innovators in the business community.

So, read on.

CATALYTIC CONVENING AND NETWORK BUILDING

I've used something like the following statements half a dozen times so far in this chapter.

> *Obviously, xxx has just scratched the surface when it comes partnering with other national networks.*
> *So, read on.*

I did so in order to point you toward the two ideas I will use to end it.

We in the peacebuilding community have a long way to go. We

have just begun building a network of people-like-us and turning them into a reasonably coherent political force that would have made the likes of Chuck Tilly or Etienne Lantier proud because we will then be able to scale upward and change the world. That is not something AfP and its Peacebuilding Starts at Home initiative can hope to do on its own. The same holds for Weave or the New Pluralists or Search for Common Ground or any other national network.

At the same time, everything you have seen in this book points toward a strategy that I inherited from and then helped spread with Dick O'Neill.

In the twenty years we worked together, we adapted the model of catalytic convening he had developed through the Highlands Forum which he used in advising senior leaders in the Pentagon. Over the years, he held fifty full forums in which he brought together small groups of thoughtful leaders who would not have met each other under normal circumstances. They would spend an intense two or three day workshop discussing topics that military leaders needed to pay more attention to. Most dealt with long-term strategic problems that often got lost in the shuffle given the need to respond to crises in the moment. Highlands became the place where military leaders and people from outside that world first considered climate change, technological innovations like self-driving vehicles, scenario planning, and the like.

One that I attended in 2005 brought military and NGO leaders together to consider how they could and should work together in the post-9/11 world. I spent a weekend with people I would have never met under any other circumstances who then became friends for life. It wasn't just me. The Highlands Forum alumni network grew to about 1,200 very smart people, many of whom found ways of working together above and beyond the network's own initiatives.

Unfortunately, Dick got too sick to continue working in 2019 at a time when we had already come up with two ideas that AfP could use to take its work to a new level, including through what would become Peacebuilding Starts at Home.

The first is what I now inelegantly call catalytic convening. In September 2024, AfP with the help of two of my Highlands colleagues brought together twenty-five peacebuilders and people in other fields who had begun pivoting in our direction. Many were in Washington for our annual PeaceCon. A few decided to come to Washington only for our event. You have met many of them in the first six chapters of this book. More importantly, the very fact that we met has begun spawning other projects, including one that includes four of the youngest people in the room who are exploring new ways of taking our work to scale. Similarly, because my libertarian friend and former student Sam Staley was there, we finally made contact not only with the libertarian community but with the New Pluralists.

Not everyone I invited was able to attend. I also forgot some people I should have invited, including the Weave project, whose office is around the corner from AfP's! We have since been part of several other less formal convenings, not all of which we organized. And, we have met dozens of new partners with whom we will be developing new projects, including the YMCA, networks of librarians, and even policy experts whom you will meet in the next chapter.

Therein also lies the second side of Dick's work that we will adapt for our own purposes. We will be creating a network of Peacebuilding Starts at Home activists that can coordinate our work along with the likes of the New Pluralists.

Until we can also take our work to scale upward.

EXERCISE 6.3: THE BIG LUNCHPAIL F***ING JOB

I doubt that you have the time or resources to do the kind of catalytic convening and network building that I learned how to do with Dick O'Neill. But, you can do some of it by expending your own network that the exercises in the first six chapters have been helping you identify.

So, think about your own network and ask these three questions:

Who else could I bring into that network?

How could I help the people I know work more effectively together?

And how can I keep them motivated for the long haul?

CHAPTER 7
REDESIGNING THE ROOM WHERE IT HAPPENS

I've gotta be in the room where it happens.

LIN-MANUEL MIRANDA

Once people I meet find out that I am a political scientist who lives in the DMV (as we locals call the Washington DC metropolitan area), my soon-to-be-friend typically reacts with pity or scorn or both. Although I am not embarrassed by either what my PhD is in or where I live, I nod my head or shrug my shoulders or otherwise let my body language suggest that I get it.

For most people I know, politics has become a four-letter word to be avoided at all costs, at least in the kind of polite company Emily Post wrote about. I find myself echoing those sentiments—albeit subtly—in my own writing when I mention that living inside Washington's (in)famous Beltway often makes me clinically politically depressed. I rarely look forward to opening the *New York Times* app every morning or watching the PBS News Hour in the evening.

Then, assuming that I remember to remind myself of what I wrote about in the first six chapters of this book and everything else I've learned over the last half century, I try to steer a conversation or redirect my own thoughts in a more constructive direction and make some version of these four points.

- Politics doesn't have to be a dirty word.
- We couldn't escape politics even if we wanted to.
- In good paradigm shift fashion, we should try to transform it.
- Finally, I get to my controversial best and say that we know how to do just that.

At which point, the people I'm talking with tend to roll their eyes even more vigorously.

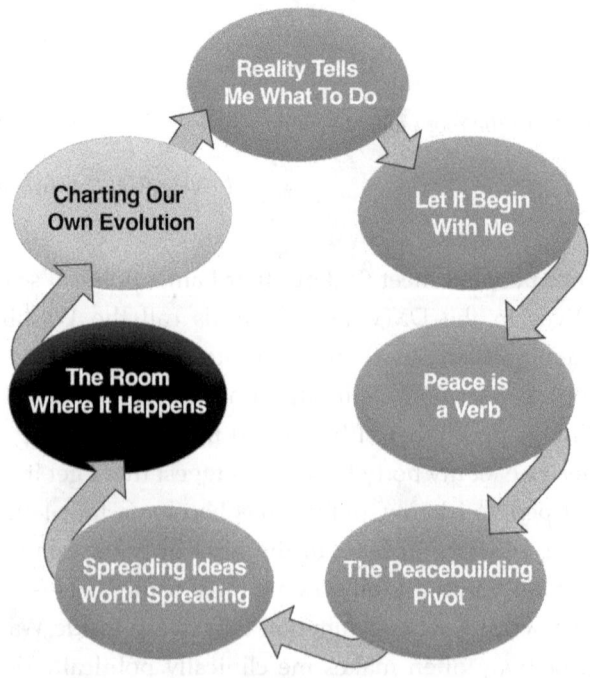

Figure 7.1: The Peacebuilding Starts at Home Loop

But believe it or not—and I know you don't—we do actually know how to turn those four bullet points into reality. The real question is whether or not we can summon up the political will to make it happen, which is why we have to move on to the next stage of the Peacebuilding Starts at Home Loop.

HAMILTON AND PARADIGM SHIFTS?

That's why this chapter starts with *Hamilton*.

No one has made the point about how hard it is to pull off a political paradigm shift more eloquently than Lin-Manuel Miranda did in his hit play, especially in its show stopping song, "The Room Where It Happens."

If you are skeptical, you are in good company.

No one expressed his doubts better than President Barack Obama when he hosted a performance of the play at the White House in 2014. It turns out that Miranda had been invited to a White House poetry jam early in Obama's administration and announced that he was working on an album "and I quote, 'about the life of somebody who embodies hip hop, Treasury Secretary Alexander Hamilton.' So we all started laughing. But Lin-Manuel was serious. So, who's laughing now?"[1]

I would have been among the people laughing with Obama had I been at the poetry jam. Until I left for college, my mother would drag me to musicals, which I hated. *The Sound of Music. The King and I. Oklahoma! The Music Man* (despite the fact that I played the trombone). Nothing like *Hamilton*. Even the seemingly revolutionary plays of my early adult years like *Hair, Jesus Christ Superstar,* or *Grease* were cut from a familiar and still not all that appealing mold.

Now consider *Hamilton*. Miranda often refers to the fact that he knew from the outset that the play itself would spark a theatrical paradigm shift because it broke all the rules of what a musical should be like. A story about the birth of our nation with a cast made up of people of color and women who couldn't have been in the room when it actually happened? Or listened to hip hop? Or played a banjo?

---

1. Obama's introduction is worth watching. https://www.bing.com/videos/riverview/relatedvideo?q=president+obama+hamilton&mid=FA9A5E0FAAD309337FF5FA9A5E0FAAD309337FF5&FORM=VIRE

More importantly for our purposes, the play is about the paradigm shift that saved the young United States. The real-life Hamilton was one of the three authors of the *Federalist Papers* that got the new Constitution ratified which, as we all learned in school, was one of those major turning points in our country's history because it helped the Founders solve what had been a seemingly unsolvable set of problems.

That part of the paradigm shift is so well known that I can leave out the first act of the play which covers the revolutionary war, the *Federalist Papers*, and all that.

When Act II opens, the new constitution has been ratified, but many of the issues that divided the Founders remain unsettled, including the location of the new country's permanent capital and its financial future. The (in)famous dinner took place the next year when (from Burr's point of view) Hamilton caved in to Jefferson and Madison by agreeing to a compromise that placed the new capital city in the slave holding South while giving the Secretary of the Treasury (who happened to be Hamilton) sweeping economic powers.

Furious, Burr then launches into:

But decisions are happening over dinner
Two Virginians and an immigrant walk into a room
Diametrically opposed
Foes
They emerge with a compromise
Having open doors that were previously closed
Bros
The immigrant emerges with unprecedented financial power
A system he can shape however he wants
The Virginians emerge with the nation's capital
And here's the pièce de résistance
No one else was in the room where it happened
The room where it happened
The room where it happened
No one else was in the room where it happened
The room where it happened
The room where it happened

PEACEBUILDING STARTS AT HOME

No one really knows how the game is played
The art of the trade
How the sausage gets made
We just assume that it happens
But no one else is in the room where it happens

By the end of the play, Burr and his friends have lost that battle to create a new paradigm while Hamilton has lost his life.

But none of the melodrama that led to their duel at the end of the play need concern us here.

What does matter is that, like Burr, those of us who care about paradigm shifts and the fate of our nation can't ignore politics and the room(s) where it happens. John Bolton understood that when he used the phrase as the title for his memoir about the first Trump administration which truly was about "how the game is played, the art of the trade, how the sausage gets made."

Miranda may have tapped into our negative stereotypes about politics and politicians. But he got the main point about political life right. Like it or not, you do have to be in the rooms where it happens when it happens. Whether you're Aaron Burr then or American peacebuilders today. Unfortunately, we aren't always there, and when we do get to the table, the rules of the game seem designed to thwart us.

In other words, peacebuilding starts at home involves more than just spreading good ideas. At least on the kinds of "big ticket" items covered in this book, we have to redesign the room. It may be that its metaphoric walls (the constitutional order) are structural and thus can't be replaced. But everything else could and should be up for grabs.

Who gets invited. The "seating plan." What they talk about. How the people who get invitations make up their minds. Whether their decisions see the light of day.

Or once again—how the game is played, the art of the trade, (and) how the sausage gets made.

In short, assuming that we have succeeded in building a movement strong enough to get us into the room where it happens, what happens in the room has to happen differently. Not only do you have to have different people (the women and people of color in Miranda's cast) but they have to think and act differently, too. Going to scale upward means continuing the paradigm shift until it is complete—or as close to complete as a paradigm shift can ever be.

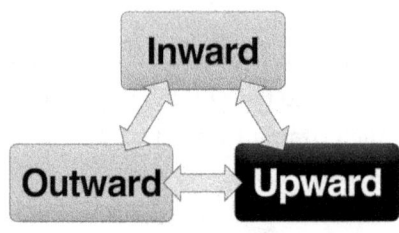

Figure 7.2: Going to Scale Upward

THE POLITICS OF THE COMMONS

Earlier, I suggested that we actually know what it will take to think and act differently when (and if) we get into those rooms. Whenever I say something like that to political scientists and political insiders, they do more than roll their eyes in disbelief. My British colleagues, in particular, go further and use one of my favorite phrases used in their version of our not always common language and accuse me of living in cloud cuckoo land.

This is not new. It has been happening ever since I started graduate school in 1969.

Then and now, orthodox social scientists make the case that only the left hand column of my table matters in the rooms where it happens—at least in the real world. That's true of realism in international relations or rational choice theory in comparative politics or neoclassical economics. Even left of center analysts like Chuck Tilly, whom you met in chapter 6, accepted most of the current paradigm's tenets as a given—even if they didn't like them.

Current Value	New Value
Thinking in terms of "us v. them"	Thinking in terms of "us with them"
Focus on short-term self interest	Focus on shared interests in the medium- to long- term
Expect a zero-sum or win-lose outcome in which I would like to win but definitely do not want to lose	Work toward a win-win outcome that benefits everyone
Assume that one side will have to use power over the other	Redefine power as something we exercise with others
Understand that conflict is bad for everyone involved	Understand that conflict can be an opportunity for growth for everyone involved

Table 7.1: Contrasting the Two Paradigms

Then and now, I was convinced that they took that assumption way too far. To be sure, the conventional wisdom did describe how most people acted most of the time especially when they were confronted with wicked problems. Phrases like it's a dog-eat-dog world or when the going gets tough, the tough get going resonate for a reason.

However, the more I learned about what the rapidly changing reality was telling us to do, the more I realized that there are alternatives to the status quo. They also weren't just theoretical options. They may not have been used in the most important rooms where the most expensive sausage gets made, but decision makers did have enough experience using these new tools and techniques to make them plausible alternatives to the business as usual that isn't working very well. In other words, they just might provide us with a way out of the mismatch that led me to write this book in the first place.

In other words, there is no escaping the fact that peacebuilding starts at home has to be political but with a different understanding of what the word political means. As paradigm shifters, we "know" that the answer does not lie primarily in playing "the game" as it is played today because its "rules" themselves are a key part of the problem.

In fact, there is no shortage of alternative paradigms for making key decisions in the public and private sector. Here, I will focus on just one of them—the Core Design Principles (CDP) as defined by Elinor

Ostrom and modified by ProSocial World. I chose them because Ostrom developed the CDPs in direct response to one of the most powerful arguments mainstream social scientists make about the staying power of the values in the left-hand column of the table.

The easiest way to see that is to start with the argument that troubled Ostrom the most, in part because the data supporting it seemed so compelling. Mainstream economists and their counterparts in the other social sciences have long worried about what they call public goods and collective action. Even the most devoted libertarian recognizes that "public goods" or things we all want that the freest marketing operating as rationally as one could possibly imagine cannot provide, including general education, national defense, and environmental protection. Without oversimplifying economic theory too much, once a society decides it wants to or has to provide these kinds of goods and services, it pretty much has to turn to government because only it can compel its citizens to take action by levying taxes or even using force — physical or otherwise.

One of the most forceful presentations of that point of view can be found in Garrett Hardin's article, "The Tragedy of the Commons," which has been—and should be—a staple of graduate education since it was published in 1968.[2] It is one of the most powerful and depressing things I have ever read, in large part because Hardin was right about so many things. But, as Ostrom and others have pointed out, analyses like his are both shortsighted and misleading because they assume that we are stuck with institutions and leaders who embody the values in the left-hand column of my table.

Hardin showed why shared resources can easily get overused, create vicious cycles, and all too often lead to a system's collapse. As an ecologist, he focused on the "classic" commons, which was a plot of land in a village in England or New England. Everyone in the town used it for everything from grazing their animals to training their militias. Using the logic of traditional economic theory or any other variation on the dominant paradigm, no one in their right or rational mind would pay to maintain the commons because it wasn't in their imme-

---

2. Garrett Hardin, "The Tragedy of the Commons." *Science*. 162 (1968): 1243–1248.

diate self-interest to do so. That is, unless you taxed them or otherwise compelled them to do their part, which violated both Hardin's personal libertarian beliefs and the principles of neoclassical economics.

From there, it was easy to extrapolate from the real world commons to all public goods for one simple reason.[3] We do frequently take commons-like resources to and beyond a tipping point after which they collapse.

Fishers in the North Atlantic almost drove the once super abundant cod to extinction. At one point in my youth, no river in my native Connecticut was safe to swim in. Public schools around the country could not survive without tax dollars supplied by local, state, and federal authorities.

And it's not just common resources. Economists and their intellectual cousins in the other social sciences have a hard time figuring out how to provide for public goods like education or transportation system infrastructure. It is just as hard to factor in the cost of other externalities, including plastics or the so-called forever chemicals, on the environment. And that's before we get to the negative impact of free riders and others who aren't willing to pay their "fair share" of what it costs for them to prosper.

There is an irony here. The same professors who introduced me to systems theory also made me read Hardin's article. They did not see that thinking holistically provided a way of getting beyond his tragedy of the commons. That was true of me as well. At the time, even though I chafed at Hardin's argument and others like it, I couldn't come up with an alternative.

Luckily for me and the peacebuilding starts at home community, Ostrom did just that in a body of research that won her the 2009 Nobel Prize in Economic Sciences—despite the fact that she was a political scientist. While she is by no means the only person to have developed a new paradigm for governing public and private institutions under the kinds of conditions I outlined in chapter 2, I chose her Core Design

---

3. The classic here is Mancur Olson. *The Logic of Collective Action*. (Cambridge: Harvard University Press, 1971).

Principles because they are among the easiest for skeptics to accept. In particular, the CDPs retain and in many ways expand on the individual freedoms that are at the heart of liberal democracy and market economies.

In the process, they do redefine those freedoms somewhat given the realities of life on our interconnected and densely populated planet in which our actions affect everyone and everything else. In other words, individual freedom and collective responsibility inevitably go hand in hand. Ostrom also understood that not all humans are angelic or even trustworthy which led her to include ways of enforcing decisions that were made for managing the commons. Last but by no means least, it is not hard to see how her ideas could be taken to scale and implemented in a wide variety of constitutional structures, some of which could conceivably be more democratic than anything we know of today.

Growing up in southern California, Ostrom was fascinated by the way people allocated one of the region's scarcest common resources, water. Eventually, that led her to earn a PhD in political science and a career at the University of Indiana where she and her husband and life-long collaborator conducted their research.

Ostrom then spent her career studying how communities of all sizes successfully governed a commons and provided public goods without collapsing or resorting to the draconian use of force.[4] As a product of another Big Ten political science department, I had known about and liked her work for decades. However, it was only after I met David Sloan Wilson and started working with ProSocial that I realized that her ideas could serve as the key to taking peacebuilding starts at home to scale upward and turn the new paradigm into reality in those rooms where it happens.

While they are still ideals when it comes to countries and national governments,[5] Ostrom derived them from real world experiences in which communities and, occasionally, larger units of government

---

4. Elinor Ostrom. Governing the Commons: The Evolution of Institutions for Collective Action. (Cambridge: Cambridge University Press: 1990).

5. For a hint of what could happen at the national level, see Jacinda Adern. *A Different Kind of Power: A Memoir*. (New York: Crown, 2025).

successfully managed the kinds of resources Hardin and conventional economists properly drew our attention to. Note that these are not idealistic goals but reflect how the real world systems Ostrom studied governed themselves. Note, too, that most of what she and ProSocial World propose can be done by "working within the system" and would not require the kinds of dramatic institutional changes that some of my progressive friends believe will be necessary—a point I will return to toward the end of this chapter. Note, finally, that they include enforcement mechanisms for authorities to use when and if people do not play by the new rules.

As is true of any system, there is no obvious place to start a discussion of the eight CDPs as you can see in this chart. What follows starts with the principles that grow most clearly out of what you have already seen. Then I will take you into new territory about what we political scientists call governance, which is our jargon term for how we make all decisions that matter, whatever the room where it happens to happen.

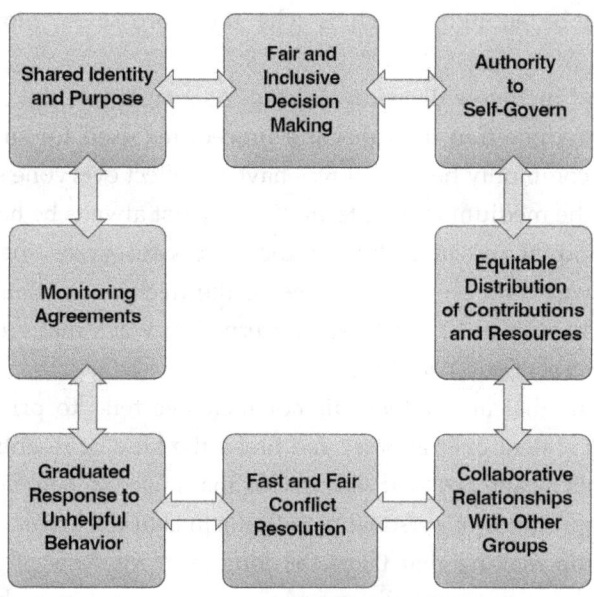

Figure 7.3: The Core Design Principles

Shared Identity and purpose. The first principle should be familiar because it reflects what reality is telling us to do. It actually goes farther than anything I've covered so far, adding the word "purpose" to our sense that we are living in an increasingly interdependent world. We also have to include what we plan to do about its problems, whether we focus on the entire planet or smaller systems like a workplace or a product's supply chain.

While I have at least implicitly raised the importance of purpose when it comes to individuals or movements, it is also important for decision makers and other elites to begin thinking in terms of adopting a new intent or purpose, too. They do talk this way from time to time as we saw, for instance, when leaders on both sides of the Atlantic began using the phrase build back better to sum up their aspirations for a post-COVID world. Occasionally, we even see signs of it being put into practice as the Biden administration was able to do to a limited degree in the Inflation Reduction Act and other measures that addressed climate change. But to be honest, American elites are nowhere close to thinking in these terms. And even if they did, that would not be enough, which is why there are seven more design principles.

Fair and inclusive decision making. As a systems thinker, Ostrom went on to argue that the rules and procedures used for successfully allocating commonly held resources have to reflect everyone's interests at least in the medium to long term. We may not always be happy with each individual outcome, but in the successful cases she studied, everyone was represented somehow in the decision making and the results were seen to be fair to all concerned in ways that are reminiscent of Rotary's Four-Way Test.

Decisions that are neither fair nor inclusive tend to privilege one part of the system over another and breed the kind of resentment that my students recalled in their discussions that I used to help you see the general importance of personal paradigms in chapter 3. Fair and inclusive decision making that takes the long-term interests of the entire system into account normally produces something akin to the kind of win-win decision making I also talked about in earlier chapters.

The authority to self-govern using the first two principles.

Successful systems manage their affairs effectively. I don't need to remind any reader who is paying even the slightest bit of attention to our public life that what Ostrom and ProSocial World call good governance is easier said than done. To have any chance of successfully governing itself, the members of any system—including its leaders—have to endorse the first two principles even if they can't apply them perfectly on every single issue they deal with.

Using the term authority here is significant because it takes us beyond political life to include all key decision making systems, a point that I was only able to hint at when I introduced the chart of the political system in chapter 2. This third principle does suggest that successful decision makers have to balance all the factors that shape the systems which they help lead. And as the term "self-govern" suggests, both Ostrom and ProSocial World understand that we are all decision makers in an interdependent system—not just those holding governmental office or sitting in a corporate C suite.

Equitable distribution of contributions and benefits. For a system to survive and thrive, its members have to believe that it is fair. That's true not only of what it actually does (as Ostrom's prose suggests) but also of people's subjective feelings about its performance. Ostrom was by no means a socialist who wanted an all but completely egalitarian society. Nonetheless, leaders do have to strike a balance between the contributions and sacrifices we make and the benefits we receive from the decisions made by those at the top. If we don't we are likely to end up with the extremism most of us find so troubling today.

Monitoring agreed behaviors. The final four principles do the most to take peacebuilding beyond anything that could be labeled pie-in-the-sky idealism. Decisions have to be implemented, and decision makers have to be held accountable. Neither is easy to do in any kind of decision making system. The ability to enforce the law and hold authorities accountable are all the more important when there is a deep distrust of leaders. Accountability requires more than the rhetoric we see during election campaigns. If nothing else, everyone who wishes to has to be able to track what decision makers do. Whether they did it intentionally or not, the organizations Ostrom studied all built in ways of measuring, for example, the number of fish that were caught so that they could maintain the stock available for the next generation of fishers.

Graduated responses to unhelpful behavior. For our purposes, the fifth and sixth principles blend into each other. It's not just the ability to know what leaders do. Members of the system also have to be able to effectively take action when and if people in positions of authority do something that does not reflect their shared values. Indeed, there is every reason to assume that a system run under the new paradigm will have its share of scofflaws and will need enforcement mechanisms of its own. The new paradigm will have to build in tools to allow decision makers to deal with individuals and organizations that don't play by the rules. This principle incorporates Ostrom's equivalent of feedback in systems analysis. Yet, as we also see every day in the news, few systems in the real world have fashioned ways of effectively using feedback to turn them into what management expert Peter Senge calls learning organizations.[6]

Fast and fair conflict resolution. In the event that the interests of the common are violated and conflict ensues, the system has to have effective mechanisms for settling those disputes. This is, of course, a skill set that the peacebuilding community is well prepared to bring to the clichéd table in the clichéd room. In this case, seeing this principle in ProSocial World's list helped convince me that we need to pivot and help other organizations reach their goals so that, together, we can take advantage of the final principle.

Collaborative relationships with other groups. International peacebuilders know that living up to this final principle is easier said than done. Still, the first seven principles lend themselves to this eighth one which applies whether other groups are our literal neighbors around the corner or our global neighbors everywhere around the world. Here, too, imagine what the world would be like if we applied these principles to foreign as well as domestic life—we found and pursued a common identity, made decisions together that sought to benefit everyone in the system, and used feedback to enforce those

---

6. Peter Senge, *The Fifth Discipline: The Art and Practice of the Learning Organization*. (New York: Currency, 1990).

decisions and make them better the next time we had to deal with a problem.

EXERCISE 7.1: AMERICA REMADE

> Start with the core design principle that interests you the most. Jot down the four or five features an America reMADE would have to have in order to live up to that criterion. This may seem like a simple assignment because this is the smallest such box in this entire book.
>
> Trust me. It's anything but simple.

POWER AND THEN SOME

Make no mistake. The new paradigm will be different.

At the same time, the old paradigm will not completely disappear. As was the case with the Copernican revolution, it will keep its equivalent of moons revolving around planets. Thus, it is hard to imagine getting rid of what almost all of us see as the gains of the last few centuries including voting, individual freedoms, and the rule of law.

But reality is telling us to adopt something like the mindset that informed Ostrom's work starting with her childhood fascination with the water supply in Southern California. The world as a whole is becoming more like a common, which means that most of its problems revolve around public goods which will require widely agreed upon solutions that take our long term security and prosperity into account. That makes the reality that is telling us what to do focus us on new behaviors based on the kind of new cultural norms that I am asking you to consider.

In other words, a lot will have to change, including many of the ABCs of social life. In particular, we will have to change our working definition of power which is the central concept in political science, because our colleagues still all but universally use some version of Robert Dahl's definition:

> *A has power over B to the extent that he can get B to do something that B otherwise wouldn't do.*[7]

I focus on the last four words in his definition because they are both all-important and we take them for granted. The B's of the world aren't going to do something they don't want to do voluntarily. All too often, getting them to go along requires at least the threat of some kind of force. It may not involve violence. The force may not have to be used. Remember that I ended chapter 1 with a form of power I used with my students. I *threatened* to reduce their grades if they handed their papers —or you handed in your homework for this book—late. I almost never had to carry out the threat, because my students (my equivalents of Dahl's B) complied, and I didn't get many late papers.

In the new paradigm, power looks very different. Sure, I could still use power over my students who don't meet their (my) deadlines. However, when I think in terms of systems and feedback loops and the long term, exerting power over you (oops, I mean B) comes at a cost. Like my students, you aren't likely to be happy when I use power in this way. If I keep doing so, you will begin to hold a grudge and eventually you will want to use power over me to "get" me in one form or another. In this case, think back to all the critical course evaluations you wrote in your own student days....

It is easy to see that "power over" is not the only viable definition if you have ever studied a romance language. The French *pouvoir*, Spanish *poder*, and Italian *potere* do not necessarily come with the "power over" implications we take for granted in English. It can simply mean to be able. *Je peux. Puedo. Posso.*

Power can also have the same connotation as the word empower. It becomes something I exert with you to make a dent in one or more of those wicked problems or reach one of those superordinate goals that we share literally in common.

---

7. Robert A. Dahl. "The Concept of Power." *Behavioral Science* 2 (1957): 201-215.

(EVEN TINIER) GLIMMERS OF HOPE

Make no mistake about it one more time.

There will not be and cannot be a clean, rapid transition from the current paradigm to the new one. Elements of the one we use today will survive. There will be times when the two comfortably coexist but there will be times when they clash.

The most I can say is that the transition to the new one is under way and that it is progressing in fits and starts. When I'm being honest, I also have to admit that right now the fits are dominating the starts.

That leads to another good news/bad news situation.

This time, the bad news has to come first. We are almost never in the rooms where it happens in Washington. Definitely not as I wrote these lines during the first six months of the second Trump administration. But I'd make the case that supporters of a new paradigm rarely had a seat at the table when Obama or Biden lived in the White House. However, on foreign policy issues, we have had enough of an impact to be invited into those (in)famous rooms on a regular basis. We have influenced legislation and budgetary appropriations under both Democratic and Republican administrations. However, when it comes to the kinds of values Ostrom raised or a paradigm shift in general, we have a very long way to go.

Still, as you are about to see, there are some hopeful signs. To begin with, there is the evidence from chapter 6 about the shifts that are taking place in the private sector. But, if I'm going to convince you that there is a chance that this paradigm shift could successfully scale upward, I do have to make the case for the public sector as well. Here, not surprisingly, the evidence supporting my case is a lot more limited than it was in any of the earlier steps along the peace building starts at home loop.[8]

The best evidence actually comes from other countries where both

---

8. There are a lot of books on this subject. My two favorites are Jeremy Heimans and Henry Timms, *New Power: How Power Works in our Hyperconnected World—And How to Make it Work for You.* (New York: Doubleday, 2018) and Moisés Naím, *The End of Power: From Boardrooms to Battlefields and Churches to States, Why Being In Charge Isn't What It Used to Be.* (New York: Basic Books, 2013).

cultural norms and institutional arrangements have made it easier to start the transition. Twelve of the one hundred sixty-two members of the Australian parliament were elected as independents and have endorsed at least some of what Australia reMADE advocates. Not all of them are on the left. A right of center German government began its *energiewende* or energy transition in 2010. By 2030, fully half of the country's total energy needs will come from renewable sources. In a process initiated by a Conservative government, the Canadian Indian Residential School Settlement Agreement create a truth and reconciliation commission to deal with that issue and more.

I am not about to claim that these governments have adopted anything even vaguely resembling the Core Design Principles. All I am saying is that they demonstrate that governments in countries not all that different from our own have made a start on this step along the Peacebuilding Starts at Home Loop.

More importantly for the purposes of this book, there are promising signs of progress in the United States, too.

Convergence Policy. For reasons that literally go back to the debates in Hamilton's day and that also go far beyond the scope of this book, we should not expect the most promising experiments to start at the national level. Nonetheless, when I was at Search for Common Ground in the early 2000s, we helped launch one of the few bright spots as far as scaling upward in Washington is concerned.

The results of the 2000 election were the most acrimonious ever (until 2020 that is) because victory in the electoral college came down to a few thousand contested votes in Florida. After the Supreme Court's decision about the recount there gave George W. Bush the victory over Al Gore, our team at Search was approached by two veterans of the partisan wars who had a novel idea. Former Democratic member of Congress Dan Glickman had gotten to know and like Montana's former Republican governor Marc Racicot. Racicot, in particular, had seen the cost of the election firsthand as head of President Bush's campaign. More importantly, he had created something called a consensus council while he was governor and knew of similar bodies in South Dakota and Delaware. The two of them asked us to help them create one at the federal level.

Basically, consensus councils use trained conflict resolution professionals to convene interest group leaders for a series of meetings that take place over a number of months. They are not looking for major breakthroughs on the big questions of the day. Rather, they work on the assumption that if facilitators can get policy advocates away from the television cameras and let them get to know each other, they can find ways of hammering out agreements on controversial but relatively narrow policy questions. Once all of the major groups have gotten behind the proposal, they could do an end run around the usual gridlock in the legislature and easily get their draft enacted into law.

So, my colleagues worked with Racicot, Glickman, and a team of prominent leaders from both sides of the proverbial aisle and drafted a bill that would create a United States Consensus Council. It came close to becoming a law in 2002 when it was attached to a larger bill that was working its way though Congress. At that point, a Democratic senator put what is known as a hold on the bill which kept it from passing.

Shortly thereafter, Rob Fersh, who had headed the project at Search decided to create Convergence as a separate organization to promote consensus-based policy making, on the assumption that we were not likely to get a law creating a council any time soon. Fersh and his team also made a subtle but important distinction by using the word convergence rather than consensus. They understood that getting all but universal agreement would be all but impossible on such "big ticket" items as overall health care policy. Instead, they could make progress by helping advocates converge around general goals from which they could develop concrete proposals. Those agreements might only lead to minimal policy changes in the short term but could lay the groundwork for more paradigm-shift-like steps later on.

Since then, Convergence has been a one of a kind organization bringing cutting edge conflict resolution skills to the policy making community in Washington and, at times, state capitals. As Fersh and his successor as president of Convergence Mariah Levison put it in their recent book, they believed that:

> *Something was missing from our capacities as a nation to take on issues of consequence: the ability to skillfully integrate the wisdom*

and experience of people with differing backgrounds and vantage points.[9]

They knew from the beginning that not all issues were what conflict resolution experts call "ripe" for resolution. If, for instance, too many minds of too many leaders are too closed, their tool kit probably won't be all that helpful.

But on controversial issue after controversial issue, Convergence has demonstrated that they can make a difference on issues like health care, immigration, prisoner reentry, and the budget.

They never ask participants to abandon or even water down their beliefs. Instead, they recruit senior leaders from the interest groups (in other words lobbyists) who are open to talking with their colleagues on the "other side," many of whom they had only previously met during shouting matches on television talk shows or at congressional hearings. As would have been the case with the USCC, Convergence's staff brings them together for a series of private meetings. Behind the scenes, the staff begins exploring language and policies that the leaders could support. Even more importantly, they help the participants build personal relationships that establish trust and sometimes even friendships across ideological divides.

At first they focus on getting leaders to see the importance of adopting a mindset that emphasizes solving problems rather than scoring points, which then helps them identify building blocks around which they begin forging at least partial solutions.

Then they help the participants in the working group identify one or more general goals that they all support. The work Convergence has done on health care, for example, has included a commitment to expanding quality coverage for more and more Americans at an affordable price.

In the process, the facilitators draw on what global peacebuilders have learned about conflict resolution. Sometimes, they simply ask the participants to do an adult version of Daniel Tiger's request and take a

---

9. Robert Fersh and Mariah Levison. *From Conflict to Convergence: Coming Together to Solve Tough Problems.* (Hoboken NJ: Wiley, 2024), 21.

few breaths and count to four. More often, they help the participants reframe the issue so that common ground can be found.

Only then, do areas of possible policy collaboration begin to emerge More importantly, they discover that they often actually like each other and look forward to deepening their relationships over time, thereby laying the groundwork for more collaboration down the line. In short, as Fersh and Levison entitle one of their book's sections, they help the participants put "people before proposals."

If Convergence had all the answers, there would not have been any need for me to write this book. Its tools have only yielded limited results especially on big ticket issues like health care coverage or immigration. It does not even try to produce the kind of cultural change I discussed in chapter 6. It does not ask its participants to do so either.

Nonetheless, it is one building block.

Municipal democracy. Given what I said at the beginning of this section, I've actually spent more time looking for examples at the state and local level. Convergence itself has done some work in Kentucky and Minnesota, states that have long traditions of citizen involvement.

There are even more promising signs in smaller cities and towns where it has proven easier for groups of citizens to have an impact. As I was finishing this book, I attended two workshops on pluralism. At each one, I met someone who told me about a project that is building peace by making local government more democratic and augmenting the power average citizens have over decision making.

This is not a new development outside of the United States. Many European countries have experimented with randomly chosen bodies of citizens who are tasked with exploring options on pressing issues for elected officials to consider. In 2019, the French government convened a Citizens' Commission of 150 randomly selected voters to help advise its new high level commission on climate change Some Brazilian cities use citizen-led assemblies that have the power to determine basic municipal spending levels and set local tax rates. Other countries have used them to set priorities for urban renewal and developing environmental policies. I actually participated in one such convening. In 2003, the government of Western Australia asked me and a colleague to help them facilitate a meeting where 1,200 residents of the Perth metropolitan area set priorities for the region's growth over the next half century when the population was expected to grow by at least fifty percent.[10]

In the 2020s, Unify America founder Harry Gottlieb's corporate work drew him to the idea of using citizens' assemblies to address tough civic problems. The organization stumbled on the opportunity to use a citizens assembly in Montrose CO. Gottlieb was meeting with leaders of that town of about 20,000 on the western slope of the Rockies on other issues when the idea of deliberative democracy came up. After some extended discussion with local officials, the Unify America team convened a panel of sixty-four residents who were broadly representative of the town's overall population. Over the course of twelve weeks, the team facilitated a series of face-to-face and virtual meetings at which the group explored ideas that were submitted by local experts and then came up with others of its own. By the time its "term" ended, more than ninety percent of the assembly members agreed on core policy proposals as well as the creation of a non-profit—Unify Montrose—to continue its efforts. As I write, Unify America is looking for other cities that could experiment with their version of a citizens assembly.

In early 2025, when I attended the New Pluralists' workshop, Abby Rapoport of *Stranger's Guide* introduced me to her college classmate, Linn Miller of Healthy Democracy, who was facilitating a session on the organization's work on citizens assemblies, which have been used around the world in both advisory and formal policy making settings.

Healthy Democracy's work can be traced back to pioneering studies on citizen juries first conducted in the late 1970s by the late Ned Crosby. Healthy Democracy continues that work from its new base in Portland OR from which it has run at least a half dozen projects in cities and states around the country. For the purposes of this book, the ones with the most potential for peacebuilding writ large are the civic assemblies it has organized in a handful of small cities. As one example, the city council in Fort Collins CO had just acquired

---

10. Janette Harz-Karp. "A Case Study in Deliberative Democracy: Dialogue with the City." *Journal of Public Deliberation*. 1(2005), 1016.

Colorado State University's former football stadium and had to decide what to do with it. Rather than simply calling in a group of urban planning experts, it decided to use a citizens assembly to help them make their final decision.

Its twenty volunteer members were selected randomly to reflect the city's population as a whole, not just those who vote. Members are paid a modest stipend, trained by Healthy Democracy facilitators, and will spend at least two weekends during the course of 2025 meeting to come up with recommendations about the former stadium's fate. Once the assembly delivers its report after this book goes to press, the city government will make the final decision, much as Congress would have done had the US Consensus Council been created.

Even I have to admit that it is a long way from advisory commissions in small cities to major legislation passed by Congress and signed into law by the President. Like the USCC, neither of these initiatives directly built on Ostrom's ideas.

Nonetheless, they are another building block.

Police to Peace. Policing has been controversial for decades. The civil rights movement of the 1960s made inequalities in the ways police officers deal with people of color impossible to ignore. While some progress has been made, we still have a long way to go, which was driven home once again by George Floyd's murder and countless other incidents in recent years.

Without getting into the disputes over allegations of police bias or whether "blue lives matter," a number of organizations are trying to improve day-to-day interactions between police officers and citizens, especially young people of color. Among the most successful is Police2Peace, in part because it tries to create informal working relationships with police officers and their community.

The organization has a far from earth-changing origin story. After decades as a corporate executive and management consultant, Lisa Broderick was on a well-deserved vacation in 2019 when she saw a police cruiser with a "peace officer" emblem on its door. Intrigued by the phrase, she began looking around and discovered that lots of departments used the phrase or something quite like it. Yet, that is not the image most Americans have of the police, especially in minority communities.

So, entrepreneur that she is, Broderick began reaching out to police departments and to citizens groups across the country. By the time George Floyd was killed, an embryonic version of Police2Peace was in place.

In the five years since then, it has worked formally and informally with police departments around the country around what it calls the Golden Rule of policing.

> *The PEACE OFFICER Initiative is rooted in this simple idea: The police as part of the community, and the community as part of the police. This rule embodies what it means to be a PEACE OFFI-CER: to prevent conflict; if there is conflict, help resolve it; diffuse situations; and aid the defenseless. By operationalizing what it means to be a PEACE OFFICER, departments can bring about cultural change, procedural change, operational change, and departmental alignment.*[11]

All of its programs are based on a simple assumption. The vast majority of police officers want to do the right thing. Many relish being called peace officers. They just don't have the training to be the kind of officer they or their communities want them to be.

Police2peace also works with local leaders outside of the police departments, including the Rotarians in Portland whom you met in chapter 6. But its core mission is to use current and retired officers to train serving police personnel in the country's roughly 18,000 police departments and sheriff's offices. Its staff can provide a wide variety of services, ranging from short training videos to intense, lengthy in person workshops. Some are purely informational; others can be used for certification and continuing education purposes.

Police2Peace is not alone. I know of similar initiatives seeking to gradually transform the way other local institutions like libraries, sports leagues, and social service providers operate. The YMCA,

---

11. https://police2peace.org/about-us/ (Accessed March 4, 2025).

Habitat for Humanity, Catholic Charities, and Interfaith America have combined to form the Team Up Partnership, which aims to help create civil society across lines of division and open doors for cooperation with local authorities.

Like the citizens assemblies and related municipal initiatives, none of this is going to change what happens in Washington any time soon.

Nonetheless, it is another building block.

NEXT STEPS

Let me bring this chapter to a close with an obvious mismatch which highlights just how much work still has to be done. There is a huge gap between the well developed and realistic theories like Ostrom's and the practical experiments that rarely are deeply grounded in any theory or paradigm. That has opened three more "spaces" in which the Peacebuilding Starts at Home community and its allies intend to focus their efforts both with average citizens and with our national leaders as we come closer to getting our seat at the table—at least for the occasional snack.

Intentionality. All previous paradigm shifts have one thing in common. They were unplanned. As Kuhn himself pointed out, even the scientists who were at the forefront of a scientific revolution often didn't realize that they were creating one until the paradigm shift was completed and the new interpretation had come to dominate scientific research. At that point, practitioners and analysts alike took a look back at the not so distant past and realized just how much things had changed. That is even more the case when it comes to social and political paradigm shifts, including the one retold in *Hamilton*.

In part because Kuhn's ideas took hold, our paradigm shift can be different. In fact, it will have to be different. To borrow a term from clinical psychology, we have to be intentional about it. We have to make a conscious decision to make this paradigm shift happen in a way that tracks something like the trajectory of my Peacebuilding Starts at Home Loop.

Once again, I don't want to go too far here. We will never be able to follow a step-by-step Google or Waze map for getting to our North Star.

Paradigm shifts don't change everything. They do not wipe the slate clean. In the Copernican model, moons still revolve around planets. In our own history, the United States Constitution that Hamilton helped promote still gave the states plenty of power.

The same will be true of the paradigm shift this book envisions. We will be able to keep most of what works in the current system, including civil liberties, a market economy, and our democratic institutions. What will change are the values and assumptions that we all—including key decision makers—bring to the table.

That's why I included the word redesigning in this chapter's title. We undoubtedly will have to create new decision making bodies that will enact new policies in both the public and private sectors. However, just about everything that follows can be incorporated into a modified, twenty-first century version of the system Hamilton helped create.

And they never really end. Perhaps even more than those in the natural sciences, social paradigm shifts turn out to be protracted struggles because they pit an old guard against groups of new thinkers at a time when there is a lot at stake. Again, just think about *Hamilton*.

You would also have to have slept through the last few decades to not have noticed that the social and political paradigm shifts of the last several centuries still spark plenty of controversy today. Continuing debates over what phrases like "all men are created equal" still roil the American public. To be sure, next to no one would want to return to the days of slavery or legal segregation. But, affirmative action? Civil war memorials? Wokism? Transgender rights?

It is even more useful to think of a period like the current one as a time of transition in which we live under dueling paradigms when the assumptions of the current and future paradigms both help shape what we do. That is easiest to see in the corporate world where, as you saw in chapter 6, quite a number of leading companies have adopted elements of the paradigm I've been developing throughout this book

To see that point, it is worth quoting from the Preface of a recent book by former Harvard Business School Professor, John Kotter, to which he gave the provocative title *XLR8*.

> *The world is now changing at a rate at which the basic systems, structures, and cultures built over the past century cannot keep up with the demands being placed on them. Incremental adjustments to how you manage and strategies, no matter how clear, are not up to the job. You need something very new to stay ahead in an age of tumultuous change and growing uncertainties.*

> *The solution is not to trash what we know and start over but instead to reintroduce, in an organic way, a second system—one which would be familiar to most successful entrepreneurs. The new systems adds needed agility and speed while the old one, which keeps running, provides reliability and efficiency. The two together —a dual system—are actually very similar to what all mature organizations had at one point in their life cycles yet did not sustain (and have since (been) long forgotten).[12]*

And we have to talk to them both.

EXERCISE 7.2: NAILING IT

Don't try to envision a way of "nailing it" on every aspect of governing. Pick one of the examples discussed in this chapter or another of your own choosing and ask yourself two questions. First, what would it take for my community or my country to make this way of managing our affairs the norm using the relevant core design principles? Second, what can you do to turn those dreams into reality?

---

12. John F. Kotter, *Accelerate: Building Strategic Agility for a Faster Moving World*. Boston: Harvard Business Review Press, 2014), Kindle location 30-38.

WORLD PEACE AND OTHER FOURTH GRADE ACCOMPLISHMENTS

I know that I don't have all the answers. All I can do is point to ideas and initiatives that suggest what we could do after we build the movement that gets us into tomorrow's version of Hamilton's room.

I also know these ideas are not the only ones I could have included. Adding worker ownership, corporate social responsibility, or public budgeting would just add more scattered islands in the archipelago and not do much to convince you that we can connect those metaphoric dots.

Indeed, if I were a gambler, I would not place a bet on achieving a paradigm shift unless the bookie gave me terrific odds. If anything, the prospects for pulling one off undoubtedly decreased in the two years it took me to write *Peacebuilding Starts at Home*.

At those down moments, I take heart from a mini-paradigm shift—even if it was made by a group that would have found my discussion of them mind numbingly boring. For decades, John Hunter helped his students in Charlottesville VA succeed in meeting the world's most serious challenges as discussed in his book, *World Peace and Other Fourth Grade Achievements* and a related documentary.[13]

Hunter began experimenting with what became the World Peace Game in 1978. He wanted to include a unit on Africa in his class and found that there wasn't much material available for him to use. He also knew that he wanted to foster creativity in his students and that they loved to play games. Within just a few years, the project took off beyond its roots in Africa and became the game as it has been played for decades.

In his own classrooms, he dedicates eight afternoons to playing the game. It is played in a plexiglass structure that has four levels—undersea, land and the oceans' surfaces, the atmosphere, and outer space.

---

13. John Hunter, *World Peace and Other Fourth Grade Achievements*. (New York: Houghton Mifflin Harcourt, 2013). For information on the documentary, visit https://worldpeacegame.org/the-game/the-film/ (Accessed July 20, 2024).

The game only has four countries, but it does have the World Bank, the UN, some arms dealers, and a weather god.

On the first day, he divides the class into teams with defined roles either within one of the four countries or in those other organizations. Each country starts out with a certain number of assets that are represented by typical board game tokens. On the first day, each group gets a thirteen page "secret dossier" that includes fifty global environmental, geopolitical, ethical, economic, and social issues, each of which amounts to what I have been calling a wicked problem.

The game is designed, first, to teach the children something I introduced in chapter 2. The minute you change the parameters on any one of those fifty issues, everything else changes accordingly.

Then, he tells them that they have those eight weekly meetings to play, with victory defined as finding a satisfactory solution to all fifty of the problems in a way that increases each country's assets (John Mackey's win-win-win?). He makes things harder by adding a player whose job is to be a saboteur in addition to performing their regular role.

Hunter himself doesn't do much beyond answering the occasional question. The children themselves have to find the answers.

In Hunter's experience, the children always find the creativity to win. They pull off a global paradigm shift. Like so many Americans today, they start off confused about and overwhelmed by Hunter's scenario. Because their initial attempts only make matters worse in their simulated world, they typically get more confused and overwhelmed until their collaborative creativity kicks in and—almost always at the last moment—they work it all out. As he put it,

> As the game nears its end, there is always this spontaneous, informal assessment to find out who in the world is not okay and what everyone has to do about it. I've designed the Game with that hope in mind—with "winning" defined as good conditions for everybody. They learned to think globally and to translate that concept into material reality: international agreements, budgets, environmental planning. But the fundamental collective concern— the wish for everybody to be okay, for nobody to be left out—was

there from the beginning. But it's still up to the students. They still have to decide that everyone is going to win. And they do decide that. I'm in awe every time I see it.[14]

I know that the real world has more complications than any board game written for ten and eleven year olds. Still, I want you to learn Hunter's lesson before we move on.

If fourth graders can pull off a paradigm shift, why can't we adults?

Or, as my then fourth grade grandson put it to me after he finished reading Hunter's book, "Grandpa, kids can solve problems, too, you know."

Like the citizens assemblies and related municipal initiatives, the World Peace Game is not going to change what happens in Washington any time soon although then Chair of the Joint Chief of Staff Mike Mullin was blown away by it.

Nonetheless, it is one building block.

EXERCISE 7.3: THE LUNCHPAIL F***ING JOB

My grandson can be excused for being a bit naïve. After all, he was in the fourth grade when he read Hunter's book.

Presumably, you are a lot older than he was at the time. So, ask yourself how internalizing Ostrom's Core Design Principles and/or other values discussed in this chapter can prepare you for what will undoubtedly turn into a commitment that will last for the rest of your life.

---

14. Hunter, *World Peace*, p. 25-6.

CHAPTER 8
CHARTING OUR OWN EVOLUTION

Selfishness beats altruism within groups. Altruistic groups beat selfish groups. Everything else is commentary.

E. O. WILSON AND DAVID SLOAN WILSON

Unlike good mystery novels, most nonfiction books end with a whimper rather than a bang. Like me, their authors typically reveal the equivalent of whodunnit in the first few pages and then spend the rest of the book defending their conclusion.

Rather than having some sort of "great reveal," academic authors, in particular, tend to use the final chapter to sum up their argument. Or call for more research.

All too often, that means readers skim or skip it altogether, assuming that it will an anti-climax. I know that's true, because I am an experienced final-chapter-skipper—something I probably shouldn't admit in the third paragraph of my own final chapter!

Please don't do that here. I can't promise you a surprising conclusion that will knock your proverbial socks off. I'll be satisfied if I help you see that doing peacebuilding starts at home might help us accomplish what this chapter's title and epigraph promise, which takes us beyond everything I've laid out in the first six steps of the loop.

Thinking of peacebuilding in evolutionary terms takes me back one final time to the mismatch between our country's needs and the tools we are using to meet them. It must already seem monumental. Now, I want to make it seem even bigger. (I don't know what is bigger than monumental? Brobdingnagian?) Because, when all is said and done, building peace will involve rethinking where humanity is heading.

In other words, I'm going to ask even more of you in the seventeen pages that are left. Building a society that is anchored in the values that I have outlined in the first seven chapters will demand the best of us. But if I'm right, adding this last step will make my invitation and our journey together one of the most enriching, empowering, and enjoyable things you have ever done.

I do need to make one thing clear at the outset. From where I sit, neither this chapter's title nor its epigraph is an exaggeration.

Everything I have said so far has been building to the two conclusions that are implicit in them. First, the challenge we face is huge. It is far bigger than "merely" creating a more peaceful country or planet. It involves tapping into the success story that is part of our history as a species, building on it, tackling the wicked problems we face, and coming out far better off at the end. Second, as I have said all along, we won't have a chance of pulling this off unless you and I and everyone we know does their part.

In the 1980s, the leaders of the Beyond War movement talked about how their work reflected the long story of life on earth. They even claimed that we would be ushering in the next stage in human evolution if we succeeded.

At the time, the reference to evolution felt like a throw away line. In fact, Beyond War's leadership asked me and two of my friends to write a book like this one toward the end of the 1980s. After a few months, I dropped out of the project because it felt like the kind of pie-in-the-sky idealism I have been railing against in these pages.[1]

---

1. One of my friends did eventually finish the book. While I love it, it still feels to me

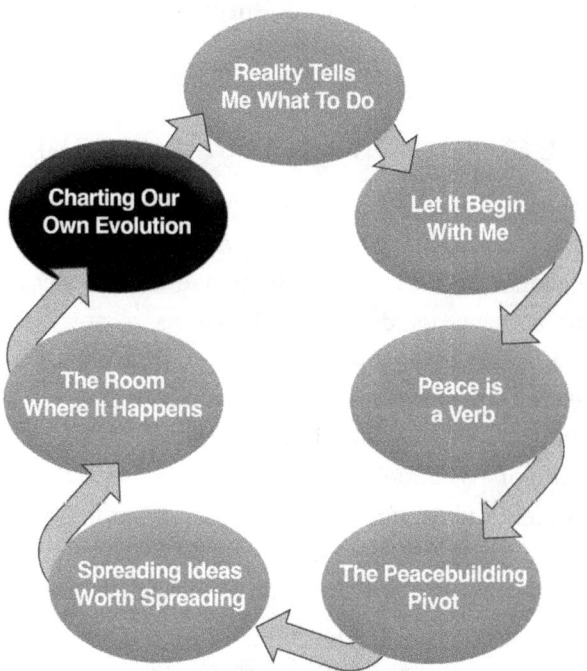

Figure 8.1: The Peacebuilding Starts at Home Loop

Now, however, times have changed. What I have covered so far could and should make what Safi Bahcall calls a loon shot and make moon shots seem realistic.[2] But, we have learned a lot about how peacebuilding starts at home can lay the groundwork for creating a better world. At the very least, I've convinced myself that we just might be able to make a quantum leap forward not only in how we deal with each but also in how we define ourselves as a species. In short, the Beyond War claim may not be so outlandish forty years later.

That means making my invitation even more daunting. If you take me up on my offer, you could help chart the next phase of humanity's evolution. You will not "just" be building peace but doing your part in creating a better world in which our children and grandchildren and

---

like pie-in-the-sky idealism. Winslow Myers. *Living Beyond War: A Citizens Guide.* (Maryknoll NY: Orbis Books, 2009).

2. Safi Bahcall. *Loonshots: How to Nurture the Crazy Ideas That Win Wars, Cure Diseases, and Transform Industries.* (New York: St. Martin's, 2019).

their children and grandchildren can thrive in ways that we can only dream of today.

CULTURAL EVOLUTION AND HUMAN NATURE

Unless you are a biologist, I have to start by casting some doubts on a key stereotype you probably have about evolution. Until recently, most scientists believed that evolutionary change is slow because natural selection unfolds across dozens and dozens if not hundreds and hundreds of generations. If anything, that understanding was reinforced once scientists discovered genetics.[3]

One simple example should help you see how pervasive this understanding of evolution has become. In Europe (but not in Asia), a genetic fluke left a handful of people able to tolerate milk-based food once they were weaned. Over the generations, that new gene came to dominate, and we now have a population of Europeans and their descendants who have "lost" their lactose intolerance.

That kind of evolution does take many generations to play itself out. The scientific obsession with the biological side of evolution made sense as recently as the turn of this century in ways that were popularized through books with titles like *The Selfish Gene*.[4]

Today, however, evolution is in the midst of a paradigm shift of its own. There is no need to go into all aspects of that scientific revolution here, including the often nasty infighting in the scientific community. Still, a handful of new findings did help me see how and why my invitation has to include a request to embark on an evolutionary quest that just might come close to fruition a lot sooner than you think.

A history of paradigm shifts. That quest starts with a new way of understanding the history of human civilization, which most scholars date from the adoption of agriculture roughly ten thousand years ago. Once our ancestors learned how to grow fruits and vegetables and domesticate animals, they could live more or less permanently in a

---

[3]. The best single source for non-scientific readers is Carl Zimmer. *Evolution: The Triumph of an Idea*. (New York: Harper, 2001).
[4]. Richard Dawkins, *The Selfish Gene*. 40th Anniversary Edition. (Oxford: Oxford University Press, 2016).

single location along with hundreds and then thousands and ultimately millions of their fellow humans.

As a result, they could build ever larger and more complex societies with ever larger and more sophisticated institutions to govern their affairs. All of them became possible because we also made quantum leaps in our ability to cooperate with—as well as fight with—each other.

The easiest way to see this point is through the work of David Ronfeldt, who was a reasonably obscure but visionary strategic planner at the RAND corporation where he focused on the future of warfare. By the 1990s, along with his colleague John Arquilla of the Naval Postgraduate School, he had come to see that the same realities that told peacebuilders what to do should reshape what national security planners did, too. From there, the two of them began exploring the noosphere or the notion that we were moving into a period that would be defined by the growing unification of who we are and how we think as first defined by the French Jesuit priest and biologist Pierre Teilhard de Chardin in the 1950s.

As Ronfeldt's vocal chords were beginning to fail, the same Dick O'Neill to whom this book is dedicated recorded a twenty-three minute video in which Ronfeldt laid out his key ideas. Obviously, it glosses over lots of details. After all, it is less than half an hour long.

As was the case with the other videos I've included, you can click this link to see it if you are reading this book online. If you are reading the print edition, you will have to follow this footnote.[5] Ronfeldt is nowhere near as well known as authors like Yuval Noah Harari or Steven Pinker whose books have made the New York Times best seller list, but his video is a great place to start, at least if you don't have the time to read a lengthy book or two.[6]

As Ronfeldt saw it, that history has been marked by four main forms of social organization which he labels TIMN reflecting each phase's dominant power structure.

---

5. https://www.youtube.com/watch?v=UBulH9_04vc
6. Yuval Noah Harari, *Sapiens: A Brief History of Humankind*. (New York: Vintage, 2014). For the purposes of this chapter the most useful book by Steven Pinker is *The Better Angels of our Nature*. (New York: Viking, 2011).

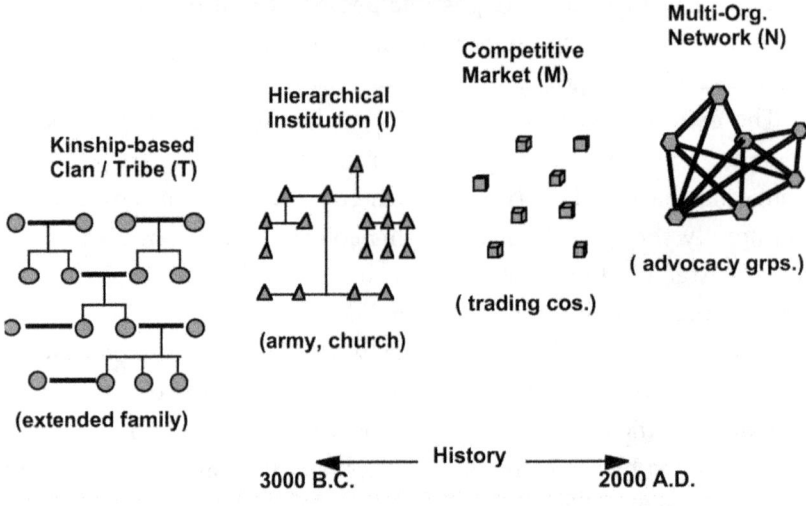

Figure 8.2: TIMN

People first came together in small groups that social scientists have variously called as tribes, clans, or kinship groups, none of which anyone likes. Whichever term you use, these were small communities, rarely including more than two hundred people, almost all of whom were related to each other. Few lived in any one place. Most were what anthropologists call hunter-gatherers who foraged for edible plants and stalked prey that they cooked over open fires.

For reasons no one fully understands, some of our ancestors created permanent settlements whose size required what Ronfeldt refers to as hierarchical institutions to manage their lives together. These were probably the first communities that, as the figure suggests, needed organized militaries, governments, and religions. These institutions and the individuals who led them were in charge of almost everything in the so-called civilized world from the dawn of recorded history until the end of the Middle Ages.

After that, hierarchical institutions began to give way to structures that revolved around markets and embraced individual liberties, democracy, and capitalism. During what critical theorists refer to as modernity and Ronfeldt called the market phase, our ancestors made the remarkable progress we benefit from today, in large part because they learned how to organize themselves in ever larger units. Even more importantly, they found ways of solving collective problems by working together. Their expansion of cooperative practices make ideas like "we are one" or Ostrom's core design principles possible.

While their actions did lay the groundwork for our current crisis, focus for a moment on their accomplishments. It is hard to imagine what life would have been like for our ancestors in the 1720s. It is even harder to imagine how most of us living today could last for long in a world without electricity, central heating, or supermarkets, let alone modern medicine, global supply chains, or the Internet.

No one made that progress easier to see than Hans Rosling did in dozens of videos that were full of data—and humor.[7] Rosling was a physician, statistician, and (I kid you not) sword swallower who used all of his skills (sometimes including sword swallowing) in his TED talks and other videos about population, health, and wealth many of which went viral. One he made for the BBC for its "Joy of Stats" series shows how people around the world have come to live longer and healthier lives since the beginning of the nineteenth century—in this case without the sword swallowing.

In it, Rosling used his visually stunning Gapminder software to trace the evolution of life expectancy and wealth in two hundred countries. The states are represented by bubbles that reflect their relative size and are color coded by region. In less than four minutes he shows how the rich countries of the west got healthier and wealthier until the middle of the twentieth century and then how the rest of the world began catching up. Rosling and his data made it clear that there still was a huge gap between the west and the rest. However, he also noted some powerful changes, such as the spread of washing machines to a billion more homes in the last decades of the twentieth century.

Rosling died in 2017. His work has continued both through the

---

7. https://youtu.be/jbkSRLYSojo?si=Q_0gBMNVrCF5nYH6

foundation he created and in the Our World in Data project which is based at the University of Oxford and has a lot more data that you can explore on your own.

Just before I wrote this chapter, I read *Not the End of the World* by Hannah Ritchie, the project's head of scientific outreach.[8] Ritchie focuses on environmental issues and rarely casts her historical net as far back as Rosling did. Building off the ideas of her intellectual mentor, she describes herself as an "urgent optimist." She does not reject what I have called Doom and Gloom 101 but wants us to understand that the world has gotten better in many ways and could get a whole lot better quite quickly. To that end, she points to data that show that we have made progress in dozens of environmental areas, including air pollution, fisheries, and agricultural production—the same kinds of issues that Ostrom focused on. Even when it comes to climate change, she identifies places which have already or soon could be "bending the curve." In particular, as prices continue to plummet, there is no reason why we cannot speed up the transition from carbon-based fuels to renewables, even if we miss the current target of limiting the increase in global average temperatures to 1.5 degrees centigrade in the next few years.

Rosling, Ritchie, and the other scientists whose research I would have included if I had enough pages left would be among the first to point out that the progress they have documented will not be enough. If what I have said so far is even close to accurate, we won't be able to get there.

We might still be able to improve our lives to some degree especially by building on the benefits of the ongoing technological revolution. But we just aren't going to be able to deal with all of the challenging realities of today's VUCA world. Indeed, there can be little doubt that some of the progress we have made also ended up reinforcing other social ills such as racism and imperialism while introducing new wicked problems of their own, most notably weapons of mass destruction and climate change.

---

8. Hannah Ritchie, *Not the End of the World: How We Can Be the First Generation to Build a Sustainable Planet*. (Boston: Little, Brown, 2024).

That's why the fourth section of Ronfeldt's chart when the network becomes the dominant organizational form in the near future is so important. Networks themselves are not new. The word itself dates back at least to 1550 when it was used to describe a collection of wires or string that looked like a net. That meaning led nineteenth century pundits to use the term in describing the growing web of canals and railroads that were spreading all over Europe, North America, and, eventually, the rest of the world. Then, the telephone, radio, television, and computers gave the term its current meaning, which is how and why I introduced it in discussing how reality tells us what to do in chapter 2.

Ronfeldt is by no means alone in arguing that the network is becoming the defining organizational structure in today's world, which he still labeled post-industrial when that video was made in 2013. If anything, its sway has only increased since then with the spread of social networks and artificial intelligence in the tech world, the speed at which the COVID-19 virus moved from continent to continent, and, of course, our realization that climate change affects everyone of us in ways that seem to become harder to ignore every day.

But notice two more things about that chart.

First, networks and network-based societies are different from all of the social structures that came before in one key way that has been at the heart of this book. They are completely interdependent. While networks have been around for centuries, it is only in the last couple of decades that they have come to define the way our lives are organized. In much the same way that feudalism and other hierarchical structures were ill-designed for a market-based society, market-based models are ill-designed for one based on networks.

Ironically, we see that mismatch in the very power that the large technology companies have accumulated, in large part because we have not yet figured out how to use tools like Ostrom's Core Design Principles in managing these new realities. In short, we have not yet figured out how to make networks operate in ways that benefit all of society rather than further adding to the wealth and power of individuals and organizations that have learned how to put them to use in the current paradigm.

Second, Ronfeldt gave an arbitrary date for the end of the transition to a networked society—the year 3000. When I asked him about it, Ronfeldt said he chose it because he had no idea when the network would occupy the role that the large corporation plays today, but that he knew it would be a lot sooner than 3000. He agreed that we also couldn't wait anywhere near that long to create a society that operates along the lines outlined by the likes of Elinor Ostrom.

EXERCISE 8.1: AMERICA REMADE

How does thinking of human history in terms of successful paradigm shifts change the way you envision America reMADE as you have developed it since chapter 1? In particular, how does your vision of a future America reflect both our past and our need to do things differently in the future?

Social evolution and the secret of our success. Another new and controversial ideas known as dual inheritance theory stresses social rather than biological evolution. The first research on the topic was published in the 1980s but only reached public attention through the work of Joseph Henrich and my friend whom you have already met a few times, David Sloan Wilson. They and their colleagues readily acknowledge that genes, mutation, and physical adaptation are all central tenets of modern biology and, hence, evolution. However, they argue that because humans are the only species that can think and plan, we evolve culturally, too, in ways that are far more important for our foreseeable future than any physical change that might be in the evolutionary cards.

Henrich's work is particularly useful here. Trained as an evolutionary biologist, his research prompted him to include concepts from anthropology and psychology in an interdisciplinary journey that led him to generate the (in some circles) famous acronym WEIRD (western educated industrialized rich democracies).

More useful here is the support he gave for one of the conclusions about our species that has been at the heart of this book. Unlike just about any other animal we know of, humans have agency.[9] We can anticipate the future and act accordingly. As he saw it, however, the secret to our success lies in our ability to work together which, in turn, has allowed us to form societies and civilizations and make the kinds of progress I've been describing in this chapter. As he put it:

> *The secret of our species' success resides not in the power of our individual minds, but in the collective brains of our communities.*[10]

Other research suggests that our social experience can affect the traits that we pass to our offspring through epigenetics. When all is said and done, Henrichs and his colleagues claim that our biological and cultural evolution build off each other in a feedback loop of their own.

You don't need to understand or accept everything Henrich, Wilson, and their colleagues have to say. I just want you to focus on two things. First, our capacity to think and work together has shaped the way humanity has evolved. Second, next to none of that evolution up to this point has been intentional.

I was drawn to Wilson's books and articles because he is convinced that we can use our intelligence as it has evolved over the millennia to steer our society's evolution in a ProSocial direction. What's more, given the stakes of life in the twenty-first century, we have little choice in the matter. If we continue on our current trajectories, we may undermine human civilization. We may not become physically extinct and

---

9. There is some debate here. Some scientists argue that a few other species have some capacity to think about and plan for the future. No one that I am aware of has argued that members of any other species come close to *homo sapiens sapiens* on this front, which is why I consigned this point to a footnote.
10. Joseph Henrich, *The Secret of Our Success: How Culture is Driving Human Evolution.* (Princeton: Princeton University Press, 2015).

go the way of the saber toothed tiger or the dodo. But, we could do irreparable damage to the civilization our ancestors created and undermine the very secret of our success.

Last but by no means least, Wilson and his colleagues understand that a successful response to our evolutionary challenge(s) won't happen if we simply tinker with the status quo. That led him to form (and me to join) a New Paradigm Coalition which is open to anyone—including you—who wants to play a part in accelerating humanity's evolution.

Human nature and psychological adaptivity. Throughout my career as a peace activist and scholar, critics have dismissed arguments like mine by asserting that our human nature will always keep us from living harmoniously with each other. For a term that is used so often and with so much certainty, human nature is amazingly ill-defined. Nonetheless, when I ask average citizens I work with to define human nature, their answers invariably reflect the pessimism of theorists like Thomas Hobbes whose ideas shaped the way most of think about human nature most of the time. I hear themes like we live in a dog-eat-dog world. Many of my academic colleagues talk about the rational individual or organization or country always "looking out for number one."That powerful but vague definition is deeply enough engrained/ingrained in our culture that when people do the exercise I first introduced in chapter 3, they often assume that most of us will always use values like those in the left-hand column of my table when dealing with most of the tough issues in life just about all of the time.

That definition is, of course, on target a lot of the time. Humans often are competitive, aggressive, and even violent. I have gotten myself to the point that I can't imagine using physical violence, Although I don't get angry and lash out very often any more, it is most likely to happen when I'm feeling threatened or ill-treated by someone I expect to treat me better. Or I forget my internal Daniel Tiger.

Yet, in the last half century, there has been an explosion of research in new interdisciplinary fields ranging from evolutionary psychology to behavioral economics to neuroscience that has shown that those interpretations of human nature that we all grew up with miss a lot. Yes, we definitely have a selfish and even aggressive side that often seems to serve us well as the first sentence of the Wilsons' statement suggests. But that's not all we are.

There is plenty of evidence that our tendency to act in these ways is to some degree "hard wired" into us both genetically and as a byproduct of the way our species has evolved culturally. After all, our ancestors had to cope with any number of threats for which things like our fight or flight mechanisms made sense. To be sure, we no longer have to worry about being eaten alive by a saber tooth tiger. But we do have to take the threats to life and limb that we face seriously. There are still times when it is hard not to react with violence, including after 9/11 in the United States or Hamas's attack on Israel on October 7, 2023.

Still, I want you to see something about human nature that would open the door to more creative ways of responding even under the most trying of circumstances. The Bush and Netanyahu governments had choices to make. Theirs was not an individual or instinctual reaction that only involved personal fight or flight instincts. They did have to react quickly and decisively. Still, those governments had the time—indeed, they took the time—to make group decisions. They could have used a grown-ups' version of Daniel Tiger's advice and used that time to question whether their gut instinct to lash out at the Taliban or destroy much of Gaza made the most-sense.

In other words, they undoubtedly had the time to consider potential medium to long term consequences of their massive military response. They still might still have chosen to overthrow the Taliban or Hamas. But did either of them have to go as far as they did? In creating the mess represented by the Spaghetti Map or all but wiping Gaza off the face of the earth?

However, it is clear that few governments and few of their citizens stop to consider options and their longer term consequences, especially when clichéd push comes to clichéd shove. Nonetheless, we should not forget that evolutionary scientists like Henrich and Wilson have shown that, over time, humans have learned to cooperate more and more often when dealing with more and more kinds of problems more and more of the time.

This approach has to include rethinking what we mean when we use terms like human nature, has been on my agenda since the Beyond War team also asked us to consider the work of a scientific panel convened by UNESCO, which tissued what became known as the Seville Statement in 1986. It read in part:

> *It is scientifically incorrect to say that we have inherited a tendency to make war from our animal ancestors.*
>
> *It is scientifically incorrect to say that war or any other violent behaviour is genetically programmed into our human nature.*
>
> *It is scientifically incorrect to say that in the course of human evolution there has been a selection for aggressive behaviour more than for other kinds of behaviour.*
>
> *It is scientifically incorrect to say that humans have a 'violent brain'.*
>
> *It is scientifically incorrect to say that war is caused by 'instinct' or any single motivation.*

Note that the Seville Statement doesn't say what human nature is. Luckily, on the day I finished this section, I had an appointment with my therapist whom you met in chapter 3 because she turned me on to the book by Emily Post's great grandchildren. So, I took advantage of the coincidence and asked her how her fellow psychiatrists define human nature. Dr. Whohasnoname shrugged her shoulders and confessed that they tend to avoid simplistic definitions. Individual behavior is complex and varies from person to person and time to time, which makes it foolish to talk about any single, simple definition. Rather, our behavior has many causes and we can almost always choose the ones we want to emphasize. Then, as she reminded me, the two of us had spent our time together strengthening my ability to be as effective a peacebuilder and human being as possible. With a smile, she pointed out that I am living proof that we have a lot of leeway when it comes to determining how we are going to act in almost any circumstance that we encounter.

Everything I've learned from first encountering the Seville Statement to reading a lot of evolutionary science to my hours with Dr. Whohasnoname has convinced me that human nature is a lot more fluid than I was led to believe when I last took a biology course in high school. Whatever the remnants of our lizard brain (a term that makes Dr. Whohasnoname cringe every time I use it), we have lots of leeway when it comes to making the tough decisions we seemingly have to make every day.

Early in this book, I hinted at a lot of this by invoking the sweeping aspirations of the serenity prayer or the cute folksiness of Robert Fulgham's reflections on kindergarten. In a way, that material all helped bring us to this point at which my invitation in the very first sentence you read asks you to join me in helping us all make better choices. These better options lead us to move collectively into the second column of the Contrasting Paradigms table and do a far better job of changing the things we can control.

I will be the first to admit that none of us can make more collaborative choices all of the time. But to repeat a line I've used in slightly different form at least a dozen times, we will all be a lot better off once most of us learn/try to deal with most of our problems more cooperatively most of the time.

Today, scientists like Henrich and Wilson make the case that our ability to cooperate helped us learn how to come up with and, more importantly, communicate our thoughts to each other. That, in turn, made it possible for us to pass what we learned from one generation to another through formal education, the socialization of children, and the adoption of common social norms. Perhaps most importantly of all, those skills are every bit as much a part of our human nature as fear, wariness, and aggression.

EXERCISE 8.2: NAILING IT

> What would it take for you to break your own habits and nail your own evolution? And those of the people you interact with regularly? And of our leaders?

CREATING OUR OWN EVOLUTION

I led you through this crash course in evolution for a reason. The principles of evolutionary science are what leads to my conviction that we all have to act and act decisively. My invitation thus ends by asking you to join me and the people you have met in addressing not just a challenge facing our generation, but one that threatens the future of our species itself. We can—and perhaps we must—lead the way into the next phase of humanity's evolution.

While it is true that it takes hundreds of generations for the genetic side of evolutionary selection to produce noticeable differences in what any species is like physically, we humans can evolve socially and do so very quickly. And because of the mismatch I've been documenting since p. 1, we have all but reached the limits of what we can accomplish if we don't take the next step in our social evolution.

There are plenty of other ideas I have picked up from evolutionary biologists and psychologists. There are, for instance, periods of punctuated equilibrium even in biological evolution that can be sped up to provoke what are known as major evolutionary transitions. Scientists who have been inspired by Elinor Ostrom's work have noticed that those transitions can occur at multiple levels at the same time in processes that resemble fractals or repetitive patterns that are more familiar to non-scientists who know about the shape of snowflakes or heads of broccoli.

We can adapt.

We can evolve.

We can overcome what may feel like some of our deeply ingrained instincts to, say, lash out or always "look out for number one." But it is a choice that requires more than one decision in which we cut away from the ways of thinking and acting that have gotten us into the bind(s) we are in today while retaining the ones that still help us solve our problems.

Our ancestors adapted time and time again in the past because they took advantage of the one skill that sets humanity apart from every other species we know about. We can think and, as Daniel Tiger also likes to say, we can use our words to solve our problems. We have evolved to the point that we have created Hans Rosling's world of growing prosperity tied to our interconnectedness. At the same time, we have created a world with climate change and nuclear weapons.

There is no reason why we can't evolve again in the days, weeks, and years to come in something like the ways I've outlined in these pages. And that no one has put more pithily or powerfully than David Sloan Wilson and E. O. Wilson in their pioneering work on social evolution that I used as the epigraph for this chapter:

> *Selfishness beats altruism within groups. Altruistic groups beat selfish groups. Everything else is commentary.*[11]

Think about that statement for a moment. If two of the leading evolutionary biologists of our era are correct, people who embrace the ethos of a supposedly dog-eat-dog world may do well when it comes to their business or even their political lives. However, when it comes to the ways societies evolve and interact with each other, those that stress the good of the whole tend to do best.

Neither of the Wilsons would claim that we have figured out how to make altruistic motivations or win-win outcomes the norm globally —given, most notably, the state of the world's climate. However, if you look at world history over the last several thousand years, the balance has definitely shifted toward bigger political units that incorporate larger numbers of people who settle a larger proportion of their disputes without the use of violence on an all but every day basis.

---

11. E. O. Wilson and David Sloan Wilson. "Rethinking the Theoretical Foundation of Sociobiology." *The Quarterly Review of Biology*, 82(2007), 327–348.

ONE LAST CLICHÉ

Before I let you go, take one last look at any of the charts I've used to illustrate the Peacebuilding Starts at Home Loop.

Ignore the words.

Just look at its structure. I experimented with other graphics but choosing a loop turned out to be a no brainer, because a loop never ends.

In other words, I have invited you onto a life time's journey. It's one I've been on since I was a teenager and went to that Pete Seeger and Joan Baez concert with Dick O'Neill.

Our thirteen year old selves had no idea that we would reunite forty years later as a career peace activist and career naval officer and find common cause in ways that led to this book.

Dick died a few months before Jon Stewart's monologue aired. But he clearly anticipated its message, which he kept coming back to as his friends and colleagues planned to keep the work of his Highlands Forum going. So, on what turned out to be our final Zoom meetings together, I showed him an early version of the loop. He realized that it was an invitation to a lifelong journey. Knowing my writing style as well as anyone, Dick sent me a chat message saying he had one more cliché that I should use to end the book. It also means that there is no need for an exercise 8.3 other than his three words.

Rinse and repeat.

STUDY GUIDE

Peacebuilding Starts at Home was written with group discussion in mind. In fact, I built suggestions for discussing it in book club, classroom, or other group settings into the text through the three exercises that appear in each chapter.

Recall from chapter 1 that I said that doing them and considering all of your answers as a whole would lead you to develop a personal strategy for your own peacebuilding starts at home strategy.

The same holds for your book club or other reading group. If you read *and* talk about the book and the exercises together, the "whole" you get to will certainly greater than the "sum of its parts" that you could reach on your own.

To that end, I have pulled them together here with an important "warning" and their overarching logic both of which were hard to include in the flow of the text in chapter 1 and, especially, in the rest of the book.

PICK IT APART

Although I make this point in chapter 1, I need to emphasize it here.

I know I don't have all the answers.

I have even reached different conclusions about what our basic strategies should be any number of times earlier in my career.

In particular, readers who are highly critical of the Trump administration (or the Biden one before it) will find the absence of anger and frustration in these pages, well, frustrating—at best.

So, feel free to whack away at any and every idea in this book.

Indeed, I would love to see your criticisms so that we can include them to improve the Peacebuilding Starts at Home movement and include them in other things my colleagues and I write.

ZIG ZAG

Remember that the three exercises in each chapter feed off of each other as do the chapters themselves. So, keep asking yourselves how defining your America reMADE helps you nail it and build a long-term strategy for whatever it was that Jon Stewart had in mind.

But then also remember to think back in the other direction. How do your new strategic insights (re)shape your tactics or even the North Star you are aiming at?

WHY THERE IS NO CHAPTER BY CHAPTER GUIDE

There actually is no need for me to repeat the exercise-by-exercise and chapter-by-chapter guide here. The questions to ask are, again, built into the book itself.

I also can't offer you a fool-proof way of recording what you and your group came up with. Some people love physical notebooks and would probably prefer doing this as a kind of journaling exercise. I did the guide myself using a basic word processing file that I kept updating as I finished editing each chapter.

HAND IT IN

Last but by no means least, my colleagues and I do want to see what you came up with. We can use it to help you find your own on ramp onto the Peacebuilding Starts at Home Loop or deepen it if you have already begun. Meanwhile, it will also help us deepen our own understanding of what and how Americans think about the issues facing our country.

The easiest way is to just send me an email at hauss@allianceforpeacebuilding.org.

ACKNOWLEDGMENTS

This book could not have been written without the help of dozens of people.

That starts with the people who are featured in it. They are its heroes. They also are mine. If I listed them by name and included how and why that was the case, the acknowledgements might have been longer than the book itself.

My heartiest and most heart-felt thanks goes to Dick O'Neill who died right after I finished the first very rough draft. Although he doesn't really appear until chapter 5, this whole book reflects our all but lifelong friendship that went back to nursery school.

Just as important is Gretchen Sandles. We have been married since 1990 and friends since we started graduate school twenty years before that. Gretchen makes a few cameo appearances in the book. But it's her behind the scenes presence that counts. To begin with, we have worked together at the Alliance for Peacebuilding (AfP) and now Rotary pretty much full time since she retired from the intelligence community twenty years ago. She also served as copy editor and lead critic for this book, skills she honed writing and editing analytic documents for American foreign policy makers.

Not far behind is Abby Rapoport. As you saw in the text, she features in chapter 5 and, that alone, would not have gotten her into the acknowledgements. But she has become one of my most trusted and valued friends ever since her father showed me *Stranger's Guide* at my fiftieth college reunion. Then, she really got her place in this section when she and her friend Nicco Mele decided to make *Peacebuilding Starts at Home* the first book that they would publish through their new venture, N/A Books (for Nicco and Abby, of course).

Not far behind her come the three people who gave me what started as vignettes to begin the book and then morphed without my quite realizing it into what became the homework assignments. I haven't actually met any of them. But that doesn't make them any less central to the writing of this book. I tell the story of how I met Kelly Corrigan in the first chapter, so I won't repeat it here. Her impact goes much deeper since her weekly podcasts made me think more often than I expected when I started listening to them. Lily Spencer got me to think about the political and social options that go far beyond her own work to include really cool political alternatives being developed in her adopted country of Australia. And, well, Jon Stewart is Jon Stewart. Need I say more?

Liz Hume, AfP's indefatigable executive director, also makes her share of appearances in the body of the book. She gets mentioned here because she has become one of our best friends whom we will see more now that we live less than a mile apart. And because she made me watch the Jon Stewart monologue.

Then there is Doctor Whohasnoname who, of course, does have a name. However, our wonderful psychiatrist/patient relationship carries with it expectations of confidentiality. Not only did she hear about the book at our weekly sessions, she actually read most of the first draft. And agreed about Jon Stewart, whose monologue she listened to before I did.

In many ways, this book would never have been written if it weren't for Patricia Shafer. She sent me an email from the Charlotte NC airport on Christmas eve 2022 suggesting that we write a book together. I agreed before she got on the plane (which says something about how both of us deal with holidays). I already had written a few thousand words with something like this book in mind, but it wasn't going anywhere. Her ideas and her confidence in me turned a vague dream into a concrete reality. In the end, our styles and our schedules meant that we couldn't finish the book together. Still, she deserves all the thanks in the world for the work she does as reflected in the fact that it appears in three different chapters and for getting me off of my rear end and in front of the keyboard.

David Sloan Wilson entered my life in early 2024. As I say in the text, I had known his work for years, but an unexpected email from a friend pointed me toward David's own work, his connection to Eleanor Ostrom's core design principles, and the whole question of evolution. Even more importantly, I've been able to help David build his projects at ProSocial World and the New Paradigm Coalition. Plus, Dick O'Neill and I had read his father's novels when we were in high school—and our teachers assigned us other books.

In 2018, Gretchen and I became charter members of the Next Big Idea Club which sends two of the best non-fiction books to its members each quarter. It also sends out lists of books that didn't become final selections, makes podcasts with its authors, and now puts out daily book bites by authors who at least made its short list. For its first six years, I could only thank the NBIC for helping me make Jeff Bezos wealthier because I bought so many of the books they recommended, including over half of the ones cited in my footnotes in *Peacebuilding Starts at Home*. In the last six months, I have begun working with Rufus Griscom and his team on two of their new initiatives, one which will turn it into more of a club and the other which is trying to create a community of creative non-fiction writers which, I guess, I have become.

Thanks, too, to Saleema Vellani and the team at Ripple Impact. They came on board after the book itself was done to help promote it and the larger Peacebuilding Starts at Home initiative. Ever since I met her a few years ago, I have been looking for an opportunity to work with her and her team. And while we are just beginning to devise our long term strategy together as I type these words, I can already see that she has enhanced my life.

Lots of other people played a role, too. Mara Zepeda and Jenn Brandel of Zebras Unite, the rest of my blended family some of whom made it into the book, and even the realtors who sold our house and helped us buy the condo we moved into while Abby and Nicco were turning my Microsoft Word files into a real book.

This book really has been a labor of love.

And I mean what I say in its first and final lines.

Charles Hauss
Falls Church, Virginia

www.ingramcontent.com/pod-product-compliance
Lightning Source LLC
Chambersburg PA
CBHW060455030426
42337CB00015B/1599

The Modern Monk © Copyright 2024 1° Publishing

All rights reserved. No part of this publication may be reproduced, distributed or transmitted in any form or by any means, including photocopying, recording, or other electronic or mechanical methods, without the prior written permission of the publisher, except in the case of brief quotations embodied in critical reviews and certain other noncommercial uses permitted by copyright law.

Although the author and publisher have made every effort to ensure that the information in this book was correct at press time, the author and publisher do not assume and hereby disclaim any liability to any party for any loss, damage, or disruption caused by errors or omissions, whether such errors or omissions result from negligence, accident, or any other cause.

Adherence to all applicable laws and regulations, including international, federal, state and local governing professional licensing, business practices, advertising, and all other aspects of doing business in the US, Canada or any other jurisdiction is the sole responsibility of the reader and consumer.

Neither the author nor the publisher assumes any responsibility or liability whatsoever on behalf of the consumer or reader of this material. Any perceived slight of any individual or organization is purely unintentional.

The resources in this book are provided for informational purposes only and should not be used to replace the specialized training and professional judgment of a health care or mental health care professional.

Neither the author nor the publisher can be held responsible for the use of the information provided within this book. Please always consult a trained professional before making any decision regarding treatment of yourself or others.

For more information, email shift@modernmonkpath.com

ISBN-13 Numbers:

Paperback 979-8-9923168-0-3

Hard cover 979-8-9923168-1-0

Hardcover with Jacket 979-8-9923168-4-1

ebook 979-8-9923168-2-7

Kindle/Amazon ebook 979-8-9923168-3-4

THE MODERN MONK

WALKING THE PATH TO AN ELEVATED LIFE

HAYDEN MCCOMAS

A STEP-BY-STEP JOURNEY TO LONG TERM HEALTH, FITNESS, AND WELL-BEING

BEGIN YOUR JOURNEY WITH *THE MODERN MONK*

Download *The Shift* for Free!

Thank you for picking up *The Modern Monk*. Before beginning this exciting journey to discovering a new version of you, we want to give you a head start!

Download The Shift: 7 Simple Steps to Transform Your Health and start implementing small but powerful changes right now.

By signing up, you'll get access to:

- **The Shift eBook** – Seven small changes that will kickstart your journey to better health, energy, and mindfulness.
- **Exclusive Resources** – Macro calculators, a monthly newsletter, and tools to help you integrate your journey through *The Modern Monk*.
- **Special Deals and Community Announcements** – Receive discounts on recommended products and stay connected with others walking the same path toward an elevated life.

Ready to make that first shift? Simply scan the QR code below or visit subscribepage.io/theshift to access your free guide and start creating positive change today.

This book is dedicated to the power and beauty of Contrast without which we could not find our way back home again.

CONTENTS

INTRODUCTION - What is a Modern Monk? 15
    1° Is All It Takes 20
    The Fallacy of Discipline 23
    Modern Monk Methodology 26

SLEEP - It All Starts Here 29
    The Importance of Sleep 31
    Poor Sleep: More Than Tired 36
    Sleep Hygiene 38
    Understanding Insomnia 50
    The Art of Napping 51
    Putting it all together: Building Quality Sleep Habits 54

MEDITATION - Cornerstone of an Elevated Life 57
    What is Meditation? 58
    Body-Centered Awareness 60
    The Benefits of Meditation 67
    How to Start Meditating 68
    Putting it all Together: Building Your Meditation Practice 70

NUTRITION - Fuel for the Meat-Suit 73
    Food Quality Matters 75
    Common Deficiencies 77
    Your 2nd Brain: The Gut Microbiome 80

Poop: Why You Should Give a Sh!t 89
PMS : Finding Flow on the Path 93
Food Toxicity.. 102
"Healthy" Foods that Aren't.. 109
Putting it all together - The Path to Premium Fuel 119

NUTRITION: Part II - Every Calorie Counts................................. 125
The importance of Meal Frequency and Timing................... 132
The Importance of Hydration 136
Calculating Your Macros.. 152
Sources of Protein.. 157
Key Nutritional Biomarkers 166
Putting It All Together - Building Weekly Menu Plans ... 178

EXERCISE - Movement along the Path.. 181
Defining Exercise 182
Forms of Exercise.. 186
Recovery 191
Essential Recovery Protocols 192
Putting it All Together – Staying Active 202

NEUROPLASTICITY - Time to Train the Brain 205
Building Skills 208
Cultivating Experiences 214
Putting it all together - Charting the Path 218

BONUS MATERIAL - Walking the Inner Path........................... 221

Final Thoughts 237

Selected Bibliography 239

Additional Resources 243

References 245

"I have not failed. I've just found 10,000 ways that won't work."
— *Thomas A. Edison*

"The purpose of life is to live it, to taste experience to the utmost, to reach out eagerly and without fear for newer and richer experience."
— *Eleanor Roosevelt*

"The greatest thing in the world is to know how to belong to oneself."
— *Michel de Montaigne*

THE MODERN MONK

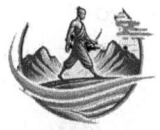

INTRODUCTION

WHAT IS A MODERN MONK?

In 2016 I thought I was living my best life. I had settled in Bali after spending the better part of a year traveling the world chasing my passions. I attended photography intensives, I studied under renowned yoga and meditation teachers, I participated in sacred healing ceremonies led by powerful *curanderos* deep in the Amazon rainforest, and at the time I was training to become a raw vegan chef with a prestigious culinary program. Every day felt like an incredible dream full of shiny, happy people, tropical fruit, and flowy clothes. At that point, I had been on a vegan diet for about 6 months at the strong recommendation of a spiritual teacher. For three of those six months, I felt incredible–energized, light on my feet, and mentally sharp. My plan, and I was convinced, my destiny, was to change the world with modern raw cuisine. Before embarking on this spiritual journey, I had been a chef in San Francisco and healing the world with food felt like the next evolution of my craft and the natural progression of my life's path. But then things in my body started changing drastically.

    The first signs of trouble were bloating and gas. Initially, these symptoms were intermittent and seemed odd but dismissable. Over time, however, the condition became increasingly persistent, painful, and unrelenting. Sleep was the next bodily function to go off the rails. I had always been a rock solid sleeper, "have pillow, will travel" was my motto. But now, I was waking up every couple of hours, partially because of the gas, but as things got worse, I would wake up with dizzy spells and my heart pounding like a jackhammer. What used to be a refuge of rest and recovery became a dreaded torture session night after night. Dark puffy bags lived under my eyes so pronounced that I was embarrassed to even go out in public without sunglasses. In just a few short months, I went from a paragon of health and vitality to someone who looked like a drug addict living in the shadows. As I wrestled with that irreconcilable reality, I became wracked with anxiety and my self-esteem disintegrated. But the downward spiral was not done yet—not by a longshot.

I graduated from college with a degree in English and although I never pursued a writing career, creative writing had always been a passion and a hobby of mine. A strong vocabulary and ability to express myself were always something I was known for amongst friends and colleagues. But "brain fog" doesn't care about English degrees and it eats ten-dollar words for breakfast. Suddenly my razor-sharp recall for all manner of words, movie quotes, and turns of phrase became buried beneath a thick impenetrable darkness. No longer was I able to call on words that had been part of my vocabulary for years—I had a faint sense of the shape of the word in my head and a notion for what I was trying to say—but the bridge between the two had collapsed.

More and more frequently I was living on the tip of my tongue and had to downshift from witty repartee to speaking in basic concepts in order to communicate. That was when I started worrying that something was very wrong with me and the beginning of my journey to recover from what turned out to be major deficiencies, bacterial imbalances, and inflammation requiring immediate changes to what I put in my body, how I exercised, my living environment; all of it. Fast forward six years and many health related side-quests later, I finally felt like my body was back in balance and full of vitality again; vitamin and key nutrient levels restored, a healthy and high functioning gut microbiome, sharp mental recall, quality sleep. The list goes on and on. This book is the culmination of that long road and my desire to offer what I've learned along the way about becoming aware of the signs your body gives you, understanding those signals, and developing the foundational building blocks to help you and your body thrive. Throughout the book I will continue to share anecdotes of my healing journey as part of the context for why certain elements have been included. Everything referenced in this book has either contributed to my healing or supports my current path to sustaining ongoing well-being. It has been a long, sometimes very dark road finding my way back to feeling great again and after traveling too far down that dark road, I can say unequivocally that if you don't have your health, you really don't have anything. Hopefully, in walking this path together, we can keep you moving continually "up and to the right" towards the light. Nothing presented here is rocket science or revolutionary in scope–but in this crazy world of convenience, consumption, and distraction, it's incredibly easy to lose sight of and become disconnected from the cornerstones that cultivate optimal health and well-being. This program is your reminder. Your healthy era has begun.

Living an Elevated Life in the Modern World

Drawing inspiration from the ancient householder traditions of Hinduism, the Modern Monk program is a path designed for those looking to elevate their lives amidst the hustle and bustle of the modern world. In Hindu philosophy, the concept of the householder, or *Grihastha*, emphasizes living a life of responsibility, devotion, and self-improvement while being fully engaged in worldly duties. Unlike the ascetics who renounce worldly life completely, retreat to a cave, and sit in silent contemplation for the rest of their days, householders find spiritual fulfillment within the context of their daily lives, integrating personal growth with the demands of family, work, and society. The Modern Monk program channels this ethos, guiding individuals to achieve continuous self-improvement that send ripples of positive change throughout every aspect of their lives and subsequently the lives of those around them.

In the householder tradition, the journey of self-improvement is seen as a sacred duty. It's a holistic approach that recognizes the interconnectedness of all aspects of life—physical, mental, emotional, and spiritual. The Modern Monk program takes this principle and adapts it for today's world, where the pressures of modern life can lead to a disconnection from understanding ourselves more fully and operating day-to-day driven largely by unconscious programming. In focusing on continuous self-improvement, the program helps cultivate optimal health, mental resilience, and a deeper sense of purpose, which inevitably radiates outward, strengthening personal relationships, energizing enthusiasm for work, and improving the overall quality and experience of life.

This ripple effect of self-improvement is a core principle of The Modern Monk program. When one commits to bettering oneself—whether through physical fitness, mindfulness practices, or intellectual growth (and ideally, all three)—the benefits extend far beyond the individual.

Improved health leads to increased longevity, more energy and a sharper mind, which enhance our ability to interact with the rhythms of life. A clearer, more focused mind leads to better decision-making and greater self-awareness, boosting our emotional intelligence (EQ) and improving our Interpersonal relationships. Over time these small, consistent improvements compound, leading to a profound transformation in the quality of one's experience. The Modern Monk recognizes that this precious journey of life is not just about personal gain; it's about creating a positive impact on the world around you, one small change at a time.

That journey starts with you, with your body, the incredibly sophisticated high-performance machine you've been gifted to navigate the world. Central to this philosophy is the idea that the body is more than just a vessel—it's a living resume for life, updated in real time. In the modern world, where wealth and material possessions are often seen as the ultimate indicators of success, The Modern Monk program looks to challenge that notion by asserting that the true measure of a person's life is reflected in their physical and mental well-being. Just as a great C.V. highlights one's professional accomplishments and skills, a healthy, vibrant body showcases self-respect and commitment to the pursuit of excellence. The body is a visible, undeniable testament to the choices one makes every day and a strong, well-functioning body is the product of living a balanced, purposeful life. Master yourself, body and mind, and material success is bound to follow. How many times have you heard stories of the singular pursuit of material success leaving someone largely unfulfilled, wishing they had spent more time nurturing relationships, taken better care of themselves or paid attention to their mental health? What person, lying in a hospital bed with a chronic or terminal illness wouldn't trade all of their material success for the opportunity to be healthy once again? By treating the body as a resume for life and committing to daily practices that enhance well-being, The Modern Monk strives to help you create a life that is not only successful by modern standards but also deeply fulfilling and aligned with your highest potential. In Hinduism, the body is considered a temple, a sacred space that should be treated with respect and reverence. The Modern Monk program embodies this principle by encouraging individuals to view their physical health as a priority, not just for the sake of appearance, but as a foundation for all other aspects of life. A strong, healthy body supports a sharp mind, a compassionate heart, and a resilient spirit—all of which are essential for navigating the complexities of modern life.

The intent of this program is not to prescribe one certain way as the only path to attaining health, happiness, well-being and self-awareness—"equanimity" in the words of the Buddhists. Although, the goal is most certainly to guide you down the path of improving all of these aspects of your life. But, there is no singular path. Each of us is literally as unique as the grains of sand or the stardust from whence we came and so, naturally then, we all require something a little bit different to help us get where we want to go. With that in mind, the structure of this program is not to give you a strict list of eat this, quit doing this, do such and such exercise, take 'xyz supplement' but rather the idea is to *meet you where you are* and provide scientifically backed guidance and scaling options for everything that we are proposing. We can't possibly know who you are, what your body is like, what resources you have available, or what your goals are in beginning this journey. What we can do is provide you with an array of options that all point in the same direction, allowing you to 'get in where you fit in' and make progress in a way that will inspire you to keep moving forward and keep taking small steps in the right direction.

1° Is All It Takes

You may be familiar with the idea that just a 1° change in your trajectory can make a significant difference in where you end up. And the longer your journey, the more that 1° makes an impact. This concept is core to the approach of this program. To put it in perspective, a 1° shift in trajectory plays out as follows: after one foot, you'll be wide of your destination by 2/10ths of an inch—maybe not a big deal. After 100 yards, you'll be wide by 5.2 feet. Okay. After a mile, you'll be 92.2 feet away from your original destination. You can see how that one degree is starting to make a difference. After traveling the 500+ miles from San Francisco to L.A., you'll be off by 6 miles. And from San Francisco to Washington, D.C., you'll end up on the other side of Baltimore, 42.6 miles away. Traveling around the globe from Washington, DC, you'll end up in Boston instead, 435 miles away. In a rocket aimed at the moon, that 1° difference will have you ending up 4,169 miles wide of your initial destination (nearly twice the diameter of the moon). And now headed for the sun, you'll be over 1.6 million miles away from your initial destination. (nearly twice the diameter of the sun). All of that, a result of shifting the trajectory of your journey by a single degree.

We presume you are reading this because you want to change something about your current destination. The fundamental concept behind this program is about shifting some basic but very important habits just 1°. If you do that, over time, you will find yourself in a totally different place, or more accurately, in a totally different body as a totally different person with a greater capacity to make another 1° shift. For everyone, however, that 1° is going to be something different. For one person it might be that getting an additional hour of quality sleep gives them the energy to want to work out an extra day during the week which means they burn more calories, which means they lose some weight they've been trying to lose. For someone else, it might be that eliminating a food that had been causing inflammation means their dry skin goes away which gives them more body positivity which leads to greater confidence and better performance at work and for someone else, developing a meditation practice might give them the self-awareness to notice a tendency towards reacting without listening which improves their relationships at home and in the office. The point is, whatever the 1° is for you, this program is designed to help you key into that and put into motion the compounding effect of better choices made consistently over time to work for you. But let's also be clear, you don't end up 1.6 million miles from where you started overnight. This is a journey, ideally one that you are continuing for the rest of your life, beginning now.

In today's health circles, biohacking has become the trend de jour in self-improvement. This program and methodology is not about biohacking, it's not about shortcuts or reductionist science pushing results in a vacuum. It's not the easy way to six pack abs or a road to riches (although it might be a fountain of youth). It's a path and a trajectory that theoretically never ends because there's always another level, another degree you can shift the direction your life is headed. And if you stick with it and develop these fundamentally life-affirming habits, we believe you'll have the mental acumen and the physical capacity to be the captain of your ship until the very end, sailing off into a sunset of your choosing. Of course, everyone's life path is unique, fraught with different obstacles and challenges. But walking this path will undoubtedly prepare you to navigate inevitably stormy seas with presence, power, and strength. Eventually, as your trajectory points you by degrees closer to your optimal state of well-being you'll be operating on momentum and it won't matter any more where you came from, (in fact that will be a distant memory) only the possibility of where you can go will remain. That's what the path of 'attainment' looks like. We are spiritual beings, or energy if you will, having a human experience. But before we can peel back the layers of the woo-woo and the esoteric to navigate the unseen we need to learn how best to drive this meat-suit, this vessel that we've been gifted to hold our conscious awareness in the physical world. It's our rocket ship, our high performance vehicle, and we only get one. It is my firm belief and personal experience that the more I have been able to fine tune the function and performance of my body, the greater my awareness and connection to everything and everyone around me has become. I don't think that's a coincidence nor do I think you need to live in a cave for the rest of your life in order to figure that out–no shade on cave dwelling, that's certainly one way to do it–it's just not the only way or the most practical, especially in modern times. In fact, I believe that by coming into harmony with our bodies, we give (gift) ourselves more of that precious time here on Earth in the human experience to actively explore the greater mysteries, or spend time with loved ones, or acquire new skills, or travel to different parts of the world, or whatever it is for you that makes living the extraordinary experience that it is.

The Fallacy of Discipline

The concept of discipline is often touted as the bedrock of achievement and success, implying that to accomplish anything worthwhile demands sheer willpower and the ability to resist temptation. I'm not so sure that's true. Discipline implies friction or resistance that must be overcome to succeed in the face of forces or behaviors that would draw or knock us off the path to achieving our stated goal or dream. If we are in choice about who we desire to be, if the possibility we hold for ourselves is already present, then we can operate from a perspective and a mindset that does not require discipline because we are already acting as the person we want to become. Actions spring naturally from the authentic clarity that comes with understanding what will best support who we desire to be. The worship of discipline overlooks a deeper, more intuitive truth: when someone is genuinely committed to something they love doing or want to become, the need for discipline becomes obsolete. Instead of forcing oneself to engage in activities out of a sense of duty or obligation, the experience transforms into one of effortless flow. The idea that discipline is essential to excel at something may actually be a fallacy, as true commitment and passion naturally drive a person to engage in and enjoy the process of learning, practicing, and mastering their craft—in this case, the craft of living.

Think about how easily people spend hours playing video games, practicing golf, gardening or playing the guitar. These activities, driven by genuine love and interest, rarely feel like they require discipline. Of course, to achieve mastery at any skill requires consistent, sustained effort. But, the time and effort invested come naturally, fueled by intrinsic motivation, by inner desire. When someone is passionate about an activity, they don't need to force themselves to engage in it; they are drawn to it because it brings them happiness and satisfaction. The excitement of playing a challenging video game, the thrill of perfecting a golf swing, the joy of discovering a newly blossoming flower, or the sense of accomplishment in mastering a guitar riff all create a sense of flow that renders the notion of discipline unnecessary.

Reframing discipline in this context allows us to shift the focus from forcing oneself to overcome resistance to using the body and mind to create a frictionless experience. When we embody the commitment to a goal or passion, we naturally align emotions, actions, and habits with that commitment. The body, in turn, becomes a tool that serves this alignment. Instead of battling against ourselves to have discipline, we can learn to operate with the harmony and natural progression of continuous action, creating a seamless integration of effort and enjoyment.

This perspective also highlights the importance of slow and gradual change—again what we might call the 1° of change concept, or **Kaizen** according to the Japanese. By making small, incremental adjustments in pursuit of habits and activities that support an elevated way of being, we can facilitate growth without the need for harsh discipline or trying to 'bite off more than you can chew' which inevitably leads to failure, frustration, and futility. But small incremental changes, made consistently over time, create positive feedback loops, reinforcing the newly acquired behaviors, making them feel natural rather than forced. Each small success builds on the last, making the journey toward the objective a smooth, enjoyable experience rather than a constant battle.

Kaizen (改善)

Kaizen is a Japanese term that means "continuous improvement" and is rooted in the practice of making small, incremental changes toward achieving long-term goals. In business. Kaizen is often associated with efficiency and productivity improvements, but in the Modern Monk context, it represents the idea of daily progress in developing the best version of ourselves. Whether it's committing to consistent exercise, refining a skill, or deepening mindfulness, the principle of Kaizen encourages steady, consistent growth through intentional, small steps that compound over time. It emphasizes that excellence is achieved through commitment to gradual, consistent effort. Our development is a process and like every good process, continuous improvement will inevitably lead to the best possible outcome.

Make no mistake, there will always be struggles, setbacks, and self-doubt in the process of becoming someone different—this is an inevitable consequence of the ego's natural inclination to protect our developed sense of "self", but with patience and deliberate action, the transition to a new way of being is subtle enough that the ego incorporates the new way being without triggering a fear of change. Inevitably, it becomes harder and harder for that little voice in our heads to argue its way out of choices that undeniably make us feel better when compared to the choices that leave us tired, bloated, stiff, and stagnant.

I know from my own experience, this isn't always simple. We all have traumas and emotional programming that makes choosing something in our highest good maddeningly difficult and a process in and of itself to overcome. Part of this process for you may be in first discovering where the roadblocks lie and where your conditioning is limiting your capacity to act in your own best interest—whether its a hangup around eating, a fear of failure, a sense of overwhelm that prevents taking action—there are many flavors of limiting beliefs. Hopefully this process can and will help tease those out. With awareness, you take the first step towards overcoming them by understanding the framework, the boundaries of the prison you've created for yourself. In the *Bonus Material* chapter at the end of the book, we explore some of the alternative healing modalities that I have used and continue to use to explore, heal, and overcome my own limiting beliefs. Truly the process of unfolding into the best version of ourselves is never-ending. There is always another level. This is a sign on the road pointing you in the right direction.

Modern Monk Methodology

The Modern Monk program is designed to guide you on the path to an elevated life by integrating principles of self-mastery, physical health, and mental well-being. At the core of this program is the concept of *meeting you where you are* recognizing that everyone's journey is unique and requires a personalized approach. This approach was inspired by my experiences training in CrossFit, where scaling options across a wide range of capabilities and levels ensure that everyone, regardless of their entry point, can participate fully and make meaningful progress. For me, this approach has been invaluable and deeply inspiring, particularly as I developed the strength and skills to perform complex movements. When I first started CrossFit, the bar muscle-up (a challenging move that combines elements of a pull-up and dip into one fluid motion) seemed not just daunting but nearly impossible. However, by breaking the movement down into its component parts, I worked slowly towards mastering it, and a year after starting CrossFit, I completed my first unassisted muscle-up. The sense of accomplishment was profound and it drove home the concept of breaking complex difficult goals into a progression of manageable steps.

The Modern Monk program applies this same philosophy to the broader pursuit of an elevated life. By breaking down complex skills and concepts into smaller, manageable sequences, each participant can find their edge and push it just enough to foster growth without feeling overwhelmed. This methodology ensures that participants understand not only what they're doing but why each step is important. Whether the focus is on physical fitness, developing proper nutrition, or acquiring a new skill, the approach remains the same: break down complex goals into smaller, achievable steps, and provide support and guidance as people work at their own pace. such that no one is left behind.

The Modern Monk program is not intended to be comprehensive or irrefutable; rather, it is a compilation of the ideas, methods, and rationale that have been demonstrated to yield great results, drawing from my personal experience trying (and failing) at all sorts of protocols, as well as knowledge and recommendations culled from leading experts I have followed, studied, and learned from over the years. All the evidence mentioned is cited for reference and a *Selected Bibliography* has been added to the end if you want to dive more deeply into any of the topics or source material mentioned.

This program is designed to walk you down a path, through a progression of practices or pillars, that we've identified as fundamental to living an elevated life. Each pillar contains its own set of increasingly more substantive practices to help you attain a level of proficiency within it. There is a logic and a design with regard to the order they are presented but as we've discussed, one of the core tenets of this program is meeting you where you are. If your sleep is already dialed-in, then by all means, move on to another area where you feel you need (or even better, are excited) to focus your time and attention. The path as it's laid out is merely a suggestion based on personal experience and contemplation. In many ways, the path of attainment is a circle or more accurately, a spiral, anyway—the more we come to understand about our bodies, the more our awareness of ourselves expands, the greater the depth we can explore these topics—we move up the scale of understanding like octaves of a musical note and there is always more to learn. It is my hope and metric for success that when you have successfully 'walked this path' you will be in a place of greater personal inquiry with such a nuanced understanding of what makes you specifically look and feel your best that you will become your own guide on this path forward and more than likely, new experts and mentors will appear who can help direct you along the road that lies ahead.

By meeting participants where they are, the program makes the journey of self-improvement accessible and achievable for everyone. Each small victory builds on the last, creating momentum and confidence that carry participants forward, eventually leading them to the full expression of their potential. Just as the muscle-up is mastered one movement at a time, the path to an elevated life is traveled one step at a time, with each step tailored to the individual's current capabilities and future goals making sure no one gets lost along the way.

SLEEP

IT ALL STARTS HERE

Paradoxically, the path to living an elevated life starts with mastering the time that we are the least active all day. If we have mastered the art of sleeping, we will be spending 30% of our days in rest and repair mode. Done consistently, this will literally supercharge how we are able to approach the remaining 70% of our waking days. I used to be a huge proponent of the mantra, 'sleep when you're dead'–always opting to stay out later, stay up longer, never wanting to miss even the last little bit of 'experience' in whatever I was doing but there is nothing further from the path of wellness and well-being than putting off sleep for another day. We literally can't make up for lost sleep. Our bodies don't work that way. Behind breathing, which is involuntary, and perhaps warmth, which most of us take for granted but is essential for normal bodily function, sleep is the most important activity we do all day. And cutting corners or compromising the quality of our sleep with habits or activities that undermine its due process is quite simply self-defeating. So don't think of sleep as time lost, think of sleep as the first threshold to becoming the best version of yourself.

How Much Sleep is Enough?

Determining the optimal amount of sleep for the average person involves understanding both the quantity and quality of sleep necessary for maintaining health and well-being. The recommended sleep duration for most adults is between 7 to 9 hours per night. It's not arbitrary; those numbers are supported by extensive studies on sleep patterns and health outcomes. Research has shown that consistently sleeping less than 7 hours per night is associated with an increased risk of various health issues, including cardiovascular disease, diabetes, obesity, and impaired immune function.

Conversely, regularly sleeping more than 9 hours may also be indicative of underlying health problems. One notable study conducted by the National Sleep Foundation analyzed data from multiple sleep studies involving thousands of participants. This meta-analysis found that adults who slept within the 7 to 9-hour range had the lowest rates of morbidity and mortality, underscoring the health benefits of adhering to these guidelines.

Defining Quality Sleep

We are going to talk a lot about getting 'quality sleep'. But naturally, if we are sleeping, it's hard to determine exactly what that means. Quality sleep refers to sleep that is *uninterrupted*, *deep*, and *restorative*. Sleep quality is just as important as sleep duration. Achieving quality sleep involves progressing through the different stages of the sleep cycle, including light sleep, deep sleep (slow-wave sleep), and REM sleep.

To determine if you are getting quality sleep, consider the following metrics:

Sleep Efficiency: This is the ratio of time spent asleep to the total time spent in bed. A sleep efficiency above 85% is generally considered good. For instance, if you spend 8 hours in bed but only 6 hours sleeping, your sleep efficiency would be 75%, indicating poor sleep quality.

Sleep Latency: This refers to the amount of time it takes to fall asleep. Ideally, it should take between 10 to 20 minutes to fall asleep. Taking significantly longer may indicate insomnia, while falling asleep almost immediately could suggest sleep deprivation.

Wake After Sleep Onset (WASO): This measures the amount of time spent awake after initially falling asleep. Frequent awakenings and prolonged wakefulness during the night can reduce sleep quality. Ideally, WASO should be minimal, with the sleeper spending most of the night in continuous sleep.

Sleep Stages: Progressing through the different stages of sleep is crucial for restorative sleep. Deep sleep (slow-wave sleep) is essential for physical restoration, while REM sleep is vital for cognitive function and emotional regulation. Using sleep tracking devices that monitor these stages can help provide insight into your nightly sleep quality.

Daytime Functioning: Feeling refreshed and alert during the day is a good indicator of quality sleep. Persistent daytime sleepiness, mood disturbances, or cognitive impairments suggest that sleep quality may be inadequate.

Quality sleep, characterized by high sleep efficiency, appropriate sleep latency, minimal wakefulness during the night, balanced sleep stages, and good daytime functioning, is essential for reaping the full benefits of sleep.

The Importance of Sleep

Sleep is the unsung hero in the grand symphony of our lives, a maestro orchestrating the delicate balance of our mental and physical health. Sleep is the bedrock upon which optimal functioning of the body and mind is built which is why we have positioned this pillar at the beginning of the path.

Brain Function: The Nightly Housekeeper

Think of your brain as an expansive library. Each day, new books (memories and information) are added haphazardly to the shelves. Without the librarian—our nightly sleep—these books remain scattered and disorganized strewn about the library and hard to find or access. Sleep, particularly REM sleep, serves as that diligent librarian, sorting through the day's influx of information, filing away memories for short-term and long-term storage. This process of memory consolidation is akin to weaving a complex tapestry, where threads of experience are intertwined to create a coherent narrative. Without sufficient REM sleep, our ability to integrate, access, and make sense of new information is significantly impaired.

Nemuri (眠り)

From the Japanese perspective, **Nemuri**, or sleep, is more than just rest: it is viewed as essential for maintaining harmony between mind, body, and spirit. Quality sleep is crucial for physical recovery. mental clarity, and emotional stability, allowing one to approach each day with renewed energy and focus. During deep and REM sleep, the body repairs itself, releases growth hormones, and the mind processes emotions and consolidates memories, aligning with the Japanese value of balance in all aspects of life. The practice of Nemuri involves creating a peaceful environment, following calming rituals, and honoring rest as a key part of overall well-being. In this way sleep becomes a deliberate act of self-care, ensuring sustained health and a clear mind essential for fully engaging with life's responsibilities and joys.

Cognitive performance, much like a finely tuned orchestra, relies on the precision of every note.

Adequate sleep sharpens our problem-solving skills, enhances creativity, and fortifies decision-making. It clears the mental fog, allowing for clarity and focus. Quality sleep improves learning efficiency and retention by up to 40%, making it a critical component of our cognitive arsenal. Interrupted or incomplete sleep on the other hand, impairs cognitive performance to such an extent that *operating on less than four hours of sleep can reduce motor skills to levels comparable to those of a drunk driver.* A study showed that after 17-19 hours without sleep, individuals performed tasks worse than those with a blood alcohol concentration (BAC) of 0.05%. After longer periods, their performance deteriorated to levels equivalent to a BAC of 0.1%—legally drunk in many countries.

It seems to be widely accepted that as we get older, the quality of our sleep declines. I would assert that part of the reason for this is that as we get older our bodies become more sensitive and fragile to some degree–less able to 'power through' and get a good night sleep, especially if we've been drinking or staring at phones and computer screens right before bed or doing any number of things that can impact a good night's sleep. And after weeks, months, and years of poor nights of sleep here and there, the hours of lost sleep begin to compound. Over time, our internal sleep librarian is unable to keep up with the backlog of integrating, filing, and organizing our short term and long term memories. So is it surprising then how often when we get older, many of us start to discover gaps in our memory? It's not because there's no more room in our mental library and new memories have somehow squeezed out the old. In fact, I'm sure we all know someone whose ability to recall minute details of distant memories seems astonishing in comparison to our own.

And I'd venture to guess that if you asked that individual about the quality of their sleep, 99 times out of 100 that person will say that they sleep soundly night in and night out. I think the correlation between cognitive function as we get older and proper sleep is VASTLY underestimated. And once you realize how these two things are connected, it (should) become increasingly difficult to choose activities that are going to impact sleep. Becoming aware of and understanding the cause and effect relationship between our actions and their impact on our quality of life is a large part of what walking the path of The Modern Monk is all about. Ignorance might be bliss until you realize that 'bliss' is coming at the expense of the quality of your daily living experience.

Physical Health: The Invisible Armor

Sleep is your body's invisible armor, fortifying you against a myriad of health issues. During quality slumber, the body produces cytokines—proteins that act as the knights of the immune system, battling infections and inflammation. It's no wonder that a good night's sleep often precedes recovery from illness, as these cytokines ramp up their defense mechanisms while sleep deprivation weakens the immune system, making us more vulnerable to common colds and infections. Sleep is also the guardian of our emotional well-being. It enhances our ability to regulate emotions and interact socially. Without sufficient sleep, our mood darkens, anxiety increases, and depression can take hold, like shadows lengthening at dusk. Research indicates that sleep-deprived individuals are more likely to experience emotional volatility and have difficulty managing interpersonal relationships, opening the door to a whole host of coping mechanisms (e.g., alcohol, prescription medications, caffeine) that are likely suboptimal for living an elevated life.

Similarly, the cardiovascular system operates most efficiently when well-rested. Quality sleep regulates blood pressure and mitigates stress on the heart. Chronic sleep deprivation, however, is akin to running an engine without oil—leading to hypertension, heart disease, and an increased risk of stroke. Individuals who consistently sleep less than six hours per night are at a 200% higher risk of having a heart attack or stroke. This statistic alone underscores the critical role sleep plays in maintaining heart health. As you may already be aware, the leading cause of death in this country is heart disease—aka heart attacks and strokes. Although there are obviously many factors that play into the cause of this disease, It's clear that poor sleep has an important role to play in the epidemic of heart disease right along with nutrition, exercise, and other pillars we will discuss here. Our goal is not dwell in the negative but to shine a light on just how critical these pillars are to the optimal function of our meat-suits and further how all of these functions work in concert and should not be considered separate independent functions of the body.

Hormonal Balance: The Silent Conductor

As you are probably picking up by now, sleep is much more than just down time; it's also a crucial period for maintaining hormonal balance, which is the conductor orchestrating the symphony of your body's physiological processes. Among the key players in this nocturnal concert are growth hormone and cortisol, each playing vital roles in growth, repair, and stress regulation. Deep sleep (different from REM sleep) triggers the release of growth hormone (gH or hgH), essential for growth, cell repair, and muscle development. This hormone is a first chair starring instrument of your body's nightly symphony, ensuring that each cell plays its part in maintaining and repairing the body's tissues. Without adequate sleep, this instrument falters, and the harmony of growth and repair is disrupted. This hormone is especially vital for children and athletes, as it's promotes muscle recovery and overall physical development.

Cortisol, the primary stress hormone, is another featured player in this nocturnal symphony. It is beneficial in short bursts but detrimental when persistently elevated. Elevated cortisol levels are akin to having a constant alarm bell ringing in your head, preventing you from achieving a state of relaxation and peace—while sleep is the silencer that restores calm and tranquility. Cortisol follows a diurnal rhythm, peaking in the early morning to help you wake up and gradually decreasing throughout the day. The relationship between cortisol and sleep is delicate and when not well managed, can easily create a vicious cycle. Consistently elevated cortisol levels lead to increased stress, anxiety, and even depression which impacts the ability to get quality sleep. Sleep deprivation in turn raises cortisol levels, and elevated cortisol further disrupts sleep. This cycle can lead to chronic stress and a host of related health issues. Chronic stress and elevated cortisol disrupt the neural circuits in the prefrontal cortex and hippocampus, areas crucial for memory and learning. This disruption can lead to difficulties in concentration, decision-making, and memory retention.

Poor Sleep: More Than Tired

Now imagine your brain and body as a high-performance sports car. Sleep is the fuel that powers this finely tuned machine. Without it, you're running on empty, and no amount of high-octane fuel additives will make up for the lack of a full tank. Poor sleep isn't just an inconvenience; it's a full-scale breakdown waiting to happen, impacting every system and function you rely on to navigate your daily life.

Hypertension

Cortisol plays a significant role in regulating blood pressure as well. Under normal conditions, cortisol helps maintain cardiovascular function. However, when cortisol levels remain elevated, it can lead to sustained increases in blood pressure. This condition, known as hypertension, increases the risk of heart disease, stroke, and other cardiovascular issues. Poor sleep and stress-induced high cortisol levels force the cardiovascular system to work harder, straining the heart and blood vessels over time. Studies have shown that cortisol causes blood vessels to constrict, which raises blood pressure and, if chronic, can damage the arteries and heart.

Weight Gain

Elevated cortisol levels are also linked to weight gain. Cortisol disrupts the balance of hunger hormones—ghrelin (which stimulates appetite) and leptin (which signals satiety)—leading to increased hunger and reduced satisfaction from eating. Cortisol increases appetite and cravings for high-calorie, high-fat foods, and ultimately to overeating. It also promotes the storage of fat in the abdominal area, which is associated with a higher risk of metabolic diseases. This hormonal imbalance, coupled with a higher propensity to crave unhealthy foods, contributes significantly to weight gain and obesity.

Weakened Immune System

Cortisol also has immunosuppressive properties, which means that prolonged high levels can weaken the immune system. In the short term, cortisol helps manage the immune response and reduce inflammation. However, chronic elevation of cortisol suppresses the production and function of white blood cells, which are vital for fighting infections. This suppression makes the body more susceptible to infections and slows down the healing process. Individuals with high cortisol levels due to chronic stress or sleep deprivation are more likely to suffer from frequent colds, infections, and have prolonged recovery periods. So, if you suffer from frequent colds, infections or it seems to take forever for you to get better when you do get sick, take a look at the quality of your sleep. Could it be improved?

Put bluntly, disrupted sleep can set off a cascade of imbalances in the way our bodies are meant to function that contribute to a whole host of conditions that can make our waking life experience less than optimal. Unfortunately, modern society has developed in such a way that isn't necessarily conducive to getting a great night's sleep, encouraging habits that might require a conscious effort to rewire, lest we sabotage our own sleep quality unknowingly (I'm looking at you, coffee and alcohol). If your objective is better sleep on a nightly basis, then developing solid sleep hygiene is the first place to start.

Sleep Hygiene

In the intricate song of sleep, certain habits and practices can act as unwanted instruments, disrupting the rhythm and harmony needed for a restorative night. The more we've come to know about how to get a good night's sleep, the more important "sleep hygiene" has become. Good sleep hygiene involves avoiding the conditions that we know impact a good night's sleep. But, you have to know what those things are first and once you know, then you can make informed decisions about how to ensure you get the best night's sleep you can possibly get.

Heavy Meals at Night

Eating heavy meals before bed is like ramping up a factory just before closing time; it forces your digestive system to work overtime when it should be winding down and paying overtime is expensive. While a large, hearty meal might leave you feeling content and maybe even a little bit sleepy, it can significantly disrupt your sleep quality, leading to a night of tossing and turning rather than restful slumber. When you consume a heavy meal late in the evening, your body is diverted from its primary nighttime function of rest and repair to focus on digestion. Digestion of a heavy meal can elevate your core body temperature, which is counterproductive for sleep. Our bodies are programmed to cool down as we prepare to sleep, and this cooling is essential for the onset of sleep. By raising your internal temperature, a heavy meal delays this process, akin to keeping a furnace running on a hot summer night.

Late-night eating can also lead to acid reflux, a condition where stomach acid flows back into the esophagus, causing a burning sensation and discomfort. Lying down shortly after eating can exacerbate this condition, as gravity no longer helps keep the stomach acid in place. This discomfort can wake you up multiple times during the night, preventing you from achieving deep, restorative sleep. Eating late at night also impacts the hormonal balance that regulates sleep.

Consuming a large meal can spike insulin levels and affect the production of melatonin, the hormone that signals to your body that it's time to sleep. The disruption of melatonin production can interfere with your circadian rhythm, the body's internal clock that dictates when you feel sleepy and when you are alert. This disruption creates a domino effect of less than ideal choices. Poor sleep quality leads to increased hunger and cravings for high-calorie foods the next day, potentially resulting in consuming foods that are processed or high in sugar and fat with little nutritional value. Who hasn't chased a cheeseburger and fries or a plate of chilaquiles after waking up hungover?

To minimize the impact of heavy meals—and all digestive functions on sleep, aim to finish eating **at least 3-4 hours before bedtime**. This allows your body to complete the majority of the digestive process before you lie down, reducing the likelihood of discomfort and sleep disruption. Opt for lighter, easier-to-digest foods in the evening, and save heavier meals for earlier in the day. There is an old adage, "eat breakfast like a king/queen, lunch like a prince/princess, and dinner like a pauper" that seems like a pretty good rule of thumb to guide your daily meal planning if you don't have a specific program you are already following. And as it turns out, there is even scientific evidence to support that this way of distributing calories throughout the day can result in increased weight loss (given you are in a caloric deficit, of course) when compared to a similar number of calories consumed in the opposite way (pauper, prince, king).

Alcohol

For me personally, understanding the negative impact of alcohol on my sleep was one of the single biggest discoveries in trying to improve and restore my quality of sleep. Alcohol is a trickster, offering a temporary sense of calm and relaxation, only to rob you of a peaceful night's rest once you've passed out. While it might initially help you fall asleep, alcohol significantly disrupts sleep patterns and reduces sleep quality, leading to a fragmented and unrefreshing sleep experience.

Alcohol acts as a central nervous system depressant, sedating you and helping you fall asleep faster. However, this sedation is not the same as natural sleep. Alcohol suppresses REM sleep, which is crucial for emotional regulation, memory consolidation, and overall mental health. REM sleep is often referred to as "dream sleep," and it is essential for cognitive processing and emotional resilience. The suppression of REM sleep can leave you feeling unrefreshed, despite having spent hours in bed. Moreover, alcohol fragments your sleep, causing you to wake up multiple times during the night as the body processes alcohol's metabolites, such as acetaldehyde. These micro-awakenings are often not remembered but prevent you from achieving deep, restorative sleep, reducing the overall quality of rest. This disruption sets off a vicious cycle. The lack of restorative sleep leaves you feeling tired and groggy the next day, which can lead to increased caffeine consumption as a "pick me up" in the morning and alcohol consumption as a means to unwind in the evening after what was undoubtedly a less than optimal day. This cycle of reliance on alcohol further impairs sleep quality and exacerbates daytime fatigue. Alcohol also exacerbates sleep disorders such as sleep apnea. Alcohol relaxes the muscles of the throat, increasing the likelihood of airway obstruction and apnea events. This not only fragments sleep but also decreases oxygen saturation in the blood, leading to more severe health consequences over time.

For those who enjoy a drink, it's crucial to time alcohol consumption wisely. To minimize its impact on sleep, **avoid alcohol at least 3-4 hours before bedtime**. I've come to adopt a little mantra that I use if I'm out and about enjoying adult beverages these days – "sun's down, cups down".

Giving yourself this window between your last drink and when you go to sleep allows your body to metabolize the alcohol and reduces its disruptive effects on sleep architecture. By moderating alcohol intake and timing it appropriately, you can enjoy its social benefits without significantly sacrificing the quality of your sleep. Understanding the effects of alcohol on our bodies, and making mindful choices can help break the cycle of disrupted sleep and reliance on alcohol, leading to better overall health and well-being.

Caffeine

Here's a big one. Caffeine is probably the world's most beloved stimulant. But, caffeine is a mischievous sprite, bestowing a burst of energy while secretly plotting to steal your precious slumber when your eyes are closed. Acting as a stimulant, caffeine blocks adenosine receptors in the brain, effectively delaying the onset of sleepiness. This might seem like a gift when the afternoon slump hits, but it becomes a curse as night approaches. What's important to understand is that the half-life of caffeine in your system is approximately 5 to 6 hours, meaning that half of the caffeine you consume lingers in your system well into the evening. This prolonged presence can be likened to leaving a light on in a dark room, disrupting the tranquility needed for restful sleep.

Caffeine significantly alters sleep architecture, reducing the amount of deep sleep you get each night. This deep sleep, or slow-wave sleep, is crucial for physical restoration and cognitive function. When you don't get enough deep sleep, you wake up feeling groggy even if you 'slept the entire night'. This disruption is akin to attempting to build a house on a shaky foundation; without deep sleep, the body's ability to restore itself on a nightly basis is compromised. Caffeine, consumed even six hours before bedtime, can reduce sleep by more than an hour. The stimulant effect of caffeine keeps your brain wired, preventing the natural process of winding down and leading to fragmented sleep. This continuous disruption not only affects sleep quality but also impacts overall health, increasing the risk of cardiovascular issues and metabolic disorders. The danger is how this cycle can become self-reinforcing, as poor sleep quality drives the need for more caffeine the following day. Imagine starting your day in a fog, struggling to stay awake, and reaching for a cup of coffee to kickstart your brain. This reliance on caffeine to combat sleep deprivation leads to further disruptions in sleep architecture, particularly in reducing REM sleep, which is essential for emotional regulation and memory consolidation. As a result, you wake up feeling groggy, perpetuating the cycle of caffeine dependence. Put alcohol and caffeine together and you've effectively eliminated the possibility for a good night's sleep with both REM sleep and deep sleep being fragmented.

For those who insist on indulging their caffeine fix, it's advisable to limit consumption to the morning hours, drink plenty of water (caffeine is a diuretic), and avoid it after 2 p.m. This timing ensures that most of the caffeine has been metabolized by bedtime, allowing adenosine to perform its natural function of promoting sleepiness. By respecting the powerful influence of this stimulant and breaking the cycle of dependence, you can enjoy its benefits without sacrificing the sanctity of your sleep. Prioritizing good sleep hygiene and managing caffeine intake are crucial steps toward restoring and maintaining a healthy sleep architecture. Personally, having been off caffeine for over a year now, I actually can't imagine being on the energetic yo-yo caffeine creates. I wake up refreshed and never look back, relying solely on my body to signal when it's time for rest again. If you are looking to kick the caffeine habit, I found it extremely helpful to "step down" slowly. I moved from lattes to cappuccinos to chai lattes and from chai lattes to decaffeinated tea. Reishi makes a fantastic turmeric ginger tea that explodes with flavor and has become my go-to warm morning wake-up beverage. I'm convinced that part of the caffeine addiction, like smoking, is the ritual. The brewing, the warm steamy liquid, the mug. There's no need to give up these important and comforting habits while filtering out the caffeine.

Cannabis

Cannabis, much like alcohol, is often used for its sedative effects. However, its overall impact on sleep quality is complex and multifaceted. Cannabis, like caffeine, is a double-edged sword, offering upfront benefits but potentially disrupting the deeper stages of sleep that are crucial for restorative rest.

THC: Dream Suppressor

THC (tetrahydrocannabinol), the primary psychoactive compound in cannabis, can help you fall asleep faster by inducing a sense of relaxation and drowsiness. However, this benefit comes at a cost. Studies have shown that THC reduces the latency to sleep onset but at the cost of REM sleep suppression. This suppression can lead to cognitive impairments and emotional instability due to the lack of restorative dream sleep. Although not technically addictive, the long-term use of THC can lead to dependence. When regular users discontinue cannabis use, they often experience a "rebound effect", where REM sleep returns with a vengeance, leading to vivid dreams or nightmares and overall disrupted sleep. This phenomenon is akin to a dam bursting, where the suppressed REM sleep floods back, causing an overwhelming and often distressing experience.

CBD: Calming Agent

On the other side of the cannabis spectrum is CBD (cannabidiol), a non-psychoactive compound known for its anxiolytic and calming properties. CBD is often touted for its potential to aid sleep onset by reducing anxiety and promoting relaxation. Unlike THC, CBD does not seem to suppress REM sleep, which is a positive aspect. CBD's anxiolytic properties have been supported by research indicating its potential to reduce anxiety and improve sleep onset. However, more research is needed to fully understand how CBD interacts with sleep stages over prolonged use. The use of cannabis for sleep is paradoxical. While it can help individuals fall asleep faster, the alteration of sleep architecture—particularly the reduction in REM sleep—can compromise overall sleep quality. This disruption can lead to a cycle of dependence, where the initial relief provided by cannabis use is offset by long-term disturbances in sleep patterns.

For those considering cannabis for sleep, it is essential to weigh these factors and consider the potential for dependence and sleep disruption. By understanding the nuances of cannabis's impact on sleep, you can make more informed decisions and seek alternative methods to improve sleep quality if needed. In the context of TMM, our recommendation would be to use THC or CBD as a last resort. That is, work on improving your sleep hygiene first–eliminate all the other factors that might be negatively impacting your sleep quality *before* taking an exogenous substance that will obscure the impact of other proven ways of improving your sleep.

Irregular Sleep Schedules

Your body operates on a circadian rhythm, an internal clock that thrives on regularity. Going to bed and waking up at different times each day is like changing time zones without ever leaving home; it confuses your internal clock and disrupts your sleep quality. Imagine trying to follow a schedule where your work hours change unpredictably every day. Your productivity and mood would likely suffer. The same principle applies to your sleep schedule. Inconsistent sleep patterns throw off your circadian rhythm, making it harder for your body to know when to feel sleepy and when to wake up. Maintaining a consistent sleep schedule anchors your circadian rhythm, aligning your body's internal processes with the natural environment. Whereas, an erratic schedule can lead to "social jetlag," a state where your body's internal clock is perpetually misaligned with your social obligations leading to chronic sleep deprivation and its associated health risks. To maintain a consistent sleep schedule, try to go to bed and wake up at the same time every day, *even on weekends*. This regularity helps stabilize your circadian rhythm, making it easier to fall asleep and wake up naturally, without the need for alarms or groggy mornings… or caffeine.

Circadian Rhythms

Interestingly, not everyone's circadian rhythm is the same. Some people are naturally "morning larks," who wake up early and are most alert in the morning, while others are "night owls," who prefer to stay up late and are most alert in the evening. This variation is influenced by genetics and is known as chronotype. Research by Till Roenneberg, a leading chronobiologist, suggests that these chronotypes are deeply embedded in our biology and affect how we function best at different times of the day.

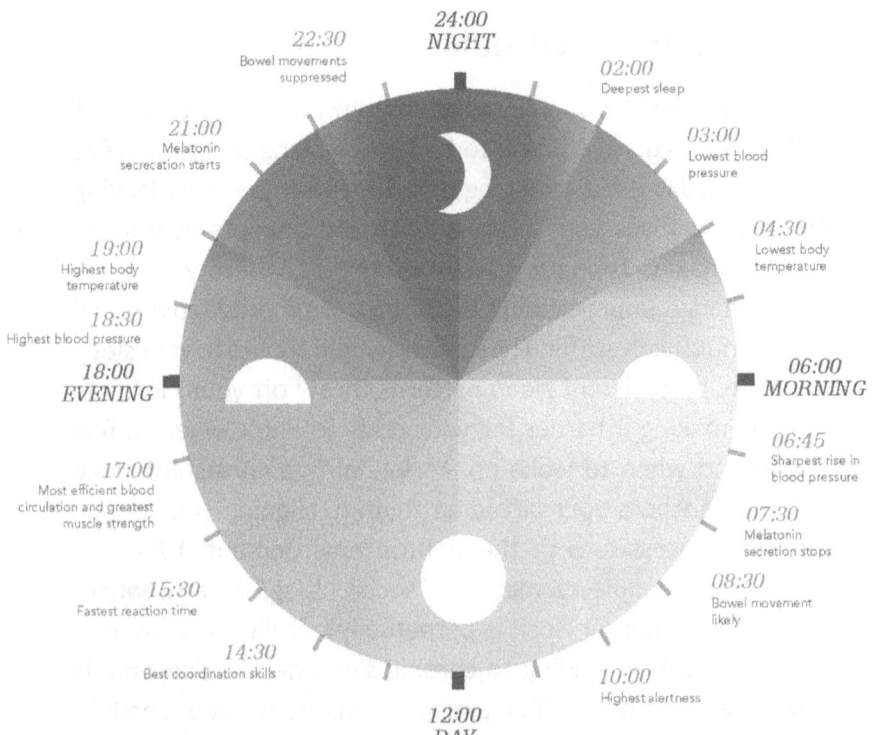

Morning larks and night owls each have their own optimal schedules. For morning larks, a consistent early bedtime and wake-up time align with their natural inclination, enhancing their sleep quality and daytime functioning. Conversely, night owls might struggle with traditional early morning schedules, leading to conditions of "social jetlag" when their natural sleep preferences are out of sync with societal expectations. Forcing people to conform to a standard 9-to-5 work schedule can be detrimental, particularly for those whose circadian rhythms do not align with these hours. Data indicates that insufficient sleep costs the U.S. economy up to $411 billion annually due to reduced productivity, increased absenteeism, and higher healthcare costs. By understanding and respecting your circadian rhythm and chronotype, you can optimize your sleep schedule and attack your waking hours with peak energy and focus. Regularity and alignment with your natural sleep patterns are key to achieving restful and restorative sleep. Restorative sleep is crucial for your body to function optimally. Cultivate awareness around your body's needs—notice if your current routine has you trapped in a cycle of dependence on other substances to stay alert or fall asleep—and start to (re)align your daily life to support the best version of you.

Lights at Night

In our modern society, artificial evening lights are ubiquitous. But, if you are having difficulty getting quality sleep and falling asleep in particular, then it's important to understand all the potential causes that might be impacting your body's natural sleep functions and artificial light at night can be one of those factors. Bright lights in the evening are a modern-day saboteur of sleep, stealthily disrupting the natural processes that prepare your body for rest. While blue light from screens often gets the most blame, it's essential to recognize that all bright lights, particularly those within the blue spectrum, can interfere with your sleep quality.

Imagine bright lights as an artificial sun, extending the day into the night and confusing your internal clock. This exposure can significantly delay the onset of sleep by interfering with melatonin production. Melatonin is the hormone responsible for signaling to your body that it's time to wind down. The brighter the light, the greater its impact on delaying sleep onset. This delay can reduce the amount of REM sleep, the critical stage for emotional regulation, memory consolidation, and cognitive function. Dimming lights in the evening and creating a low-light environment can help signal to your body that it's time to prepare for sleep. Blue light, specifically, is particularly potent in its ability to suppress melatonin. The screens of phones, tablets, computers, and TVs emit blue light that penetrates the eyes and signals the brain to stay awake.

One effective strategy is to implement a digital curfew by turning off all screens (including TV) **at least one hour before bedtime.** For those who need to use devices in the evening, utilizing blue light filters or the "night mode" setting can help minimize blue light emission. Changing the tint on your screens to reduce blue light can also be beneficial, but it's not a complete solution. While night mode or blue light filters on devices do reduce blue light exposure, the overall brightness and content you're engaging with also play roles in sleep disruption. Engaging in stimulating activities, like work or intense gaming, can keep your brain alert and delay sleep onset, regardless of the light emitted.

Dimming the lights in your home as the evening progresses can also signal to your body that it's time to wind down. Opt for lamps with warmer, dimmer bulbs instead of bright overhead lights to create a more sleep-friendly environment. Engaging in a low-light bedtime routine, such as reading a book with a soft, amber light or taking a warm bath with candles, can help prepare your body for sleep without the stimulating effects of bright lights. Furthermore, using warm-colored lights (yellow, orange, red) in the evening is less likely to interfere with melatonin production compared to cool-colored lights (blue, white). By being mindful of these triggers, you can better navigate the challenges posed by artificial evening lights and signal to your body when it's time to rest.

Just as darkness signals to our brains and bodies that it's time for rest, Exposure to morning sunlight is essential for signalling that its time to fire up the engines again for another day. Natural light early in the day boosts mood, focus, and energy levels by triggering a healthy increase in cortisol, a hormone that enhances wakefulness and immune function. It also helps synchronize the body's internal clock, improving sleep quality and metabolic health. Morning sunlight reduces residual melatonin, promoting alertness and reducing sleepiness (and the need for caffeine!). Consistent exposure to morning sunlight is linked to better overall health and enhanced mental and physical performance. Even on cloudy days, the benefits remain significant, though extended exposure may be necessary to compensate for reduced light intensity.

Lights, Temperature, Action!

Creating the right sleep environment plays a crucial role in the quality of rest we achieve each night but it's not limited to dimming the lights before bedtime. One of the most important factors is the *light in the bedroom itself.* Our bodies are deeply attuned to natural light cycles through the regulation of our circadian rhythm. Exposure to any kind of light before or during sleep—whether from street lamps outside or the small glowing LEDs on electronics in the bedroom—can disrupt the body's natural production of melatonin, the hormone responsible for making us feel sleepy. A truly dark room signals to the brain that it's time for rest. Blocking out all sources of light, from heavy curtains or blackout blinds to covering electronics, helps maintain this natural balance. Even seemingly insignificant lights, like those from alarm clocks or charging devices, can subtly disrupt sleep quality over time. Equally important is temperature. The ideal room temperature for sleep typically falls between **60 to 67°F (15 to 19°C)**. Our body's core temperature naturally drops during sleep, and a cool environment facilitates this process, promoting deeper, more restorative sleep. Overheating can lead to restlessness and frequent awakenings, as the body struggles to maintain an optimal temperature. Investing in breathable bedclothes (or foregoing them altogether!) and lightweight sheets made from natural fibers like cotton or linen can also help regulate temperature, keeping the body cool throughout the night.

Understanding Insomnia

I had always been an incredibly sound sleeper, able to fall asleep almost anywhere at a moment's notice and wake up the next morning refreshed and bounding with energy. Then something started happening in my gut (although I didn't realize it at the time) and I began tossing and turning all night, having terrible nightmares. These symptoms persisted and became more acute to the point that I basically didn't sleep more than 1-2 hours a night for the better part of 4 years. I went from loving sleep to dreading getting in bed knowing that another 6-7 hrs of torture awaited me.

Deep dark bags developed under my eyes, big holes started showing up in my memory and I lost muscle mass. There were many interrelated factors that caused my insomnia and they are largely the reason I wrote this book—the journey to solve my insomnia led me down many different pathways of healing imbalances and inflammation that had developed over time but it was insomnia as a leading symptom that was the tip of the investigative spear. If you are suffering from insomnia, I feel for you. I know your pain and frustration and while there are many different reasons why people suffer from insomnia, it is my sincere hope that by traveling the path laid out by this program, you will be able to eliminate or greatly reduce many of the contributing factors which will help you to narrow down the root cause.

Insomnia is more than just the occasional sleepless night; it's a chronic condition that can severely impact your quality of life. Defined as the persistent difficulty in falling asleep, staying asleep, or achieving restorative sleep despite adequate opportunity, insomnia can lead to significant daytime impairment. Imagine your brain as a computer that can't shut down, continuously processing worries and fears. High levels of cortisol, the stress hormone, can make it difficult to relax and fall asleep. A racing mind filled with anxiety prevents the transition from wakefulness to sleep, keeping the body in a heightened state of alertness, further disrupting sleep.

Medical conditions and medications can also play a critical role in insomnia. Chronic pain, gastrointestinal problems, or hormonal imbalances can be formidable barriers to sleep. Certain medications have side effects that disrupt sleep, creating a vicious cycle of sleeplessness and discomfort. Addressing these underlying health issues with a healthcare provider is crucial. Psychological conditions such as depression and anxiety are both causes and symptoms of insomnia. Sleep disturbances exacerbate these mental health issues, creating a feedback loop of sleeplessness and psychological distress. Additionally, genetic predisposition can mean that some individuals are naturally more susceptible to insomnia, much like a hereditary trait passed down through generations. This genetic component can make insomnia a particularly significant challenge to overcome.

If you find yourself struggling with insomnia despite good sleep hygiene and other lifestyle adjustments, we strongly recommend seeking professional help. A sleep specialist can provide a thorough diagnosis and tailor a treatment plan to address the specific causes of your insomnia, helping you achieve the restorative sleep you need and deserve.

The Art of Napping

Napping offers a myriad of benefits that extend far beyond just catching up on lost sleep. Studies have shown that naps can significantly improve learning, memory, and emotional regulation. For instance, a 90-minute nap can enhance learning capacity and help overcome the post-lunch dip in alertness, making it an effective strategy for sustaining productivity throughout the day. The Fatigue Countermeasures Program, in which NASA studied the effects of naps on pilot and astronaut performance, found that a 40-minute nap improved performance by 34% and alertness by 100%. Additionally, naps can reset emotional responses, reducing sensitivity to negative emotions like fear and anger, and enhancing positive emotional reactions. From a physiological perspective, napping can lower blood pressure and improve cardiovascular health. Regular short naps have been associated with better immune function and reduced stress levels, making them a valuable addition to a healthy lifestyle.

Nap length is crucial to reaping its benefits without experiencing the downsides. The ideal duration for a nap clocks in right around 20 minutes. This duration is long enough to enhance alertness and concentration but short enough to avoid sleep inertia, the grogginess that can occur when waking from a deeper sleep stage. For those who have more time and can afford a longer nap, a full 90-minute nap can be beneficial as it allows for a complete sleep cycle, including REM sleep, which can improve memory and emotional regulation.

Timing is everything when it comes to effective napping. The best time to nap is generally in the early afternoon, typically between 1 PM and 3 PM (assuming you are a daytime oriented person). This timing aligns with the body's natural circadian rhythm, which includes a dip in alertness during the early afternoon. Napping too late in the day, however, can interfere with nighttime sleep by reducing sleep pressure—the build-up of adenosine that creates the feeling of sleepiness.

A Note on Sleep Tracking

To track or not to track, that is the question. And I don't know if there is a right or wrong answer. If you are chronically not sleeping well though, I'd say you don't need a sleep tracker to tell you what you already know. Waking up groggy and not feeling refreshed to a digitized score that confirms you aren't well-rested creates a negative feedback loop that can lead to incremental and unnecessary anxiety. Personally, I don't use a sleep tracker. I did for a while and it gave me said anxiety about trying to reach a certain score each night only to come up short no matter what I did, over and over again because I hadn't yet addressed the root cause issues of why I wasn't sleeping well (in my gut). Beyond that, I'm not a proponent of electronics in and around my body while I'm sleeping, however small they may be. Having said that, they can be a valuable tool to quantify and confirm how changes to diet, alcohol consumption, cannabis intake, or improvements to sleep hygiene are impacting your sleep. Certainly, some people find motivation in the gamification aspect, trying to improve their scores night after night. If that's you, then by all means, invest in a tracker and dance with the data. The technology is at the point where you will get fairly accurate readings and meaningful information if that's your thing. But try not to rely on gadgetry to tell you what you already know intuitively. That is how we become disconnected from ourselves in the modern world. How you feel when you wake up (Am I refreshed? Do I feel rested? If not, why not?) is the best tracker you can use and you don't need an app for that.

Guarding the Sanctity of Sleep

Sleep is not a luxury; it's a necessity, a sacred process, essential for your physical and mental well-being. Sleep is the very fuel that keeps your brain and body running smoothly. From cognitive function to emotional stability and physical health, every aspect of your being relies on quality sleep. Without it, you're not just running on empty—you're heading towards a breakdown.

As you navigate the path to better sleep, remember that sleep is an active and dynamic process that rejuvenates and restores your body and mind. By understanding and avoiding detrimental habits and practices, you can protect and enhance the quality of your sleep. Whether it's limiting alcohol consumption, avoiding heavy meals before bed, reducing screen time, maintaining a consistent sleep schedule, or being mindful of cannabis use, each small 1° of change contributes to moving closer to a healthier, more restful night.

Putting it all together: Building Quality Sleep Habits

In the introduction we talked a bit about the idea of providing scaling options to 'meet you where you are'. For every pillar, we have created levels or scaling options that are designed to allow you to assess where you are and begin taking action. If you need to start at the beginning, great, Level 1 provides options for you to start shifting 1° towards a new horizon. If you have some experience and awareness, Level 2 has options that can challenge you to move forward from there and if you consider yourself a subject matter expert, Level 3 is where you might choose to begin. Wherever you choose to engage, we recommend you look at the previous levels with "a beginner's mind" and see if there are options or recommendations you haven't previously considered. This is your journey and no one is watching (although we're here to support you) so there is no shame in starting wherever you feel most appropriate or even backtracking to re-establish good habits and build from there.

Level 1: Good Sleep Hygiene

- **Consistent Schedule:** Go to bed and wake up at the same time daily to ensure 7-9 hours of sleep per night. *Even on the weekends.*
- **Practice the 3-2-1 rule: 3hrs** before bed - **no food / 2hrs** before bed - **no liquid / 1 hr** before bed - **no screens**
- **Sleep Environment:** Create a dark, quiet, and cool (around 65°F or 18°C) sleeping area.
  - Ear plugs / White Noise
  - Face mask / Blackout shades
  - Cotton bedding
- **Morning Light Exposure:** Get 5-15 minutes of sunlight on your (closed) eyes and skin within the first hour of waking up *every day* to help reset your circadian rhythm

Level 2: Eliminating Detrimental Factors

- **Pre-sleep routine:** Habitually signal to your body that it's time to wind down
  - Practice activities like reading, taking a warm bath, or practicing meditation.
  - Lower bright overhead lights after sunset
- **Limit Stimulants:** Avoid caffeine and nicotine in the hours leading up to bedtime.
- **Eliminate Alcohol:** 4-6hrs before bedtime, aka 'sun's down/cups down'
- **Eliminate THC:** 4-6hrs before bedtime
- **Physical Activity:** Incorporate regular exercise into your routine, but not too close to bedtime.

Level 3: Good Sleep above All Else

- **Behavior Adjustments:**
    - Practice eating meals like a King/Prince/Pauper throughout the day
    - Avoid alcohol consumption, especially in the evening.
    - Eliminate Caffeine
- **Sleep Tracking:** Use a sleep tracker to monitor how changes are impacting your sleep quality.
- **Professional Help:** Seek help from a sleep specialist if experiencing persistent sleep problems or disorders.

Sleep - subscribepage.io/sleepresources

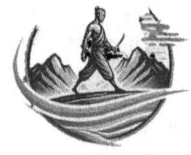

MEDITATION

CORNERSTONE OF AN ELEVATED LIFE

By choosing to walk this path, you are embarking on a journey where each step you take enhances your well-being, a path where each small change contributes to a larger more complete transformation. The practice of meditation is a fractal of this larger journey. Far from being just a stress-relief tool or another 'woo-woo' buzzword, meditation is a practice that can profoundly change our brains, improve our lives, and help elevate our experience of existence.

Meditation is one of the cornerstone practices of TMM because by cultivating this practice you will naturally increase your capacity for self-awareness. Self-awareness is a fundamental skill we are trying to develop with the TMM program across a number of dimensions. For thousands of years schools of meditation throughout the world have touted the notion that consistent practice leads to the development of a stronger sense of self-awareness. Even just 5 minutes of daily meditation, when done consistently, over time, will yield significant benefits. This single degree of improvement can ripple out to elevate almost every aspect of your life, making you more mindful, compassionate, effective, and aware. And practicing it couldn't be more simple; it literally costs nothing, other than a fraction of your day, requires no physical skills or equipment other than a small amount of space, and your own internal dedication to practicing.

With the rise of social media and the short attention span culture, we live in a world that is increasingly single-use, shallow, and disposable. We are constantly distracted by fads and trends—music, diets, clothing, ways of speaking, dating apps, TV shows, hairstyles, dance challenges, cars, the list goes on forever. As something that has been part of the human experience dating back thousands of years, it's safe to say that meditation is more than just a passing fad, it's a practice that has transcended time and culture. From as far back as there are records, meditation has illuminated a path to deeper emotional balance and mental clarity. At its core, meditation is about cultivating mindfulness—a state of present-moment awareness that is both focused and non-judgmental. This awareness allows us to observe our thoughts, emotions, and sensations in the body as they arise, providing insight into the workings of our mind and fostering a sense of peace and equanimity. If you took nothing else from this entire program, sitting in quiet contemplation for five or ten minutes a day would be that thing that would yield the most lasting and long term impact on your well-being.

What is Meditation?

Meditation teaches us to be fully present in the moment. It is a practice of being in the here and now, fully engaged with whatever we are doing. This presence allows us to experience life more deeply and authentically, free from (or probably more accurately) *aware of* our inner monologue that anticipates what's going to happen next as a function of experiencing what has happened in the past. The concept of "being present in the moment" at its core, involves fully engaging with and experiencing what is happening now without distraction from preconceived ideas, past memories, or future anxieties. This state of awareness is embodied by a heightened sense of reality, where one's focus is entirely on what is happening in this instant, allowing for a deeper connection with oneself and the world—in the modern day optimization movement, this is often referred to as being in a "flow state".

Mushin (無心)

Mushin translates to "no mind" or "empty mind" and is Zen concept frequently referenced in martial arts. It refers to a state of mental clarity where the mind is free from distractions, fear, and ego-fully present and responsive. In the context of the Modern Monk, Mushin represents the goal of training the mind to reach a state of flow, where actions are performed naturally and effortlessly without overthinking. Whether in meditation, physical practice or creative endeavors, Mushin is the cultivation of mindfulness and presence, allowing for optimal performance and a calm, centered approach to life's challenges.

Philosophically, the notion that the past and future do not exist in the present moment is rooted in the understanding of time and consciousness. The past is a collection of memories—events that have already occurred and are stored in our minds. These memories can shape our perceptions and influence our emotions, but they have no tangible bearing on the present. Similarly, the future is a realm of possibilities and projections, consisting of events that have not yet occurred. The future literally exists only as a sense of anticipation around events in our minds that have yet to actually take place. The present moment is the only time that can be experienced directly. The ancient Greek philosopher Heraclitus famously stated, "You cannot step into the same river twice," and I believe there is similar wisdom in Indian traditions regarding the Ganges river. We are not the same person who experiences the river each time we step into it nor is the river, in a constant state of flow and change, the same body of water we engaged with before.

Meditation provides a means to explore and become aware of how our minds, our thoughts, and our emotions influence our experience of reality. By observing our thoughts, and feelings without attachment, by "letting go", we can begin to understand that our sense of self is not as solid or as permanent as we might believe it to be. Our sense of self is more like the river, constantly moving and changing and meditation can help us become aware of how we are experiencing the flow of our river in any given moment. At a fundamental level, meditation offers an awareness of how we react to the way life unfolds. And at its most sublime, we can experience moments of transcendence, where the boundaries of the self dissolve completely, leading to a sense of unity and interconnectedness with all life.

Body-Centered Awareness

Connecting deeply with the body is a fundamental aspect of meditation and also to the TMM program as a whole. The body holds inherent wisdom and information that can be accessed through meditation. By focusing on bodily sensations and the breath, we can ground ourselves in the present moment and experience a profound state of being that transcends mental constructs—the patterns of thoughts, beliefs, and narratives that our minds create to bring structure to our perception of reality. While these constructs can be useful in navigating day-to-day social interactions, they often disconnect us from our direct experience of the present moment and our true selves. Think back to the last time you drove home from work. What color were any of the cars around you? How many dogs did you see? How many children? Can you remember the faces of anyone you noticed? Chances are, you don't remember any of those details because your mind was not in the present moment but somewhere else–possibly replaying a past memory or anticipating an interaction you planned to have later that day. Regardless of what it was that captured your attention, it was some kind of "signal noise", a construct that took you out of present moment awareness. Persistent self-criticism, future anxieties, past regrets, social comparisons, and rigid beliefs are just some of the mental constructs that create "signal noise" and interfere with our awareness. These constructs overshadow our intuition, cause unnecessary stress, trap us in cycles of guilt, create feelings of inadequacy, and limit our adaptability, all of which compromise our capacity to listen to our bodies and frequently to those around us as well.

The body possesses an innate wisdom that, when accessed, can guide us toward making better choices in a number of different ways. "Gut Feelings" or instincts are a great example of our bodies sending us information about our external environment. We've all had an experience of meeting someone for the first time and, for no obvious reason, feeling an instant connection or, on the flip side, an unease you can't quite put into words. In the fast pace of daily life, we often brush these feelings aside, focusing on the task at hand, the next action item, or the problem that needs to be solved. But if we take a moment to slow down and be more present with ourselves, we can better take these signals into greater account. Our bodies pick up on subtle cues—tone of voice, body language, or even energy—that our minds may not immediately bring to conscious awareness. By becoming more attuned to these sensations, we can make better decisions, trust our instincts, and avoid situations or people that may not be aligned with our best interests. This awareness often leads to greater confidence and helps us navigate life with a deeper sense of clarity. Another way to tap into your body's wisdom is known as intuitive eating. Since everyone's body is unique, with a different gut microbiome and different sets of bacteria, nobody knows better than your body what foods are best for it. It's purely speculative for someone to tell you that by eating certain foods you will be 'healthy' or that eating certain other foods will help you 'lose weight'. We are all different by intelligent design and thus have different needs. Intuitive eating means paying attention to how different foods make us feel and how our body reacts to them, learning to discern which ones nourish us and which ones deplete our energy, ultimately creating our own personalized playbook for promoting physical health and well-being. In some ways, we are already intuitive eaters—think about cravings. Where do cravings come from? They are effectively our bodies' gut microbiome signaling the brain to give it more of something that it's either lacking (e.g., craving a steak is likely signaling an iron deficiency) or that it wants more of (sweet tooth, anyone?). These are basic examples but with practice, we can begin to feel how the morsel of food we consume is making us feel or what our bodies are trying to tell us they need. However, before we can do that effectively, it's important to learn to quiet the incessant chatter of the mind (known in meditation circles as the 'monkey mind') and practice tuning into our bodies and the messages it is sending us.

As human beings, we are a contained energy system (the body) moving through a larger energy system (nature) connecting everything on the planet and beyond (the universe). When we become cognizant of the interplay between these energy systems, there is a vast amount of information to access about how to move within these systems in greater harmony. Unfortunately in the hyperactive and distracted states of mind most of us spend our time in (which is by design in an economy based on consumption), it is very easy to overlook or bypass.

Being present with our bodily sensations can also heighten our sensitivity to the emotions and experiences of others, fostering empathy and compassion. When we talk about someone's "vibe" what we are really speaking about is the quality of the energy that they give off and that we are picking up. Recall a time when you walked into a party and were immediately hit with a palpable sense of excitement and joy or when you worked out in a group or with a team and you had 'extra energy' to work harder. Whether you realize it or not, in these scenarios, you are tapping into the collective field generated by the group. This works both as an external and internal source of information. By developing a meditation practice that helps us build awareness of our own emotional state, we can also begin to expand our awareness to emotional states of those around us, which in turn allows us to connect with others on a deeper level. As we become more attuned to our own emotions, we can better understand and support others, even when there is not a strong collective field being generated.

We all generate a field (aura) that reflects our emotional state of being. Grounding ourselves in the body helps us become more aware of that field and manage our emotions more effectively. By observing the emotions arising within us we can address them before they escalate, leading to greater emotional resilience and stability. Regularly connecting with our bodies sharpens our intuitive abilities, allowing us to sense subtle shifts in our environment and relationships and enabling us to respond with greater wisdom and insight, with thoughtfulness rather than blind reactivity. By observing our thoughts and emotions without judgment, we also cultivate a sense of self-compassion and understanding. Knowing the source of your feelings and emotions empowers you to release behind the bondage that comes in believing that external events "make" us feel a certain way. With meditation you gain the wherewithal and the discernment to maintain sovereign and creative control of your own experience; that is, you can choose how you feel in any given moment and nothing—no person or circumstance has the power to dictate your emotional response. This empowerment allows us to face our fears and anxieties with greater acceptance and creates a level of awareness within us that can help us overcome or "dial down" those fears and anxieties in the moment, allowing the best version of ourselves to emerge even under pressure.

The practice of meditation at the most basic level, involves embracing silence and stillness. By first identifying or witnessing our own incessant mental chatter, we begin to separate our 'awareness' or consciousness–the thing that is observing the noise from the noise or chatter itself. Once we can see there are levels to our awareness, that there is an observer present, we can release the chatter—anxiety about an upcoming meeting, plans we've made, work stress, unpleasant memories—and let it drift along like clouds across the sky, returning our awareness once again to a place of stillness and inner quiet. In these moments, we can connect with the deeper reality of our existence. This stillness and silence provide a sanctuary for the mind, where true peace and insight can emerge. And eventually, this is an awareness that we "take with us" into everyday life. It is not relegated to the time and place where we practice meditation. Rather our meditation becomes the place we practice building the muscle of awareness and every day, we head into the world with that muscle stronger than the day before and by extension 1° closer to catching an emotional flare-up or an unconscious reaction in the moment.

There is something subtle but very powerful about having the capacity to "catch oneself" and step back from *automatic reaction* in favor of *thoughtful response*. By way of personal observation, I have been meditating fairly regularly for over ten years now but there are times when my practice falls off and I convince myself I am "too busy" one day and then another and before I know it, it's been a few weeks since I sat and meditated. And then, without fail, every single time I come back to it within days of restarting my practice I am stunned by how much easier life seems to be. How the intrusive and debilitating thoughts in my head seem to disappear or 'pass on by', how much easier it is to eat well, to exercise regularly, to stay focused, to remain calm in stressful situations, and how much more easily I seem to find and drop into a creative flow state. I have also kept a journal—for longer than I have been meditating and sometimes I have to laugh at myself because I've noticed more than once that I've written almost the same entry verbatim in those few days after resuming a regular meditation practice.

9/19 - Back in the Saddle

I wonder how many times I've made this observation through the years: when I'm consistent in my daily meditation practice (~20min/day) every aspect of my life improves demonstrably. I am more focused, more motivated, more consistent, my penmanship improves, my sleep becomes deeper, and my connection with the energetic flow of the universe increases such that new opportunities appear, unexpected allies emerge, and the path forward becomes unmistakably clear. Practicing is like training a muscle, an ability to surrender - to let go of having to 'know' what comes next and instead trust that whatever comes, I will have the capacity and the calm to choose, in that momentt of arrival, what is best for me. Put simply, meditation creates or cultivates ease and continuity in my life like no other practice I've ever encountered

Meditation cultivates insight and wisdom by revealing the transient nature of thoughts, emotions, and sensations. By observing these phenomena with mindfulness, we can develop a deeper understanding of the true nature of reality—that is, that *we are in control of how we choose to react to any given situation.* There is the instinctual reaction—the sense of injustice or unfairness or not being heard or impatience or whatever triggered emotion emerges trying to hijack the mind with an immediate response—but with a bit of presence, a bit of self-awareness, we can step back and decide how we want to react, to consider the situation, the other person, and what course of action might yield the best results for everyone involved. This level of insight and awareness helps us navigate life with greater clarity and purpose, making informed decisions and responding to challenges with wisdom rather than with blind, raw emotion. But this isn't limited to confrontation or conflict. Cultivating compassion and goodwill enhances our happiness and strengthens our relationships, leading to a more connected and joyful life. A study in *The Journal of Positive Psychology* found that loving-kindness meditation increases positive emotions and overall life satisfaction. This type of awareness becomes extremely valuable as we simply observe our own behaviors and patterns. We can become aware of certain habits around food or patterns of procrastination or nervous tendencies in moments of social anxiety where the only interactions we are having are with ourselves and our internal monologue. With meditation we can begin to separate our experience of reality from the patterns and habituated behaviors we've all developed along the way in some form or another to take a more active role in *choosing* how we want to be in any given present moment. Even becoming 1° more aware of ourselves, catching ourselves once each day in 'reactive mode', day over day will lead to a stronger ability to witness and choose how we experience reality.

Meditation is not just a practice confined to a specific time or place; it is about integrating mindfulness into every aspect of daily life. We may train in a specific place, the same way we train our muscles in a gym but our awareness travels with us everywhere we go and so does our practice.

Practicing mindfulness in everyday activities, while walking, eating, washing dishes, and even breathing, helps maintain a continuous state of awareness. This integration makes mindfulness a part of our daily routine, enhancing the quality of our lives and fostering a deeper connection with the present moment.

> "Being aware of your breath forces you into the present moment—the key to all inner transformation. Whenever you are conscious of the breath, you are absolutely present. You may notice that you cannot think and be aware of your breathing. Conscious breathing stops your mind. But far from being in a trance or half asleep, you are fully awake and highly alert. You are not falling below thinking, but rising above it. And if you look more closely, you will find that those two things—coming fully into the present moment and ceasing thinking without loss of consciousness—are actually one and the same: the arising of space consciousness."
>
> - Eckhart Tolle (A New Earth)

The Benefits of Meditation

Meditation activates the body's relaxation response, which counteracts the stress response and lowers cortisol levels. This reduction in stress hormones leads to a calmer state of mind and reduced physical tension, helping to navigate daily challenges with greater ease.

Developing greater emotional resilience is essential for self-actualization. By approaching our inner experiences with kindness and patience, we build emotional stability. Meditation sharpens the mind by training it to stay present. This heightened focus and cognitive clarity improve attention span and concentration, making it easier to engage fully in tasks and avoid hasty decisions made in emotionally charged states of mind.

How Meditation Changes the Brain

If sleep is your nightly librarian, meditation is your mental gardener tending to the mind's landscape. Scientific studies have shown that regular meditation practice can lead to measurable structural changes in the brain. A study in *Psychiatry Research: Neuroimaging* found that meditation increases gray matter density in the hippocampus, which is crucial for memory and learning. It also enhances the connections between different brain regions, promoting better communication and cognitive function. Additionally, it helps counteract the age-related shrinkage (shrinkage!) of the prefrontal cortex, which is essential for attention and decision-making. These changes not only boost mental clarity but also provide long-term protection against cognitive decline. This neuroplasticity demonstrates the profound impact meditation can have on our overall mental framework. Building a meditation practice is like setting out on an adventurous journey. It requires patience, dedication, and a willingness to explore the unknown. But the rewards—a calmer mind, a more compassionate heart, and a bigger brain—are well worth the effort. So, take a deep breath, embrace the journey, and discover how meditation can elevate your life.

How to Start Meditating

At the most fundamental level, all you need to begin your practice is a quiet, comfortable space to minimize distractions and a cushion or chair. You don't need to be able to sit in any kind of special posture, wear any specific clothing, or chant any particular mantra (although those are all things that can support your practice). Understanding your intention, such as reducing stress or improving focus, can help provide motivation and direction but your willingness to sit quietly with your eyes closed for a few minutes is all you really need.

For absolute beginners, guided meditations available on almost all of the most popular apps can offer structured sessions to get started. Focus on your breath and practice mindfulness by paying attention to the present moment without judgment. Patience is key, as meditation is a skill developed over time. Accept your thoughts and feelings without judgment, practice watching them come and go like clouds floating across the sky, recognizing that the goal is to observe the mind rather than empty it.

4-7-8 Breathing

The 4-7-8 breathing technique, developed by Dr. Andrew Weil, is a powerful relaxation method designed to manage stress, anxiety, and promote relaxation by following a specific breathing pattern: inhaling for 4 seconds, holding the breath for 7 seconds, and exhaling for 8 seconds. This technique is beneficial because it activates the parasympathetic nervous system, which is responsible for the body's "rest and digest" functions, helping to counteract the effects of the sympathetic nervous system, or the "fight or flight" response. By promoting relaxation, 4-7-8 breathing can reduce anxiety, improve focus, and help with concentration, redirecting attention from stressors to a calmer state of mind. If you have trouble falling asleep at night, 4-7-8 Breathing is a great technique for calming the mind and body, easing the transition into a restful state, and lowering heart rate and blood pressure through controlled breathing, which improves oxygenation and lung capacity.

To practice 4-7-8 breathing, find a comfortable position and begin by inhaling quietly through your nose for a count of four, holding your breath for seven seconds, and then exhaling completely through your mouth for a count of eight. This pattern should be repeated for at least four cycles, but build the practice over time. Start with a few cycles once a day. As you become more proficient, add cycles. gradually increasing to eight cycles per sitting as you become more comfortable with the technique. After a few weeks, if you feel a noticeable sense of calm after completing all 8 cycles, consider practicing this breathing method twice daily-first thing in the morning to set a calm tone for the day and again before bed to promote sleep.

Putting it all Together: Building Your Meditation Practice

Because we are walking forward on a path, our location on that path is constantly going to change—remember we're aiming for the Sun here! Throughout your journey, it's critical that you reflect on your progress regularly, noting changes in stress levels, focus, and overall well-being, and be open to adjusting your practice as needed. Initially, it may be finding the right guided meditation, the right duration that fits with your schedule, or maybe finding the best time of day for you to practice regularly. Give yourself the space and have the patience to find what works for you but above all, remain consistent. It's truly astonishing how quickly you will establish a strong and effective meditation practice that enhances your mental and physical well-being starting with just 5 minutes a day.

Level 1: Building the Habit

- **Start Small:** Begin with 5 minutes a day. Sit comfortably in a quiet space, close your eyes, and focus on your breath.
- **Set a Routine:** Meditate at the same time each day to build a consistent habit. Ideally, this is in the morning after you get up (**Pro Tip:** combine with morning sunlight exposure) but before you've picked up your phone to start scrolling through emails and social media.
- **Use Guided Meditations:** There's no need to 'fly blind' into the depths of your consciousness. We've listed some of the more popular meditation apps in the additional resource section. All of them have great (and free) beginner's paths

Level 2: Enjoy the Silence

- **Increase Duration:** Gradually extend your meditation sessions to 10-20 minutes daily.
- **Explore Different Techniques:** Try body scans, loving-kindness meditations, walking meditations or mindfulness of thoughts.

Level 3: A Deeper Unfolding

- **Increase Duration or Frequency:** Aim for 30-45 minutes of meditation daily either in a single session or two sessions, morning and evening.
- **Retreats and Workshops:** Attend a meditation retreat (like Vipassana - 10 day silent retreat) to deepen your practice and learn from experienced teachers.
- **Share the Gift:** Sharing the benefits of a meditation practice can deepen your understanding and commitment and create a ripple effect in building a more mindful, self-aware world.

Meditation - subscribepage.io/meditationresources

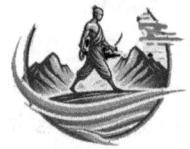

NUTRITION

FUEL FOR THE MEAT-SUIT

Our "meat-suits", the physical vessels we've all been gifted to hold our consciousness during this grand adventure called life, are actually intricate, highly complex machines that function across multiple systems working in concert to create a (mostly) smooth way to travel through life. But just as a high-performance vehicle requires the right kind of fuel to operate efficiently, our bodies need the same kind of high-performance nutrition to function optimally. Nutrition is much more than satisfying the feeling of hunger and once we begin to fully grasp what high quality nutrient dense food really means, it becomes clear that food is not really about pleasure either. In total transparency, I'm absolutely a 'foodie' and love nothing more than to sit down to a delicious multi-course extravaganza for the senses, but I've come to understand that eating to nourish the body and eating for experience are two very different activities with different purposes. Proper nutrition is about supplying the body with the necessary components to achieve peak physical and mental performance while keeping the body flush with the vitamins, amino acids, and nutrients it needs to feed muscles, actively repair itself, and simultaneously ward off diseases. That kind of multifaceted work requires energy and resources that we are responsible for supplying.

We have to begin to see our bodies as the essential equipment that enables us to interact with the world, pursue our goals, and experience life. As it is with all essential and valuable equipment, we need to take care of it and maintain it, even as we put it to continuous use. Think about wild animals in nature... they live to their last breath in a body that is nearly indistinguishable from that of their youth. Animals maintain their vitality and their ability to run, jump, fly, and hunt right up until the time they expire. The bear doesn't stop roaming the forest for the last few years of its life sitting around in a bear nursing home. It's in a state of vitality up until the last breath. And there's no reason why we as a species should be any different. By being intentional with how we nourish these bodies, our meat-suits, we begin to understand that vitality is a sense and a sensory experience of harmony within our own finite bodies, and in maintaining that harmony, we find the ability to live our lives much more vigorously and much more completely regardless of how many breaths we've been given.

With this in mind, the importance of nutrition in achieving optimal performance cannot be overstated. Nutrients are the building blocks of our body, supporting everything from cellular repair to energy production. Macronutrients, consisting of proteins, fats, and carbohydrates, provide the energy needed for daily activities and bodily functions, and micronutrients like vitamins, amino acids, and minerals are crucial for maintaining metabolic processes, immune function, and overall health.

While there is plenty of room for enjoying the sensual pleasures of an elegant meal, one of the goals of this program is to shift your paradigm of thinking around food from eating to satiate an urge or a craving to eating with absolute purpose. This doesn't mean your food has to be bland or without variety, but almost every bite should have some intrinsic nutritional value.

We'll get into meal planning in the second section on Nutrition when we discuss creating meals with specific macronutrients in mind. For now, we are going to focus on food quality as a way of ensuring the food we do eat has high nutritional value. In order to make quality meals, we first need to understand how to identify the optimal building blocks–what has the most nutritional bang for the buck. The reason being, nutritional deficiencies can lead to a host of health issues, impacting various bodily functions and the fact is that the modern American diet (based on the very outdated food pyramid, now called 'my plate') is largely devoid of nutrient dense foods and worse, often contains trans fats, seed oils, dyes, chemicals, and preservatives that are toxic and harmful rather than nourishing and energizing.

Food Quality Matters

At the most basic level, consuming lean proteins, healthy fats, fruits, and some vegetables ensures that the body receives a balanced array of essential nutrients. Proper nutrition supports focus, memory, and overall mental clarity, which are all essential for both personal and professional success. We keep coming back to the ideas of mental clarity, focus, and aspects of our experience that at first glance may not seem like they have anything to do with food, but the systems of the body from the gut to the brain are completely interrelated and it's not uncommon to experience a decline in mental acuity due directly to the consumption of foods that are disrupting your gut microbiome. These are the types of signals we want you to tune into and rather than reach for Advil or another cup of coffee to suppress that signal or artificially boost your energy, understand that your body may be telling you that the fuel you're putting in your body isn't premium and your internal engine doesn't thrive on burning it. The information provided in this chapter draws on the latest research, personal experience, and expert insights to help you make dietary choices that put you on a new course for a level of well-being and longevity a few degrees in a new direction.

To truly elevate one's nutrition, it is imperative to understand and prioritize food quality. High-quality food is typically *nutrient-dense, free from harmful chemicals, and produced through methods that support environmental sustainability and the ethical treatment of animals*. When we speak about nutrient density, we're referring to the amount of essential nutrients per calorie.

> ### Washoku (和食)
>
> **Washoku** is more than just traditional Japanese cuisine; it embodies the principles of balance, harmony, and respect for ingredients. Washoku emphasizes using fresh, seasonal, and locally sourced ingredients, highlighting the importance of high-quality nutrition. This culinary philosophy is centered on achieving nutritional balance and variety, often through the principle of "ichiju-sansai" (一汁三菜), meaning "one soup, three dishes." This principle reflects a balanced approach to nutrition, incorporating grains, vegetables, proteins, and fermented foods that support a healthy gut.

Nutrient-dense foods provide vitamins, minerals, and other beneficial compounds that are vital for health. Those foods are also minimally processed, and free from synthetic additives, pesticides, and genetically modified organisms (GMOs). Generally whole foods don't come in packages with laundry lists of ingredients that are difficult to pronounce and are largely unrecognizable.

Regenerative grass-fed beef, fresh squeezed orange juice, local honey, pasture raised eggs, raw milk, unpasteurized almonds. These are examples of whole foods that come from sustainable farming practices prioritizing soil health, biodiversity, and animal welfare.

Common Deficiencies

Studies have shown that micronutrient deficiencies are often overlooked in discussions about health, despite their critical role in preventing chronic diseases. Here are some of the more common nutrient deficiencies that can be easily corrected with a small shift in our thinking about what are considered 'good foods'. We'll also talk about supplements further down the line but here we want to establish a baseline of quality ingredients that are going to get us 85% of the way to meeting our micronutrient needs on a daily basis. Supplements are, as the name implies, *in addition to our regular daily intake* and shouldn't be the major source of daily nutrients.

Vitamin B12 deficiencies are particularly concerning as they can result in anemia, fatigue, neurological issues, and cognitive impairments. B12 is crucial for nerve function and red blood cell production and is typically found in animal products, making this deficiency common among those on plant-based diets or with poor absorption. Recent studies indicate a rise in vitamin B12 deficiency, especially in older populations and those following strict vegan or vegetarian diets. This increase is linked to factors such as reduced dietary intake (especially among vegetarians) and the use of certain medications (e.g., metformin or proton pump inhibitors).

Iron deficiency, another common issue that can lead to anemia and is characterized by fatigue, weakness, and impaired cognitive function. While iron is available in plant foods like lentils and spinach, the non-heme iron found in these sources is less readily absorbed than the heme iron in animal products. Vitamin C can enhance the absorption of nonheme iron, but careful dietary planning is essential.

Omega-3 fatty acids are vital for brain health, reducing inflammation, and supporting heart health. Deficiency can lead to cognitive decline and increased cardiovascular risk. Plant-based sources like flaxseeds and walnuts provide alpha-linolenic acid (ALA), but the conversion to EPA and DHA is inefficient in the body. Algal oil supplements can help provide these essential fatty acids.

Vitamin D is essential for bone health and immune function, with deficiency leading to bone pain, muscle weakness, and increased fracture risk. While sun exposure aids vitamin D synthesis, dietary sources are limited, especially in plant-based diets, often requiring fortified foods or supplements.

Calcium deficiency impacts bone health, muscle function, and nerve signaling, leading to osteoporosis and brittle bones. While plant-based sources exist, the bioavailability can be lower due to inhibitors like oxalates and phytates.

Zinc, crucial for immune function and wound healing, can be less bioavailable from plant sources, leading to weakened immunity and delayed healing.

Animal-based proteins naturally provide all these key nutrients, making them an essential part of a nutrient dense diet. And for those that are committed to a plant-based diet, it is imperative that you get regular blood work to determine what kind of supplementation you might need to maintain a healthy and balanced nutritional profile because the simple fact of the matter is that for the vast majority of people, plants simply don't provide the necessary nutrients in sufficient quantity to maintain optimal levels.

When we last left my personal story I was battling insomnia, finding it impossible to stay asleep for more than an hour or two at a time. And my insomnia, at the most surface level was being caused by awful and constant bloating and gas. It was not only embarrassing but after a while, it became exhausting too. At the time, I was living in Bali, training to be a vegan raw chef, convinced I was going to change the world with a cuisine that was not only cruelty free but supremely nutritious and delicious all at the same time. I was eating massive amounts of kale and cashews and soaked legumes and coconut aminos and fermented foods—all the foods the gurus and influencers insisted made for a healthy and vibrant microbiome and yet, my gut was a mess. My heart was racing in the middle of the night and I was having dizzy spells (often a precursor signal to heart attacks). These symptoms were becoming slightly overwhelming and yet here I thought I was being the healthiest person on the planet eating all fresh fruits and raw vegetables. I simply could not reconcile the idea that somehow what I was eating was causing my body to basically, for lack of a better word, fail. In fact, I was completely in denial about it. And on top of that the perception of myself held up in comparison to the cognitive dissonance of how I actually felt began to spin me into a depression that was very unfamiliar. For a while I just hoped (and prayed) it would go away. I held firm to the belief that my previously indomitable gut (which I literally nicknamed "Mr. Fusion") would prevail and whatever was percolating inside would just burn itself out. But when weeks turned into months without any relief, I started trying to find some answers. I did enemas and juice cleanses and parasite tests—because, again, I couldn't fathom that it was my 'healthy' diet that was causing my problems and yet, nothing I tried did anything to change the loud and constant protestations of my gut. The technician who performed one of my enemas did comment that I must eat a fair amount of kale but beyond, nothing was revealed. Next, I decided I needed to get bloodwork done to see if there was something else that might be out of balance. And that's when I discovered that I was massively, dangerously deficient in a number of critical vitamins and nutrients. The blood test results read like some nightmarish alphabet soup– K2, K3, B12, D, Potassium, Zinc, LDL, T3, T4. My system was on red alert!

That was when I learned that my particular meat-suit simply couldn't nourish itself effectively by eating plants alone. And this was after only 6 months on a purely vegan diet (with no supplementation). At least I now had visibility into the "low hanging fruit" that could be fixed through proper nourishment. This was also the beginning of my understanding of just how significant a role the gut microbiome plays in our overall health and the importance of bloodwork.

What I really took away from that experience more than anything was that there is no 'one way' of nourishing the body that is superior to any other way. When I see influencers pushing keto or carnivore or plant-based eating while showing off their abs and muscles with posts that say 'here's what I eat in a day to look like this' I have to laugh. We are each individual systems that require individual care and specific nourishment to flourish and only you can determine what works best for your system. A big high-five to those that are able to thrive on a plant-based diet, but that is definitely not me (and frankly, it's probably not you, either). It wasn't until quite a bit later that my nutritionist finally figured out that these deficiencies had created an excess of 'bad' bacteria in my microbiome leading to a condition pleasantly named Small Intestinal Bacterial Overgrowth (SIBO). And SIBO had hijacked not only my gut (and intestines) but my brain and my heart right along with it as collateral damage.

Your 2nd Brain: The Gut Microbiome

Home to trillions of microorganisms, the gut microbiome is a vibrant city of bacteria, viruses, fungi, and other microbes that work tirelessly to keep you healthy. Just like a well-functioning city, a diverse and balanced microbiome is crucial for maintaining various bodily functions, including digestion, immunity, mental health, and metabolism. An imbalanced microbiome, or dysbiosis, is linked to chronic inflammation and all manner of autoimmune diseases.

Common Signs and Symptoms of Dysbiosis

Digestive Issues: Bloating, gas, diarrhea, constipation, and abdominal pain signal an imbalanced microbiome.

Frequent Infections: A weakened immune system leads to more colds, flu, and other infections.

Chronic Inflammation: Joint pain, skin issues like eczema or rosacea, or chronic fatigue indicate persistent inflammation.

Mental Health Problems: Anxiety, depression, mood swings, memory, and cognitive issues (i.e., "brain fog") reflect disruption of the gut-brain connection.

Metabolic Disturbances: Weight gain, obesity, and difficulty losing weight are linked to an unhealthy microbiome.

While signs like abdominal pain, bloating, and gas may seem obvious, being aware that inflammation of the gut can also lead to skin flare-ups, mood swings, brain fog, disrupted sleep, and increased susceptibility to colds and flus are all examples of why it's so important to develop a greater sense of body awareness. We want to be able to tune into how changes in what we consume impacts how our bodies respond. The less variables in play, the easier it becomes to recognize what causes changes in our wellness.

Once again, this is a lesson I had to learn the hard way. After my dear nutritionist friend (we should all be so lucky to have one) brilliantly diagnosed my SIBO condition where several general practitioners had been completely stumped, the next step was treatment. Incidentally, it was the 'brain fog' that keyed her into the SIBO diagnosis and up until that point I certainly had not made nor was I aware of any connection between the brain and gut. (TMI sidenote: On top of the brain fog, relentless gas, and disrupted sleep, SIBO also manifested as an insatiable rectal itch that made me have real compassion for when I see dogs dragging their bums along the carpet. For the better part of two years, that's what I wanted to do every single day– drag my bum across sandpaper to cure an itch that would not subside. Not only was it maddeningly irritating and fairly gross, I sure didn't feel very confident or sexy knowing that bacteria had decided to set up shop in my backdoor. I mention this not only out of transparency but also in solidarity with anyone who might read this and be experiencing something similar with no idea what is causing the condition). Over this timeframe I'd also begun to experience increasingly frequent rosacea breakouts on my face. Bright red patches on either side of my nose and along my brow and chin. Itching and redness followed by dry skin flaking off my face and scalp. It would clear up and then start back up all over again. I tried to grow a beard to cover up as much of it as I could but no one in four generations of my family has had a beard–I just ended up looking vaguely homeless. So even though by now I had restored the key vitamins and nutrients my body needed to normal levels through adjusting my diet to a more nutrient-dense selection, I was still dealing with the collateral damage of my body being severely out of balance for a few years. Internally I was a dumpster fire burning out of control and externally, I was withering. These conditions were so personally embarrassing that I began to withdraw socially, unable or unwilling to go out in public because I would see people, complete strangers, avert their eyes when walking towards me on the street and it was devastating. During that period of time, my phone was filled with selfies, day after day, hoping and praying that somehow this horrible condition that had sapped my vitality and left me looking like the walking dead had begun to subside. Some days were better than others and I would spend hours agonizing over what was it that I was eating or coming into contact with that could be causing this to happen, thinking that by eliminating this or that from my diet for a day or two, I might find the answer but my personal inquiries did not provide an answer. As it turns out, the major step in eliminating something like SIBO is literally to starve the bacterial overgrowth while refeeding the helpful gut bacteria that have become overwhelmed and let the internal inflammation die down. To do this effectively required adhering to a very strict elimination diet for several months along with some targeted pre and probiotics for refeeding the good bacteria in my microbiome. Now that I knew what had been causing my misery and torture, I fought with my nutritionist for months, pleading for antibiotics as an instrument of vengeance to 'unleash hell' on the enemy within but she was adamant about being more gentle with my already very fragile internal ecosystem. As she reminded me on several occasions, the gut microbiome is very good at bringing itself back into balance when fed the proper catalysts and she was right. Within 3 months, all of the conditions that had been plaguing me for the better part of the last 3 years began to subside. However, with even the slightest sign of remission, I would break the restricted diet and try to eat something that was forbidden and like clockwork, my symptoms, the product of inflammation, would flare up and return—itching, skin irritation, dry scalp oh and hair loss; let's not forget about hair loss. While I may have prolonged the process of restoring my gut microbiome, I became very sensitive to understanding how certain foods were impacting my body and now, I can tell almost immediately if I've ingested something my body doesn't like or want by keying into even the slightest signs of inflammation.

    The gut and brain are like two best friends constantly texting each other through the gut-brain axis, using neural, hormonal, and immune pathways. This tight connection explains why gut health impacts mood and behavior so significantly. So, the next time 'you just feel off', seemingly out of nowhere, take a minute to consider if you've eaten something 'interesting' or unusual in the past 12-48 hours, that might have your gut working overtime. Studies have shown that changes in gut bacteria can alter levels of neurotransmitters like serotonin, influencing our mood and cognitive functions as well as affecting their ability to extract energy from food efficiently. Longitudinal studies show that individuals with a diverse microbiome have a lower incidence of chronic diseases and better overall health. Additionally, a balanced microbiome contributes to healthy aging, with research indicating that older adults with diverse gut microbiomes experience better health outcomes and longevity. Diet is obviously a major factor shaping overall gut health and balance. High-fiber diets are like daily maintenance, increasing beneficial bacteria and producing short-chain fatty acids (SCFAs) that promote gut health. While high-fat, high-sugar diets disrupt the microbial balance. Lifestyle factors such as stress, sleep, and physical activity also play crucial roles, with regular exercise having been shown to boost microbial diversity.

To keep our gut city flourishing, in the simplest terms, we need to feed it the things it likes and avoid the things that throw it out of balance. Intake of fiber-rich foods, fermented foods (like yogurt and sauerkraut), and prebiotics can be helpful. While supplemental probiotics and prebiotics can support gut health, whole food dietary sources should be prioritized for their comprehensive benefits and it should be noted that in some cases while trying to heal the or rebalance the gut, prebiotics and probiotics may not always be what is needed. Depending on the severity of the issue, consulting a nutritionist who can help guide the rebalancing process is highly recommended. Talking to a nutritionist was crucial in my own process for diagnosing the SIBO I was dealing with when several general practitioners could not make heads or tails of what was causing my problems.

Prebiotics, Probiotics, and Antibiotics

Prebiotics Prebiotics are non-digestible fibers that nourish beneficial bacteria in the gut, supporting a healthy microbiome and promoting overall well-being. Prebiotics act as a food source for the beneficial bacteria of the gut, particularly *Bifidobacteria* and *Lactobacilli*. Studies show that regular prebiotic intake resulted in improved digestion, enhanced immune function, and a reduced risk of certain diseases such as colorectal cancer and inflammatory bowel disease. Getting prebiotics from whole foods is considered the most effective and reliable way to achieve these health benefits due to the synergy of nutrients that accompany the fiber content.

Research suggests that consuming around 3-10 grams of prebiotics daily is sufficient to promote the growth of beneficial gut bacteria. To put that in whole food terms, consuming about 2 tablespoons of chia seeds or flaxseeds daily can provide around 5 grams of prebiotic fiber. 1 cup of cooked lentils or chickpeas contains about 2-3 grams of prebiotics, 1 whole kiwi has 2-3 grams of prebiotics, and chicory root is exceptionally high in inulin, a powerful prebiotic, and just a small amount (about 1-2 tablespoons) providing up to 4 grams of prebiotics.

Probiotics Probiotics are live microorganisms, mainly bacteria and yeast, that promote the growth of beneficial bacteria and inhibit the growth of harmful ones. However, it is important to recognize that a healthy and well-functioning gut does not necessarily need additional support in the form of probiotics. The gut microbiome is inherently balanced in a healthy state, and its equilibrium is largely maintained by a diverse diet rich in fiber, whole foods, and adequate hydration.

Probiotics are generally used to 'refeed' the gut when building up healthy bacteria in a damaged gut, after taking antibiotics for example, which disrupt the gut by killing off beneficial bacteria along with harmful ones. Research published in the *Journal of the American Medical Association (JAMA)* shows that taking probiotics after antibiotics can help restore gut balance and reduce the risk of antibiotic-associated diarrhea by 42%. Similarly, for individuals suffering from digestive disorders like irritable bowel syndrome (IBS) or inflammatory bowel disease (IBD), certain strains of probiotics, like *Bifidobacterium infantis* and *Lactobacillus rhamnosus*, have been shown to alleviate symptoms by promoting a healthier gut environment. Probiotics can also be useful in preventing traveler's diarrhea, particularly when exposed to unfamiliar bacteria in new environments. Studies indicate that strains like *Saccharomyces boulardii* can help maintain gut balance and reduce the incidence of diarrhea while traveling. And in situations where the immune system is compromised, such as during cold and flu season, certain probiotics have been shown to reduce the duration and severity of respiratory infections. However, for those with a well-balanced and diverse diet, the gut microbiome often regulates itself effectively *without the need for additional probiotic supplementation.*

Regular consumption of probiotic-rich foods like yogurt, kefir, sauerkraut, kimchi, kombucha, and certain aged cheeses can provide natural sources of these beneficial bacteria without the need for supplements. The general recommendation is to aim for 1 to 10 billion colony-forming units (CFUs) per day, depending on individual health needs. However, for most healthy individuals, a diet that promotes a balanced microbiome through diversity, fiber, and whole foods is often sufficient to maintain optimal gut health without the need for regular probiotic use.

Taking probiotics should be considered mainly when there is an indication of imbalance or specific health concerns.

Antibiotics Antibiotics, while life-saving in many situations, can also indiscriminately destroy both harmful and beneficial microbes in the body. They are powerful tools in combating bacterial infections and have revolutionized medicine by significantly reducing mortality from infectious diseases. However, **antibiotics should be used with caution and only in severe situations where their benefits outweigh the risks.**

When antibiotics are used, they do not selectively target only the harmful bacteria causing an infection; it's more like blanketing your entire gut with napalm. A study published in the *Journal of Clinical Investigation* found that even a single course of antibiotics can significantly alter the gut microbiome, reducing its diversity and disrupting its balance for an extended period. This disruption can lead to various issues, including digestive problems, weakened immunity, and an increased risk of infections.

Our society's infatuation with antibiotics has led to their overuse, often in situations where they are not necessary, such as for viral infections like the common cold or flu, against which antibiotics have no effect. This overuse has contributed to the rise of antibiotic-resistant bacteria that makes infections harder to treat. Antibiotic resistance occurs when bacteria mutate and develop the ability to survive exposure to drugs that would normally kill them, rendering these treatments less effective over time. The Center for Disease Control and Prevention (CDC) estimates that at least 2.8 million antibiotic-resistant infections occur in the U.S. each year, resulting in more than 35,000 deaths.

In cases where antibiotics are required, make sure you have a recovery plan in place to restore the balance of your gut microbiome, such as consuming probiotic-rich foods or taking probiotic supplements to help mitigate some of the negative effects on gut health.

Hand Santizer Public Service Announcement

Daily use of hand sanitizer has become a widespread accepted practice since the onset of COVID-19, providing a quick and effective means to reduce the transmission of germs, particularly when soap and water are unavailable. While hand sanitizers are valuable in preventing infection, their frequent (daily) use can have several downstream consequences. One major issue is the disruption of the skin's microbiome. Hand sanitizers, especially those containing alcohol, strip the skin of its natural oils and beneficial bacteria, which are essential for protecting against harmful pathogens and maintaining overall skin health. Believe it or not, allowing some level of dirt and bacteria to exist on the skin is crucial for maintaining a healthy skin microbiome, which serves as the body's first line of defense against harmful pathogens. The skin microbiome consists of a complex community of microorganisms, including beneficial bacteria that help protect against infections, maintain the skin barrier, and regulate the immune system. Over-sanitizing or frequently using harsh antiseptics can disrupt this delicate balance, stripping away beneficial bacteria and allowing pathogenic microbes to flourish. Research has shown that a healthy skin microbiome can help prevent conditions like eczema, psoriasis, and acne by creating an environment that inhibits the growth of harmful bacteria while supporting the skin's natural defenses while excessive use of sanitizer products can lead to skin irritation, dryness, and even dermatitis, as reported by the American Academy of Dermatology (AAD) and a study published in the *Journal of the American Academy of Dermatology*, which found a significant increase in hand dermatitis among people due to heightened hand hygiene practices during the pandemic.

In addition to skin health concerns, regular use of hand sanitizer can contribute to other health issues. The U.S. Food and Drug Administration (FDA) has warned that some hand sanitizers contain toxic chemicals like methanol, which can cause severe side effects if absorbed through the skin or ingested. Additionally, other ingredients, such as triclosan, found in some hand sanitizers, may act as endocrine disruptors, potentially affecting hormonal health. Research published in *Environmental Health Perspectives* has linked triclosan to disruptions in thyroid function and other hormonal processes. Moreover, daily use of hand sanitizers containing antimicrobial agents like triclosan or benzalkonium chloride could contribute to antimicrobial resistance, as these compounds may encourage the development of resistant bacterial strains over time.

While hand sanitizers can serve as a tool in preventing the spread of infectious diseases, their daily use, particularly when overused or containing harmful ingredients, have adverse effects on skin health, contribute to antimicrobial resistance, and expose individuals to potentially toxic chemicals. It is recommended to use hand sanitizer only when necessary, opting for alcohol-based formulas free from harmful additives, and prioritizing handwashing with soap and water to maintain both personal health and broader public safety.

Poop: Why You Should Give a Sh!t

Poop is really our gut's way of sending us (daily) status reports. By looking at both the color and constitution, you can tell quite a bit about how well you are feeding your gut microbiome or whether there might be something out of whack. A healthy bowel movement, much like every other aspect of the body's functioning, is an essential indicator of overall wellness. While each individual's digestive system operates slightly differently, there are general guidelines that most health professionals agree on when evaluating the quality of bowel movements.

First, **frequency** is key: ideally, one should have at least one bowel movement a day, though for some, anywhere between once a day and three times a week can still be considered within the healthy range. Consistency matters more than frequency—if bowel movements are suddenly more or less frequent, it can indicate a disruption in digestive health. **Duration** should be brief, ideally less than 10 minutes (5 if you stop scrolling). If it takes significantly longer to pass stool, or if there is straining involved, this could be a sign of constipation or other digestive issues. Efficient bowel movements occur when the body is adequately hydrated, and the diet includes sufficient fiber to support smooth passage through the intestines.

The **texture** and **form** of the stool are important factors too. According to the *Bristol Stool Scale*, a healthy stool is classified as Type 3, 4 or 5, which means it should be smooth, soft, and shaped like a sausage or snake. This **form** indicates a well-functioning digestive system that processes and absorbs nutrients effectively. Another dimension is **wiping**.

Ideally, there should be minimal need for wiping, with the stool passing cleanly, indicating that the body is digesting food well, and the stool has the right consistency. Excessive wiping can suggest softer stools or incomplete digestion, which might require adjustments in diet, hydration, or gut health.

In terms of **color**, healthy stool is generally medium to dark brown, a sign that the digestive system is processing bile properly. Variations in color can indicate specific issues—pale stool may suggest a lack of bile, while black or red stool could indicate bleeding and should be evaluated by a healthcare professional immediately.

Here is a chart to decode color variations:

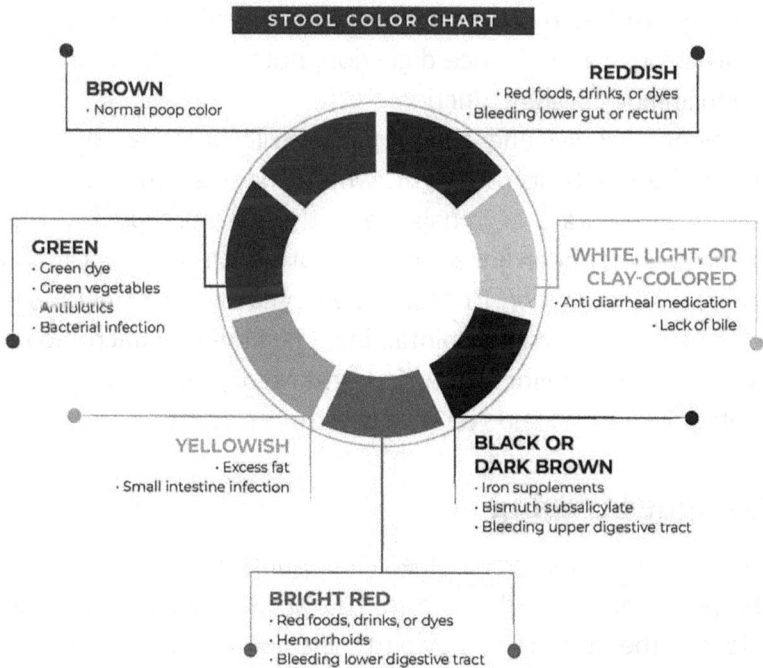

Healthy bowel movements are your daily TMM status report because they are a direct function of proper hydration, a balanced diet rich in fiber, and regular physical activity, all of which support efficient digestion and a strong gut microbiome. Maintaining regularity in these habits allows for a more balanced and elevated sense of well-being. As with all bodily functions, consistency is a reflection of harmony within, and any significant changes warrant mindful attention and adjustment.

Oral Hygiene

The mouth is the gateway to the body, and its health profoundly impacts overall well-being, particularly the gut microbiome.

Inside your mouth resides an ecosystem of bacteria, fungi, and other microorganisms that interact constantly with your digestive system. When oral health is neglected, harmful bacteria can proliferate, leading to imbalances not only in the mouth but throughout the gastrointestinal tract. These disruptions can influence digestion, nutrient absorption, and even immune system function.

Poor oral hygiene allows pathogenic bacteria to travel from the mouth into the gut, where they can contribute to dysbiosis—a state of imbalance in the gut microbiome. This imbalance has been linked to a host of health issues, including chronic inflammation, irritable bowel syndrome, and metabolic disorders. Conversely, maintaining a healthy oral microbiome supports a thriving, balanced gut ecosystem, promoting optimal digestion and systemic health.

Tongue Scraping

According to Ayurvedic medicine, tongue scraping should be performed on a daily basis. This ancient practice helps to cleanse the body by removing toxins and bacteria from your oral cavity, enhances the sense of taste by removing any coating of the tongue (i.e. 'biofilm'), which in turn enhances digestion by sending clearer signals to the brain about the types of food being consumed. Ultimately, this helps stimulate the digestive process, including saliva production and the release of digestive enzymes.

Oral health is another great opportunity for TMM self-awareness, where you can reflect on the choices of the last several days, weeks, or months, and see how those choices have affected your health. If a thick tongue coating is present, try tongue scraping along with your other oral hygiene practices and see if you notice a difference. This simple daily practice can bring more self-awareness and gives you the opportunity to make new, healthier choices.

By implementing dietary and lifestyle changes, we can ensure our gut remains diverse and resilient, leading to improved overall health and longevity. If something looks or feels off kilter, it probably is. The good news is that the gut microbiome is actually very good at healing itself once you feed it the bacteria it needs or stop feeding the bacteria causing the imbalance and with the help of a nutrition expert, healing and repair can happen relatively quickly.

But get in the habit of doing a little self-diagnosis and see what your gut is telling you about its health. What have you been eating that might be contributing to an imbalance if one exists?

PMS : Finding Flow on the Path

In the Modern Monk philosophy, your body is seen as a finely tuned instrument, capable of performing at its best when given the right inputs and care. But when something goes off-key, it sends a clear signal that there's an imbalance—often in the form of pain, fatigue, or mood disturbances. Nowhere is this more obvious than with PMS. For many women, monthly cramps, bloating, and irritability have become accepted as just "part of the deal." But what if they didn't have to be?

Just as a cracked foundation affects the integrity of an entire structure, an imbalanced cycle can throw off the harmony of your physical, mental, and emotional well-being. The Modern Monk approach challenges the notion that PMS is a permanent, inevitable aspect of being female. Instead, it views these symptoms as a *call to action by your body*, a not-so-subtle signpost pointing you toward areas that need deeper support and care. The goal isn't to mask these signals or ignore them—it's to understand and address the root causes. By dialing into the rhythms of your own body and making targeted nutritional and lifestyle shifts, you can reduce or even eliminate many of these disruptive symptoms. It's about approaching the menstrual cycle with the same mindfulness, intentionality, and self-mastery that are central to the Modern Monk ethos.

Here, you'll find guidance on how to support hormone health, reduce inflammation, and build daily practices that transform your monthly cycle from a potential disruption to a more balanced, predictable experience. True wellness doesn't mean pushing through pain—it means listening to your body, understanding its needs, and responding with the support it deserves.

The Red Flag

While PMS symptoms—cramps, bloating, irritability, fatigue—are incredibly widespread, they're not an inherent or unavoidable part of a woman's menstrual cycle. Just because something is *common* doesn't mean it's *normal*. Painful periods, intense mood swings, and debilitating cramps have been so heavily normalized by society that we tend to accept them as par for the course of womanhood. But these symptoms aren't a natural part of a healthy cycle—they're signals.

The body's natural state of balance does not include pain. Cramps are your body's way of speaking to you. Think of it like a check engine light—inconvenient yes, but meant to indicate that some area of your hormonal or metabolic health needs attention. For reasons we don't need to dive into here, many women feel resigned to just "deal with it," but at TMM we believe that with care and attention, experiencing monthly agony is *not* a given.

From a physiological standpoint, these disruptive symptoms are often linked to a few core imbalances: elevated levels of inflammatory chemicals called prostaglandins, excess estrogen, or a state of chronic low-grade inflammation throughout the body. Each of these can drive symptoms like severe cramping, heavy bleeding, and intense mood swings, making what should be a manageable, routine cycle feel more like a monthly battle.

And here's the good news—by addressing these underlying issues through diet and lifestyle, you can absolutely reduce, and in some cases, eliminate these symptoms entirely.

To be clear, a little discomfort is not cause for alarm—some mild cramping or mood shifts might occur as part of your body's normal rhythm. But reaching for painkillers just to get through the day or experiencing symptoms that disrupt your life? That's your body's way of waving a red flag. The bottom line is, you shouldn't have to suffer to be a woman. PMS is a clear invitation to pay closer attention, not a condition to silently endure. With a few mindful adjustments—supporting your body with nutrient dense foods, prioritizing hormone-balancing practices, and making lifestyle choices to mitigate inflammation—many of these symptoms can be significantly eased, hopefully turning your cycle from a monthly ordeal into a more manageable, even predictable experience.

The Science Behind PMS and Menstrual Cramps

At the root of menstrual pain are chemicals called prostaglandins—small but mighty messengers that play a critical role in regulating inflammation. During your period, prostaglandins are released to help the muscles of the uterus contract and shed its lining. A little bit of this is necessary and normal. But when your body produces too many prostaglandins, those mild contractions turn into intense cramps that radiate from your lower abdomen to your back and thighs, leaving you doubled over in pain.

Now, why would your body go into overdrive with these inflammatory chemicals? It often comes down to two key factors: excess estrogen and an inflammatory lifestyle. Elevated estrogen levels create a thicker uterine lining, which means your body has to produce more prostaglandins to expel it. This sets off a chain reaction: more estrogen → more lining → more prostaglandins → more cramping. This isn't just a nuisance—it's your body telling you that your hormones are out of balance. So what drives high estrogen in the first place? Several factors can contribute, from environmental toxins found in plastics and cosmetics (also known as endocrine disruptors) to a poor diet lacking in nutrients essential for healthy hormone metabolism. When your body is constantly exposed to these disruptors or burdened with a diet high in processed foods, sugars, and omega-6 fats, estrogen tends to accumulate, disrupting your hormonal balance. Regularly consuming foods like refined carbohydrates, alcohol, and processed meats elevates inflammation throughout the body, making it more sensitive to pain signals. Even micronutrient imbalances—such as low magnesium or zinc—can interfere with your body's ability to regulate inflammation, making cramps more severe. Meanwhile, insufficient fiber intake can prevent estrogen from being properly cleared, letting it recirculate and worsen the problem.

This deeper understanding of how diet and lifestyle impact menstrual health not only explains why some women experience more intense symptoms but also offers a roadmap for managing them. By addressing these root causes through targeted nutritional and lifestyle strategies, it's possible to reduce, or even eliminate, many of the disruptive symptoms associated with PMS and menstrual cramps.

Syncing with Your Cycle

In the Modern Monk philosophy, true wellness isn't about pushing through pain or forcing yourself into routines that leave you drained and disconnected. It's about tuning into your body's natural rhythms and aligning your lifestyle with its needs—harnessing both the ebbs and flows of energy that are unique to every phase of the menstrual cycle. That's where *cycle syncing* comes in.

Cycle syncing goes beyond basic hormonal health advice. It's a way of living that respects the complex interplay of estrogen, progesterone, and other key hormones that influence everything from your energy levels and mood to your focus and physical performance. Instead of following a one-size-fits-all approach, cycle syncing asks: "What does your body need right now?" Whether it's rest and replenishment during menstruation, high-energy workouts in the follicular phase, or stress reduction in the luteal phase, cycle syncing is about meeting your body where it's at. The goal isn't to add more complexity to your routine but to simplify it by respecting the natural cues your body is already giving you. With this approach, you're not fighting against the tide—you're learning to surf it. You can begin to see your cycle as a guide, offering a blueprint for optimizing productivity, reducing PMS, and maintaining balance in every aspect of your life. By integrating this ancient wisdom with modern science, cycle syncing becomes a powerful tool to reclaim hormonal harmony and cultivate a lifestyle that flows—literally and figuratively—in sync with your body's needs. Because the path to living an elevated life is not about conquering the body; it's about understanding it and walking the path of least resistance.

Understanding the Four Phases of the Menstrual Cycle

To implement cycle syncing effectively, it's crucial to understand the four phases of the menstrual cycle: menstrual, follicular, ovulatory, and luteal. Each phase is marked by distinct hormonal changes that influence everything from energy levels to mental clarity and emotional stability.

Menstrual Phase (Days 1-5):

This phase begins with the first day of bleeding and typically lasts 3-7 days. Estrogen and progesterone levels are at their lowest, which can lead to reduced energy, fatigue, and the need for rest. During this time, the focus should be on replenishment and gentle support:

Exercise: Opt for light, restorative activities such as yoga, stretching, or leisurely walks. These movements can aid circulation and reduce cramping without adding unnecessary stress.
Lifestyle Modifications: Prioritize rest and create a soothing environment. Incorporate self-care practices like warm baths, meditation, or journaling to help manage any discomfort and restore energy.

Follicular Phase (Days 6-14):

After menstruation, estrogen begins to rise, peaking before ovulation. This phase is characterized by a natural increase in energy, motivation, and mental clarity. It's the perfect time to focus on productivity and growth-oriented activities:

Exercise: Higher estrogen levels make your body more resilient to stress and capable of handling more intense workouts. This is the optimal time for strength training, HIIT, or cardio to build muscle and increase endurance.
Lifestyle Modifications: Use this high-energy period to tackle creative projects, set new goals, or learn a new skill. Mentally challenging tasks may feel less daunting, and social engagement can boost overall mood.

Ovulatory Phase (Around Day 14):

Ovulation, marked by a peak in estrogen and luteinizing hormone (LH), lasts about 3-5 days. This phase is the most fertile and is associated with enhanced confidence and sociability.

Exercise: Opt for moderate intensity workouts like dance, running, or circuit training. Your body can effectively handle a mix of strength and endurance during this time.

Lifestyle Modifications: This is the time to schedule social activities, public speaking, or high-stakes meetings. You may find that your communication skills and charisma are naturally enhanced during ovulation.

Luteal Phase (Days 15-28):

After ovulation, progesterone levels rise to support potential pregnancy. This phase often brings on PMS symptoms like bloating, irritability, and fatigue if hormone levels are imbalanced. To minimize these symptoms, focus on calming, supportive habits:

Exercise: Transition to gentler forms of movement like Pilates, yoga, or long walks, especially if PMS symptoms start to arise. This reduces stress on the body and helps maintain hormonal balance.

Lifestyle Modifications: Emphasize stress reduction and prioritize sleep. Incorporate mindfulness practices, limit caffeine and sugar intake, and establish a regular bedtime routine to ensure adequate rest and hormone regulation.

When it comes to implementing cycle syncing, the key is simplicity. Start by tracking your cycle—whether through an app or a journal—to notice patterns in your energy, mood, and cravings. These clues will help you anticipate changes and align your habits accordingly. Don't overhaul your entire routine at once; instead, as is the Modern Monk way, make a 1° shift —focus on small, manageable tweaks and take note of how it makes you feel. Perhaps start by adjusting your workout load to match the phase of your cycle or creating a relaxation routine in the evening when your cycle begins and then, as you become more attuned, extend these shifts to your work and social schedule, creating space for rest when needed and leveraging your natural peaks of productivity. Above all, listen to your body's signals. While there are overarching principles, each person's chemistry and therefore cycle is unique, and tuning into what feels best for *you* is where the real power of cycle syncing lies. It's not about rigid rules or "getting it right", but building a lifestyle that supports your body's natural rhythms, fosters hormonal balance, and promotes long-term wellness.

Nutritional Strategies for PMS Management

When it comes to reducing PMS symptoms, food is your first line of defense. Instead of viewing nutrition as a collection of isolated fixes, it's about setting up the foundation for balance and resilience all cycle long. That means focusing on food quality—nutrient-dense, anti-inflammatory foods that support hormone metabolism and reduce the inflammatory signals that cause cramping and mood swings.

Before Your Cycle

In the weeks leading up to your period, prioritizing foods that promote healthy estrogen metabolism and reduce inflammation is key. Load up on cruciferous vegetables like broccoli and cauliflower—these powerhouses contain compounds like sulforaphane and indole-3-carbinol, which support the liver in breaking down excess estrogen, helping to keep hormone levels in check. Also, focus on getting plenty of fiber from whole grains, seeds, and legumes. Fiber binds to estrogen in the digestive tract and helps eliminate it from the body, reducing the risk of it being reabsorbed and causing imbalances.

Don't skimp on omega-3s either—these anti-inflammatory fats are crucial for managing prostaglandin production, the very chemicals responsible for cramping pain. Incorporate wild-caught fish like salmon or plant-based sources like chia seeds and walnuts. And if cramps have been a consistent struggle, consider adding zinc-rich foods (think pumpkin seeds, oysters, and lentils) to the mix. Zinc has been shown to inhibit prostaglandin synthesis, easing the onset of menstrual pain. This phase is all about building a nutritional buffer so that your body has the resources it needs to keep inflammation at bay and hormones balanced.

During Your Period

To further support your body, opt for easily digestible, nutrient-rich foods like bone broth, lentil soups, and cooked vegetables. These options are packed with minerals that replenish what's lost during menstruation, without burdening the digestive system. And as a reminder, stay hydrated to support circulation and reduce water retention. Herbal teas or water infused with a squeeze of lemon can keep hydration levels up while adding a soothing touch.

By supporting your body's nutrition by focusing on intentional high quality foods, you set the stage for a cycle that's not just tolerable but balanced and aligned with your health goals.

Remember, the goal is not to restrict or diet, but to provide the kind of nourishment that allows your body to function at its best, month after month.

When to See a Specialist

Mild discomfort and occasional cramping are one thing, but if after eliminating the factors you can control with nutrition, exercise, and lifestyle and your periods are consistently painful or disruptive, it could be a sign that something deeper is going on. Experiencing pain that leaves you bedridden, requires strong painkillers to function, or comes with other symptoms like heavy bleeding, nausea, or pain during bowel movements could indicate a more serious condition, such as endometriosis, adenomyosis, or fibroids. Similarly, if you find yourself dealing with extreme fatigue, hair loss, or unexplained weight changes along with painful periods, it's worth checking in with a healthcare provider to rule out thyroid issues, as hormonal imbalances can significantly impact your menstrual health. If you're noticing symptoms like pain that radiates to your lower back or thighs, periods lasting more than seven days, or a sudden change in your cycle's regularity, it's your body's way of signaling that something is out of alignment. Don't ignore these signs.

Chronic and debilitating period pain is never something to just "deal with"—it's an invitation to dig deeper and work with a specialist to uncover the root cause. After all, your cycle should be a barometer of overall health, not a monthly reminder of something being off-kilter. Listen to those signals, and don't hesitate to seek out a professional to get the support you deserve.

Food Toxicity

Deficiency is one major pathway to disease and the other is exposure to toxicity. Our generic commercially produced food supply, often depleted of essential nutrients due to industrial farming practices, categorically fails to provide the body with the necessary components to maintain health. This deficiency, combined with exposure to toxins like glyphosate, a common herbicide, disrupts the gut microbiome and impairs the body's ability to detoxify, leading to increased susceptibility to diseases. Growing research has demonstrated that glyphosate exposure negatively affects the gut microbiome, leading to an increased risk of diseases like inflammatory bowel disease. Chemicals in processed foods, pesticides, and environmental pollutants accumulate in the body, causing oxidative stress and inflammation. A study in *The Lancet* revealed that chronic low-grade inflammation is a significant risk factor for heart disease, diabetes, and cancer, emphasizing the need for a diet rich in anti-inflammatory foods. Many factors contribute to each individual's susceptibility to disease from genetics to environment but the more we do to limit our exposure to toxic materials and harmful chemicals, particularly in the food we put in our bodies, the less likely we are to trigger the malfunction of cells that lead directly to disease.

As we start to put the pieces together on this path to an elevated life, it's pretty clear that improving both our sleep and nutrition even by small amounts (1°!) has a direct impact on our body's ability to ward off or prevent chronic diseases, illness, and inflammation. Then, if we can reduce the 'signal noise' of inflammation in our bodies, with mindfulness cultivated through our regular meditation practice we can begin to better 'hear' and more accurately feel what our bodies need and want to thrive.

Toxic Food Products to Avoid

If you did nothing else to change the trajectory of your food quality, becoming aware of the toxicity of certain foods that are ubiquitous in our food supply and eliminating them from your diet would be a huge shift in the right direction. Below are some of the most blatantly toxic foods, food types, and chemicals that should be avoided at all costs.

SUGAR

Over the past 50 years, the average American's sugar intake has surged dramatically. In the 1970s, Americans consumed about 123 pounds of sugar per year. By 2016, this number had increased to 152 pounds annually (U.S. Department of

Agriculture). This excessive sugar consumption is closely linked to the rise in type 2 diabetes. The Center for Disease Control and Prevention reports that the prevalence of diagnosed diabetes has more than tripled in the last 50 years, with over 34 million Americans affected today.

Refined sugar contributes to a myriad of health problems. It promotes weight gain by triggering the liver to convert excess sugar into fat, leading to fatty liver disease, a precursor to diabetes. It also spikes blood sugar levels, causing insulin resistance, which is a primary driver of type 2 diabetes. A high-sugar diet can increase the risk of heart disease by raising blood pressure and chronic inflammation levels, both significant pathways to cardiovascular problems.

Additionally, excessive sugar intake can impair brain function, leading to memory issues and an increased risk of mental health disorders such as depression. The American Heart Association recommends that women limit their sugar intake to 6 teaspoons per day and men to 9 teaspoons, significantly less than the current average intake of about 22 teaspoons daily. And The Modern Monk recommends you eliminate your sugar intake altogether. If you follow the program we have laid out, then you are eating whole foods that don't contain additives or added ingredients like refined sugar.

Not All Sugar is Created Equally

When we're talking about sugar, we're really talking about refined sugars (sucrose) and high fructose corn syrup that are extracted and processed from plants like sugar cane, sugar beets, and corn by humans with machines that use energy and create waste products. These heavily refined sugars are added to a wide variety of processed foods to enhance flavor, extend shelf life, and improve texture. Unlike the natural sugars in fruits (fructose) refined sugars lack any nutritional value and are absorbed quickly into the bloodstream, leading to rapid spikes in blood sugar and insulin levels. Natural sugars on the other hand found in fruits, come packaged with fiber, vitamins, minerals, and antioxidants. This combination slows down the absorption of sugar in the bloodstream, preventing rapid spikes in blood sugar levels and providing a more sustained energy release. Additionally, the fiber in fruits aids in digestion and promotes a feeling of fullness, which can help prevent overeating. Nature literally provides us with its own candy that is delicious beyond compare and engineered for our bodies to process In a way that makes it an optimal fuel source. I challenge you to find something more incredibly delicious or more hydrating than a cold slice of juicy watermelon on a summer day.

PROCESSED FOODS

Processed foods pose significant health risks due to their composition and the methods used to enhance their flavor, texture, and shelf life. Seed oils (more on these in a minute) and trans fats are both harmful ingredients commonly found in processed foods. Created through the hydrogenation process, trans fats are used to extend shelf life and improve texture. However, they lower good cholesterol (HDL) and raise bad cholesterol (LDL), significantly increasing the risk of heart disease. It's estimated that trans fats are responsible for up to 50,000 (~8%) premature heart attack deaths annually. Processed foods are also laden with artificial dyes and preservatives. Dyes like Red 40 and Yellow 5 are linked to behavioral issues in children and have potential carcinogenic effects. Preservatives such as butylated hydroxyanisole (BHA) and butylated hydroxytoluene (BHT) are used to prevent spoilage but are associated with cancer and endocrine disruption.

The last several decades has seen the consumption of processed foods skyrocket, not surprisingly paralleling the rise in obesity, type-2 diabetes, and a host of other chronic diseases. These foods, high in refined sugars and unhealthy fats but completely lacking in nutritional value of any kind, disrupt blood sugar regulation and insulin sensitivity, leading to an array of metabolic health issues.

SEED OILS

Seed oils, often found in processed foods, pose significant health risks due to their high levels of unhealthy fats and extensive processing. These oils, including canola, soybean, corn, cottonseed, sunflower, safflower, and grapeseed oils, undergo chemical alterations through high heat and solvents, resulting in oils rich in omega-6 fatty acids and trans fats. Excessive intake of these fats can lead to inflammation, obesity, diabetes, and heart disease. One of the main issues with seed oils is their disruption of the omega-6 to omega-3 fatty acid balance. Our bodies need both types of fats, but the modern diet tends to be overly rich in omega-6, promoting a pro-inflammatory state. This imbalance is a significant factor in the rise of chronic diseases.

For healthier oil alternatives, consider extra virgin olive oil, avocado oil, unrefined and cold-pressed extra virgin coconut oil, nut-based oils like almond and walnut oil, and beef tallow. These oils are less processed, contain beneficial nutrients, and have healthier fat profiles. Extra virgin olive oil is praised for its high monounsaturated fat content and antioxidant properties, making it a heart-healthy option best enjoyed at room temperature (applying high heat destroys the flavor and the benefits). Beef tallow, a traditional fat, is also a stable and nutritious choice for cooking at high temperatures.

GLYPHOSATES

Glyphosate, the active ingredient in many herbicides like Roundup, is now a pervasive chemical in our commercial food supply. Originally introduced by Monsanto (now owned by Bayer) in 1974, its usage has increased dramatically, especially with the advent of glyphosate-resistant genetically modified (GMO) crops in the mid-1990s. This widespread use has significantly increased glyphosate exposure in the American diet. Glyphosate is now the most widely used herbicide globally, applied to more than 70 different crops, including wheat, oats, barley, almonds, apples, beans, lentils, peas, grapes, rice, and sunflowers. The dangers of glyphosate are becoming increasingly evident. The World Health Organization's International Agency for Research on Cancer classified glyphosate as a "probable human carcinogen" in 2015. Research links glyphosate exposure to various health issues, including cancer, endocrine disruption, liver, and kidney damage. Furthermore, glyphosate's role as an antibiotic disrupts the gut microbiome, which can lead to other chronic health conditions. What's worse is that glyphosate residues are found even in non-GMO labeled foods. A study showed that 18 out of 26 such products contained glyphosate, with some having alarmingly high levels. This contamination often results from pre-harvest spraying (desiccation), where glyphosate is applied to crops to accelerate drying and harvesting. But not to worry since all of those products (most of them are granola bars, cereal, etc) would fall under the category of processed foods and we are no longer consuming processed foods, right?

A Note on Gluten

Gluten is a protein found in wheat, barley, and rye. It gives dough its elasticity and helps it rise and maintain its shape.

For most people, gluten is harmless, but it can cause health issues for those with celiac disease or non-celiac gluten sensitivity.

In the United States, the rate of gluten sensitivities and celiac disease has significantly increased. This can be attributed partly to the type of wheat predominantly grown and consumed. U.S. wheat, especially hard red winter wheat, has a higher gluten content—typically around 12-14%—compared to European wheat varieties, which range from 8-10% gluten content. This higher gluten content is due to intensive breeding aimed at increasing yield, disease resistance, and protein/gluten content. Not surprisingly, the use of herbicides like glyphosate (you, again!) is more widespread in U.S. wheat cultivation. Glyphosate as we just mentioned is often used as a desiccant before harvest, which can increase the gluten content in the wheat and potentially contribute to gluten sensitivities. In contrast, European countries have tighter regulations around herbicide use, which may play a role in the lower prevalence of gluten sensitivities. (We'll save the rant about the connection between a processed food supply and the "health care" system for a later date). Europeans also tend to consume more traditionally prepared foods, such as sourdough bread, which contains lactobacilli that help break down gluten and make it more digestible. These foods are often made with clean ingredients and without preservatives so common in our industrial food supply. But the best way is to feel the difference for yourself. Let your body be your witness, your judge, and your jury. Next time you are in Europe, see how the pasta and the pizza makes you feel compared to eating similar foods in the US (unless you have Celiac disease then don't do that please) but we'd venture to guess you'll feel absolutely fine after enjoying foods with gluten in them across the pond.

"Healthy" Foods that Aren't

Here is a list of ten foods that, while they may offer some health benefits, contain contaminants or artificial ingredients that make them potentially harmful:

Farmed Salmon: Often contains high levels of polychlorinated biphenyls (PCBs) and dioxins, which are linked to cancer. The crowded conditions of fish farms also lead to higher usage of antibiotics and pesticides.

Avocado Oil: Recent findings have revealed concerning issues with avocado oil. Many avocado oil products on the market are adulterated with cheaper seed oils. A study found that 82% of avocado oils were either rancid or mixed with other lesser quality oils. With a little research, you can find the brands that have shown to test pure.

Store Bought Honey: Often contains added sugars and high fructose corn syrup to increase volume and sweetness. Some imported honey is contaminated with antibiotics and heavy metals. Ditch the cute bear, buy local honey. The notion that local honey will help with allergies is a myth but the different flavors that emerge depending on what types of flowers the bees pollinate is astounding and delicious.

Granola Bars: Frequently contain high levels of added sugars, refined grains, and preservatives such as BHT (butylated hydroxytoluene), a possible carcinogen, as well as glyphosate. These are just candy bars in disguise.

Canned Tuna: Canned and packaged tuna is often considered unsafe due to its potential mercury content. Mercury is a neurotoxin that accumulates in large, predatory fish like tuna. Over time, these fish build up high levels of methylmercury, which can be harmful to human health, particularly affecting brain development in fetuses and young children. Consumer Reports found that some brands of canned tuna contain "dangerous spikes" of mercury, posing significant risks. Additionally, concerns exist over the use of BPA in can linings, which may disrupt endocrine function.

Microwave Popcorn: Contains perfluorinated compounds (PFCs) in the packaging, which can leach into the food and are linked to cancer and immune system issues. Plus, microwaves. No bueno. Cook it on a stovetop. It's better for you and so much fun to hear the kernels sizzle and start popping. Side note: **Movie popcorn** is also terrible. It's cooked in canola oil and the 'butter' is artificially flavored seed oil. Not to mention, the kernels themselves are from glyphosate laden GMO corn. #avoid For what it's worth, I pop my own popcorn at home now and take it to the movies.

Brown Rice: Brown rice is considered less healthy than white rice due to its higher levels of phytic acid and arsenic. Phytic acid, found in the bran, can reduce the absorption of essential minerals like iron and calcium. Additionally, brown rice tends to accumulate more inorganic arsenic, a known carcinogen, which is concentrated in its outer layers.

Meat Substitutes: While marketed as a healthy alternative, plant-based meat alternatives contain processed ingredients and high sodium levels. Additionally, these products often include unhealthy fats and additives like methylcellulose, a thickener, and soy leghemoglobin, a genetically engineered protein used to replicate the taste of meat. These additives can cause digestive issues and other health concerns.

Agave Syrup: Often promoted as a "natural" sweetener, agave syrup contains high levels of fructose without nature's fiber packaging, which can contribute to insulin resistance and liver problems. It is similar to high fructose corn syrup in its effects on the body. Another example of a food fad promoted as 'healthy' without any supporting evidence. A rose by any other name...

"The Dirty Dozen": This list, maintained and updated annually by the Environmental Working Group, includes twelve fruits and vegetables known for having the highest pesticide residues when grown conventionally. Items like strawberries, spinach, and apples often top the list, with significant levels of pesticides detected.

Pro Tip: Soak your fruit in a bowl of water with 2 teaspoons of baking soda per liter of filtered water for 15 mins to clean them of pesticides and other contaminants.

The Benefits and Misconceptions of "Organic Food"

Organic food is often touted as the gold standard for high-quality nutrition. Organic farming practices exclude the use of synthetic pesticides, herbicides, and fertilizers, as well as GMOs. This results in food that is generally more environmentally friendly and potentially more nutritious.

Studies have shown that organic produce can have higher levels of certain antioxidants and lower levels of pesticide residues compared to conventionally grown produce. However, misconceptions about organic food abound. Many people believe that all organic food is free from contamination and superior in every way to conventional food. While organic farming practices aim to reduce chemical exposure, organic foods can still be contaminated. The prevalence of factory farming and the proximity of organic farms to conventional ones can lead to unintentional contamination with pesticides and other chemicals. Research indicates that wind and water can carry pesticides to organic fields, resulting in detectable levels of these substances even in organic produce which is why it's important to try to understand where your food is coming from before you put it in your mouth.

The Importance of Knowing Your Purveyors

Sourcing high-quality food from local purveyors is ideal for ensuring optimal nutrition. Local foods often have shorter supply chains, meaning they can be fresher and retain more nutrients. Supporting local farmers also promotes sustainable agricultural practices and strengthens the local economy. Connecting directly with farmers requires effort and commitment but ensures you are sourcing high quality food.

Farmers' markets, community-supported agriculture (CSA) programs, and direct farm purchases are excellent ways to source local, high-quality food. But more important than location is connecting with farms and farmers whose ethics and agricultural practices create the best quality products. In some cases, that may mean sourcing from a farm halfway across the country. Score one for the internet!

Factory Farming

Factory farming, also known as concentrated animal feeding operations (CAFOs), are characterized by the mass production of animals in confined spaces, prioritizing efficiency and profit over animal welfare. This method often results in significant physical and psychological suffering for the animals. They are kept in overcrowded, unsanitary conditions that lead to stress, disease, and injury. Practices such as debeaking, tail docking, and castration are performed without anesthesia, causing immense pain and distress which in turn causes the animal to release all manner of hormones, cortisol, etc into their bloodstream. Let's call them "marinades" that you don't want flavoring your food. Moreover, the overuse of antibiotics in these settings fosters the development of antibiotic-resistant bacteria that invite severe public health threats. These farms also generate large amounts of waste, contaminating local water supplies and contributing to air pollution, which impacts the health of nearby communities.

In 2025, the avian influenza outbreak has cast a spotlight on the vulnerabilities inherent in industrial poultry farming. While wild birds may introduce H5N1 to new areas, the virus's establishment and dissemination among domestic chickens are closely linked to human-mediated factors such as intensive farming practices and global poultry trade. Factory farms, characterized by densely packed populations of genetically similar birds, create an environment where viruses like H5N1 can spread rapidly and mutate. This overcrowding not only facilitates disease transmission but also increases the likelihood of the virus adapting to new hosts, including humans.

In response to outbreaks, standard protocol involves culling (aka slaughtering) infected flocks to prevent further spread. Given that some facilities house millions of birds, such measures lead to significant reductions in egg production. This diminished supply has contributed to soaring egg prices, with reports indicating increases of around 44% in the U.S. compared to the previous year. Beyond economic implications, the culling process raises ethical concerns regarding animal welfare. The mass destruction of birds highlights the moral dilemmas associated with intensive farming practices.

On the other end of the spectrum, game meats like venison, bison, and elk are among the healthiest animal proteins available. These meats are not only nutritionally superior but also contribute to environmental equilibrium compared to factory-farmed beef. Nutritionally, game meats are rich in protein, omega-3 fatty acids, and essential vitamins and minerals while being low in fat and calories. Venison for instance, has 50% less fat than beef and is packed with iron, B vitamins, and zinc. Elk meat contains a higher concentration of omega-3 fatty acids, CLA, and beneficial fats that support cardiovascular health. Bison, similarly, is a lean protein source with a balanced omega-6 to omega-3 ratio, making it an excellent choice for reducing inflammation and promoting heart health.

From an environmental perspective, hunting and consuming game meat helps maintain ecological balance by controlling wildlife populations. Overpopulation of species like deer can lead to overgrazing, which disrupts ecosystems and biodiversity. Additionally, game meats typically come from animals that are free to graze in their natural habitats, which is more humane, yields more nutritional meat, and is far more sustainable compared to the confined and awful conditions of factory farms.

Supermarkets

The nutritional quality of supermarket produce often suffers due to practices designed to accommodate warehousing and long-distance transportation. Fruits and vegetables are frequently harvested before reaching full ripeness to withstand the rigors of shipping and extend shelf life.

This premature harvesting leads to lower nutrient content compared to produce allowed to ripen fully on the plant. Produce can lose up to 30% of its nutrients three days after harvest and even more during extended storage and transportation periods. The lengthy supply chain of commercial produce, often spanning thousands of miles and multiple days, exacerbates this nutrient loss, leaving consumers with food that is less nutritious than its freshly picked counterparts, and that's saying nothing about the pollution of sending large trucks back and forth across the country.

Once the products are at the market, various methods are employed to extend the shelf life of meat for example to make it appear more appetizing. One common practice is the use of carbon monoxide to maintain the meat's red color, giving the appearance of freshness long after it has begun to spoil. That is not only disgusting in and of itself—more special "marinades", but also it seems fairly unethical to sell meat on the verge of spoiling. Meats are also often treated with solutions of water, salt, and other additives to enhance flavor and increase weight, which further obscures the true (lack of) quality of the product. Another controversial practice is the washing of chicken carcasses with chlorine or other antimicrobial baths to kill bacteria. This method is used to meet food safety standards and is prevalent in the industry. However, it raises concerns about the potential health effects of residual chemicals and the impact on the nutritional quality of the meat. For point of reference, washing chicken in chlorine and other disinfectants to remove harmful bacteria was a practice banned by the European Union (EU) in 1997 over food safety concerns.

Food irradiation is also used to extend the shelf life and improve the safety of various food products. This process involves exposing food to ionizing radiation to kill bacteria, parasites, and other pathogens. While the FDA and other health organizations deem irradiated foods safe, the process can alter the texture and taste of the food, and there are ongoing debates about its long-term health effects.

Even the layout of most supermarkets is deliberately designed to drive you towards suboptimal food choices. Supermarkets allocate the majority of their floor space to processed foods, which are often less expensive but nutritionally inferior to whole foods.

Processed foods that are typically high in sugar, unhealthy fats, chemicals, and additives while whole foods such as fresh produce meats, and dairy, are relegated to the edges of the store. An article from the *Journal of Retailing* explains how supermarket layouts influence purchasing behavior. The study found that placing essential items like milk and eggs at the back of the store forces customers to walk through aisles of processed foods, increasing the likelihood of impulse buys. This layout strategy is a deliberate effort to maximize profits, not to provide access to the most nutritious food options, as processed foods have higher profit margins and longer shelf lives. The higher cost of quality food is often cited as a barrier to healthier eating. However, we need to reframe our thinking around this significantly. If we are putting this food in our bodies, it should be viewed as an investment in long-term health and well-being. Consuming nutrient-dense, high-quality foods can quite literally prevent chronic diseases, reduce healthcare costs, and enhance quality of life. While organic and locally sourced foods may have a higher upfront cost, they provide significant health benefits that outweigh these expenses over time. Achieving elevated nutrition requires a commitment to spending the time to source high-quality foods, particularly animal proteins. Understanding what makes up food quality, navigating supermarket layouts, and investing in local, organic produce are crucial steps in this journey. By prioritizing nutrient-dense, minimally processed foods and supporting sustainable farming practices, we can fuel our bodies optimally, prevent disease, and enhance our overall well-being.

Intuitive Eating

Intuitive eating is an approach to nutrition that encourages individuals to listen to their body's natural hunger and fullness cues, allowing these internal signals to guide food choices rather than relying on external diet rules or restrictions. This practice is rooted in the idea of trusting your body to know what it needs to feel nourished and satisfied. Unlike traditional diets that impose strict guidelines about what and when to eat, intuitive eating promotes a flexible, individualized approach that honors your unique physical needs. Developing the skill of intuitive eating requires patience, self-awareness, and a willingness to break free from rigid dietary patterns. One of the key aspects of this approach is tuning into hunger and fullness cues.

Hara hachi bun me (腹八分目)

A Confucian teaching which roughly translates to "Eat until you are eight parts (out of ten) full" or "belly 80 percent full". This practice encourages moderation and mindfulness, where nourishment is about energy, not excess. By consciously stopping before reaching fullness, you promote optimal digestion, longevity, and a deeper connection with your body's needs, transforming every meal into a moment of attunement and respect for your health and well-being.

Mindfulness is another crucial component of intuitive eating. This involves slowing down and fully engaging with the eating process, which allows you to better recognize how different foods affect your body. An Ayurvedic practice that complements this is the habit of chewing each bite of food thirty two (yes 32!) times before swallowing. This methodical chewing not only aids in digestion by breaking down food more thoroughly, but it also gives your body time to register feelings of fullness, further preventing overeating. Chewing food slowly and thoroughly ensures that digestive enzymes in the saliva begin the process of breaking down food, making it easier on the stomach and intestines, and enhancing nutrient absorption. Chewing thirty two times per bite is an incredibly difficult practice to cultivate and maintain. I challenge you to try if only to shed light on how quickly we tend to eat and in doing so, bypass any chance to feel how our food is making us feel.

By paying attention to how you feel after eating certain foods, you can begin to identify which foods energize you and which might leave you feeling sluggish or uncomfortable. Keeping a food journal can be helpful in tracking these patterns and determining what agrees with your individual system. At one point in my personal journey, I was still suffering from semi-regular rosacea outbreaks where certain parts of my face would break out in a red rash, my scalp would itch, and strands of hair would fall out. After doing some research and writing down what I was eating, I narrowed the root cause down to a few specific foods–alcohol, coffee, and citrus fruit. And I became so attuned to how these foods felt in my body that after just a single sip (or bite) of one of these foods, I could feel my face start to tingle, signalling an oncoming flare-up. What's even more interesting is that not only by cutting these foods out did I stop the rosacea outbreaks but the general inflammation that was being triggered (including a corresponding biofilm on my tongue) dissipated and eventually disappeared altogether. And now, I can once again enjoy these foods without fear of a flare-up but I am hyper-aware of when I eat something and some part of my body feels off which I consider a kind of superpower at this point. Another method is 'the heartbeat test'—a simple yet effective method for assessing whether a particular food is suitable for your body. This test involves monitoring your heart rate before and after consuming a specific food. To perform the test, take your pulse before eating to establish a baseline, then again at intervals of 15, 30, and 60 minutes after eating. If your heart rate increases by more than 10-15 beats per minute, the food is likely causing a stress response in your body, suggesting that it might not agree with you.

Intuitive eating is ultimately about building a trusting relationship with your body and making food choices based on what genuinely supports your health and well-being. By incorporating practices such as eating until 80% full, chewing thoroughly, and observing your body's responses to different foods, you can develop a more balanced and satisfying approach to eating that honors your unique needs.

Putting it all together – Using Premium Fuel

There's a pretty broad spectrum of engagement available here. As we've discussed, find the place where you are on the spectrum and begin by reaching to make the quality of your food 1° better. There is no need to tackle this entire list today. I wouldn't expect you to empty the refrigerator and go out hunting tomorrow (unless you already have a hunt planned!). But armed with this knowledge, there is undoubtedly something you can shift to elevate your nutrition right away. And once that change has become the new normal for you, assess how you feel then reach for the next rung on the ladder. In terms of assessing how you feel, pay particular attention to where you've had chronic occurrences—skin flare-ups, dry skin or itchy scalp, acid reflux, athlete's foot, hair loss, or bloating (all tend to be signs of inflammation of some kind). If those conditions begin to lessen or disappear altogether with time, take a minute to assess what foods you have eliminated from your diet and also note which ones you've added. Pay attention to your energy levels throughout the day and see if those patterns begin to change. When your body doesn't have to work overtime to process substances that aren't toxic or unnatural, it tends to have a lot more energy to do other things. Lastly, take a minute to congratulate yourself on "letting food be thy medicine" and healing your body by giving it the nourishment it needs (and deserves). By the same token, pay attention to new foods that you might add to your diet that don't necessarily make you feel great. We can't know exactly what foods are right for everyone but if you follow the framework for choosing quality foods that has been laid out, you should be able to find quite a few that truly make you feel great—be open to experimenting and trying new things, too. Einstein has a great quote something along the lines of "We cannot solve our problems with the same thinking we used when we created them". If you aren't feeling great, chances are you need to make some adjustments to your diet.

Level 1: Out the bad, in with the good

- **Eliminate Inflammatory/Processed Foods (processed sugars, refined carbs, alcohol):** Identify the processed foods from your pantry and refrigerator.
    - Items high in refined sugars, artificial additives, preservatives, and trans fats. Simply put: ditch almost anything in a box with more than 5 ingredients. Light a candle, say farewell, and don't buy them again. They are literally killing you.
    - For PMS: track how you feel throughout the phases of your cycle (e.g., energy, mood, and symptoms) using a journal or app.
- **Start Sourcing High Quality Foods:** Select higher-quality options for staples like dairy and proteins. Opt for organic or grass fed/grass finished products wherever possible, especially for items like milk, eggs, and meat.
    - Find your local Farmer's Market or depending on where you live, connect directly with local organic farmers in your area
        - especially for items on the Environmental Working Group's Dirty Dozen list, (https://www.ewg.org/foodnews/dirty-dozen.php) which are known to have higher pesticide residues.
    - Source your meat, fish, and poultry from a farm you can identify and know their sustainability practices (local, butcher box, maui nui, etc)
- **Start Daily Tongue Scraping:** Add a daily tongue scraping to your morning routine, right after waking

Level 2: Fill it with Premium

- **Eliminate Factory-Farmed Products:** Aka don't buy any meat or fish from the supermarket.
    - Partner with a friend(s) to buy a side of beef from a local farmer and store it in a cold freezer
    - Find fishermen at local harbors selling the day's catch.
    - Connect with hunters who will sell or give you some of their kill
- **Cook More at Home:** Increase the frequency of home-cooked meals to gain better control over ingredients and preparation methods.
    - Reduce visits to fast-food and restaurants to 1-2x/week
        - This will free up money to spend on higher quality ingredients
        - Once you are down to eating out 1-2x/week, shift the target to 1/month
    - Meal prep batches of key ingredients in advance to reduce overall time spent in the kitchen. As we get deeper into this, meal prepping will likely become a necessity, so you might as well start practicing now!
    - Learn about various cooking methods that retain the most nutrients, such as steaming, roasting, or grilling, and apply these methods to your home cooking.
- *For PMS:* Adjust your diet to support each phase of your cycle, focusing on anti-inflammatory foods like cruciferous vegetables and omega-3 sources during the luteal phase and energy-boosting foods (e.g., lean proteins and complex carbs) during the follicular and ovulatory phases.
- **Daily Diagnostics:** Pay attention to the size, shape, color, and frequency of your bowel movements. If you aren't in the 'normal zone' on the Bristol Stool Scale, think about what could be causing an imbalance and make an adjustment. The digestion cycle is generally 24-48 hours so the impact of changes can be fairly quickly assessed.

Level 3: Go To the Source

- **Hunt and Fish:** Take an active role in obtaining your food through sustainable practices. We'll talk more about this in the section on Skill Acquisition. But, suffice to say, it doesn't get any more fresh, taste more delicious, or get more environmentally aligned than harvesting your own food straight from nature.
- **Grow Your Own Food:** Start a home garden to grow your own fruits, herbs and vegetables. Again, no way is more fresh, more wholesome, more delicious or feel more rewarding than picking your own produce from your backyard.
- **Practice Food Preservation:** Learn and implement food preservation techniques such as canning, fermenting, and dehydrating to ensure a year-round supply of high-quality, minimally processed foods. Fermented foods are an important source of healthy bacteria for maintaining a balanced gut microbiome.
- *For PMS:* **Match your lifestyle and exercise routine to your cycle:** schedule intense workouts and high-focus tasks during high-energy phases (follicular/ovulatory) and prioritize rest, mindfulness, and gentle movement (yoga, stretching) in low-energy phases (menstrual/luteal).

This last level might sound way out of reach especially for city dwellers but like everything in this program, small steps 1° in a new direction will have you there faster than you think. There is obviously a learning curve involved with learning how to hunt ethically and in harmony with nature. The first step is getting your license to hunt in your state. Start there. And the reality of hunting is that a single deer or elk and a boar per season will provide you with a significant amount of meat. The same holds true with growing fruits and vegetables. Start small. Grow some tomatoes in a container one summer. Eat what you can and preserve the rest. Don't start trying to grow the garden of Eden, that will just get frustrating and likely lead you to give up the endeavor altogether. Having said that, it's pretty magical when that first fruit or vegetable appears on your plant. To think that you coaxed actual food out of the dirt with some water and a little bit of love is fairly mind blowing.

Nutrition - subscribepage.io/Nutritionresources

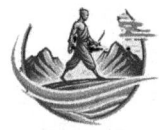

NUTRITION: Part II

EVERY CALORIE COUNTS

Macronutrients are the primary components of our diet. Proteins, carbohydrates, and fats provide the energy essential for the majority of our bodily functions. When developing an effective food plan to meet dietary goals, whether for weight loss, muscle building, or maintaining current fitness levels, understanding macronutrients is crucial. While calories measure the energy provided by food, not all calories are created equally. The way that we combine macronutrients to create a meal significantly impacts body composition, energy levels, and overall health.

Protein

Protein is a crucial macronutrient with profound impacts on both muscle building and weight loss. Metabolically, protein plays a pivotal role in muscle synthesis and repair. When you engage in resistance training or other forms of exercise, muscle fibers experience microscopic damage. Protein provides the essential amino acids necessary for the repair and rebuilding of these fibers, leading to muscle growth and increased strength (hypertrophy). This process, known as muscle protein synthesis, is stimulated by protein intake, ensuring that your body has the necessary building blocks to develop and maintain muscle mass.

In the context of weight loss, increasing protein intake is particularly beneficial for several reasons. Firstly, protein has a higher thermic effect compared to fats and carbohydrates. This means that your body expends more energy, or burns more calories, to digest and metabolize protein. This enhanced calorie expenditure can contribute to a higher overall metabolic rate, which is advantageous for weight loss and why you'll always read about increasing protein as one of the fundamental ways to lose weight effectively. Protein also aids in preserving lean muscle mass during periods of caloric deficit. When you're in a calorie-restricted state, your body may break down muscle tissue for energy. Adequate protein consumption helps mitigate this muscle loss by providing the necessary nutrients to support muscle maintenance and repair. This is crucial because muscle tissue is metabolically active and burns more calories at rest compared to fat tissue. By preserving lean muscle mass, you ensure a more efficient metabolism and a greater calorie burn, even when you're not actively exercising.

Fat

Fat is a crucial macronutrient with multifaceted roles in maintaining health, supporting energy levels, and facilitating various bodily functions. Metabolically, fat serves as a dense slow burning energy source, providing 9 calories per gram compared to 4 calories per gram from proteins and carbohydrates. This high energy yield is essential for sustaining long-term physical activity, particularly during low to moderate-intensity exercise, when the body relies more on fat stores for fuel once glycogen reserves are depleted. In muscle building, fats are integral to hormone production and cellular health. Healthy fats, such as those from avocados, nuts, seeds, tallow, and fatty fish, are essential for the synthesis of hormones like testosterone and estrogen, which are crucial for muscle growth and repair. Additionally, fats contribute to the maintenance of cell membrane integrity and support the absorption of fat-soluble vitamins (D, A, K, and E), which are vital for overall health and optimal metabolic function.

When it comes to weight loss, incorporating an appropriate amount of fat into your diet can be beneficial - wait what? Consuming fat helps lose weight?? Imagine that. Fats contribute to satiety, helping you feel full and satisfied for long periods of time, which can reduce overall calorie intake and curb unnecessary snacking. This can be particularly advantageous for managing appetite and adhering to a calorie deficit without experiencing excessive hunger. Moreover, fats play a role in maintaining a healthy metabolism. They help regulate blood sugar levels and support insulin sensitivity, which can influence fat storage and utilization. By promoting balanced blood sugar levels, fats can help prevent the spikes and crashes in energy that can lead to overeating and weight gain. Fats are also necessary for the proper function of the brain and nervous system. Essential fatty acids, such as omega-3 and omega-6, support cognitive function, mood regulation, and neurological health. This can enhance mental clarity and overall well-being, contributing to a more effective and sustainable weight management strategy.

Carbohydrates

Carbohydrates are the third vital macronutrient that plays an essential role in energy production, exercise performance, and overall health. Metabolically, carbohydrates are the body's primary source of energy. When consumed, they are broken down into glucose, which is utilized by cells for immediate energy needs or stored as glycogen in muscles and the liver for later use. This energy is crucial for maintaining optimal bodily functions and fueling various physical activities, from everyday tasks to high-intensity workouts.

In the context of muscle building, carbohydrates are equally important. During exercise, particularly high-intensity or endurance activities, glycogen stores in the muscles are depleted. Adequate carbohydrate intake replenishes these glycogen reserves, allowing for quicker recovery between workouts and supporting sustained performance. This replenishment helps prevent muscle fatigue and ensures that muscles are adequately fueled for future training sessions, which is essential for continued muscle growth and strength development. When it comes to weight loss, carbohydrates still play a supportive role. While it's important to manage carbohydrate intake to ensure it aligns with overall calorie goals, the quality and timing of carbohydrate consumption can significantly impact weight management. For instance, consuming complex carbohydrates—such as whole grains, starchy tubers, and legumes—provides a slower, more sustained release of glucose into the bloodstream. This can help maintain steady energy levels and prevent spikes in blood sugar, which can contribute to better appetite control and reduced cravings.

Often cast as the villains in the struggle against weight loss, carbohydrates are integral in preserving muscle mass during weight loss. Inadequate carbohydrate intake can lead to the breakdown of muscle protein for energy, especially when in a calorie deficit. By ensuring sufficient carbohydrate consumption, you help prevent this muscle loss, thereby preserving lean muscle mass, which is crucial for maintaining a healthy metabolism and promoting continued fat loss. Last but not least, carbohydrates impact mood and cognitive function. Glucose is the brain's primary energy source, and adequate carbohydrate intake supports optimal mental performance and mood stability. This can help maintain motivation and adherence to a weight loss or fitness program.

Adjusting Macronutrients for Specific Goals

Adjusting macronutrient ratios is crucial for achieving specific body composition goals, whether it's losing weight, building muscle, or maintaining overall fitness. Each macronutrient—proteins, carbohydrates, and fats—plays a unique role, and manipulating their ratios like levers can significantly influence outcomes.

Losing Weight

To lose weight, more than anything else, *creating a calorie deficit is essential*. That is, burning more calories than you consume in a given day. However, the macronutrient distribution within this calorie deficit can impact how effectively and sustainably weight loss is achieved. In trying to lose weight, *protein intake goes up* and *carbohydrate intake goes down*.

Protein: Increasing protein intake is vital for weight loss. Protein helps preserve lean muscle mass, which is crucial because muscle tissue burns more calories at rest. And protein takes more energy for the body to break down thereby burning more calories as a source of fuel. A typical recommendation for protein intake during weight loss is 1 gram per pound of body weight. This higher intake not only supports muscle maintenance but also enhances satiety, reducing hunger and aiding in appetite control. Protein in a weight loss phase should make up about **40%** of total daily calories.

Fats: While fats are calorie-dense, they should not be excessively reduced as they are essential for hormone production and overall health. Fats should account for around **37%** of daily caloric intake, including healthy fats from avocados, nuts, seeds, and olive oil. This balance helps maintain hormonal health and supports satiety.

Carbohydrates: Carbohydrate intake is often reduced in weight loss meal planning to manage overall calorie intake and blood sugar levels. Carbohydrates should typically comprise roughly **23%** of total daily calories. Focus on complex carbohydrates (such as whole grains, starches, and legumes) rather than simple sugars. This approach helps maintain energy levels while promoting fat loss.

Building Muscle

For muscle building, different macronutrient ratios are required to support muscle protein synthesis and recovery. The total number of daily calories goes up significantly. Our *protein intake is going to increase,* fat intake will decrease and we will be consuming *more calories in the form of carbohydrates* to feed depleted glycogen stores in our muscles.

Protein: Protein is critical for muscle growth. During muscle building phases, protein intake should be slightly increased to support muscle repair and growth. The recommendation is approximately 1-1.2 gram per pound of body weight. Protein should constitute about **30%** of daily calories. There are many philosophies out there and it's important to make your own adjustments to these ratios to optimize your results. These numbers are suggestions meant to provide guidance and set you on the path to attaining your goals.

Fats: While fats are less directly involved in muscle growth, they are important for overall health and hormone regulation. Fats should account for about **30%** of daily caloric intake This will continue to support hormonal functions related to muscle growth and recovery and provides slow-burning energy to utilize throughout the day.

Carbohydrates: Carbohydrates are essential for replenishing glycogen stores depleted during intense workouts. Adequate carbohydrate intake supports energy levels, performance, and recovery. Carbohydrates should make up **40%** of total daily calories when trying to build muscle, emphasizing complex carbs. This ensures sustained energy and enhances exercise performance.

Maintaining Fitness

For maintaining fitness, we will be consuming less calories daily than in the muscle building phase and the macronutrient ratios will stay more or less balanced, supporting a steady energy supply and overall health while avoiding weight gain or loss. In this case, protein, fats, and carbohydrates will remain in roughly equal proportion.

Protein: Maintaining adequate protein intake is crucial for preserving muscle mass and overall health. Protein should comprise about **35%** of daily calories, with a recommendation of 1.0 - 1.1 grams per pound of body weight. This ensures that muscle maintenance and repair processes are supported without excessive caloric surplus.

Fats: Healthy fats are essential for overall health, including hormone function and cellular integrity. Fats should account for roughly **35%** of daily caloric intake, ensuring sufficient energy and essential fatty acids for optimal bodily functions.

Carbohydrates: Carbohydrates should provide enough energy for daily activities and exercise without leading to excess calorie intake. Carbohydrates can make up **30%** of total daily calories. This helps sustain energy levels and supports general fitness without contributing to weight gain.

Adjusting macronutrient ratios according to body composition goals—weight loss, muscle building, or fitness maintenance—requires careful consideration of protein, carbohydrate, and fat intake.

Tailoring these ratios to your specific goals will optimize your effectiveness in achieving specific outcomes, whether by boosting metabolism, supporting muscle growth, or maintaining overall health and fitness. As always, the goal here is to help you shift your direction by at least 1° from where you might be stuck or unclear about how to move forward. And with time, you will become the master of how your body reacts to shifting macronutrient levers like protein and carbohydrates. Just remember that after a few weeks of implementing a particular plan, your body will have changed in composition and *you will need to reevaluate and reset your goals* and your macronutrient targets—you will be that much closer to the sun! Progress tracking is absolutely critical to success here. At a minimum you need to be adjusting your plan every 3-4 weeks or when you hit a plateau and stop seeing progress.

The importance of Meal Frequency and Timing

Meal frequency and timing play significant roles in regulating blood sugar and insulin levels, which in turn can have a profound impact on metabolism and overall health. Understanding how these factors influence blood sugar control and metabolic function is essential for optimizing dietary strategies for energy management, weight control, and long-term well-being. The frequency of meals throughout the day can affect blood sugar levels and insulin sensitivity. Eating more frequent, smaller meals can help stabilize blood sugar levels and avoid large fluctuations.

Consistent meal patterns (along with good quality sleep) can help regulate hunger hormones, such as ghrelin and leptin, contributing to better appetite control and preventing excessive calorie consumption. When meals are spaced too far apart, or are too large in a single sitting, the body may experience large spikes and dips in blood sugar, which can lead to increased hunger and potential overeating at subsequent meals or prevent the extremes that can contribute to metabolic issues or prevent mid-afternoon "crashes" that can lead to other suboptimal habits like afternoon caffeine.

When you consume a meal, particularly one high in carbohydrates, your blood sugar levels rise rapidly. The body needs to manage this spike in blood glucose efficiently, as consistently high blood sugar levels can be harmful to organs and tissues. To counter the spike in blood sugar, the pancreas releases insulin, a hormone that facilitates the uptake of glucose by cells for energy or storage.

Insulin's primary role is to lower blood sugar levels by helping cells absorb glucose, but when a large amount of glucose enters the bloodstream at once, the body releases a significant amount of insulin to manage it. When insulin levels are high, the body enters a "storage mode," converting excess glucose that isn't immediately used for energy into glycogen in the liver and muscles. Once glycogen stores are full, any remaining glucose is converted into fat and stored in adipose tissue. In other words, eating poorly balanced meals that trigger significant insulin release leads to more energy being stored as fat rather than being used for immediate needs. This creates systemic momentum in the wrong direction because high insulin levels inhibit the breakdown of fat (lipolysis) as the body prioritizes using glucose for energy. When insulin is elevated, the body's ability to access stored fat for fuel is reduced, minimizing fat utilization and maximizing fat storage. This effect is particularly pronounced when meals are irregular or infrequent, leading to larger spikes in insulin.

Over time, the compounding effect of irregular eating patterns and frequent large meals can negatively impact insulin sensitivity, leading to insulin resistance. Cells become less responsive to insulin, requiring the body to produce even more insulin to manage blood glucose levels. Insulin resistance is a precursor to type 2 diabetes and is associated with increased fat storage, particularly in the abdominal area. In other words, bang the insulin gong too many times by gorging on a bunch of sugar and carbs and your body begins to ignore the signal to convert the glucose to energy and simply stores it away as fat. As we touched on earlier, carbs are for energy and feeding the muscles and once you've accomplished those goals—you have energy and your muscles are fed, you don't need any more of those calories. The goal with balanced nutrition is to give the body everything it needs and nothing it doesn't.

A Note on Intermittent Fasting

Intermittent fasting (IF) has gained attention for its potential benefits in enhancing metabolic function and promoting overall health. As with so much of the 'biohacking' movement, it's important to remember that something that yields great results for one person may not be beneficial for another. IF is no exception. For individuals with an increased risk of or existing thyroid conditions, IF requires careful consideration due to its possible effects on thyroid function.

Extended fasting periods or severe caloric restriction may lead to a reduction in thyroid hormone levels, including thyroxine (T4) and triiodothyronine (T3). These hormones are essential for regulating metabolism, and their decrease can slow down metabolic rate, potentially contributing to symptoms of hypothyroidism such as fatigue, weight gain, and cold intolerance. For individuals with pre-existing thyroid conditions, this reduction in thyroid hormones can exacerbate symptoms and complicate management of their condition.

Research has shown that prolonged caloric restriction, a common aspect of some intermittent fasting regimens, can lead to decreased levels of circulating thyroid hormones. This hormonal change is a physiological response aimed at conserving energy during periods of limited food intake. While short-term fasting might not significantly affect thyroid function, long-term or extreme fasting can result in chronic low thyroid hormone levels, which could impact overall metabolic health. Intermittent fasting can influence thyroid function through its effect on stress hormones. Extended fasting or inconsistent fasting schedules can increase cortisol levels, a stress hormone that can interfere with thyroid health. Elevated cortisol may impair the conversion of T4 to T3, leading to a state of functional hypothyroidism even if thyroid hormone levels appear normal on standard tests. This disruption can contribute to symptoms associated with thyroid dysfunction and affect overall metabolic rate.

At the risk of sounding like a broken record, I only learned this the hard way. In my desperation to try and become the perfect human (*status:* still working...long way to go) I was keeping up with all the latest biohacking trends and implementing them as fast as possible, convinced that if I 'did everything', one day I would wake up and just be superhuman. Unfortunately, the exact opposite happened. I was becoming more and more fatigued and not getting anywhere near the "shred" I had been promised by the dozens of biohackers proclaiming IF to be this magic protocol. In fact, I think I was even gaining belly fat. I ended up going to a nutritionist who immediately had me back off my IF protocol, because she feared it was causing hypothyroidism and elevating my cortisol levels. She was absolutely right and within a few weeks of stopping an IF protocol, my thyroid levels began returning to normal. Another thing she mentioned really hit home and became the genesis of another core principle for this entire program. Namely, if you stack all of these protocols on top of each other at the same time, it's impossible to know what effect any of them are having positively or negatively. What you end up with is a tangled mess of practices that may be working against each other.

That is why TMM is meant to be taken as a slow and methodical process, leveled up over time as you and your body gain stability and awareness for where you are right now. It becomes much easier to notice when something makes your body feel great or when something feels off when the signal noise of trying something new has died down.

It feels a bit overwhelming when you first try to bake a loaf of banana bread, separating wet ingredients from the dry, being precise with your measurements, and understanding when the loaf is baked all the way through. But at some point, after you've done it a few times, and the basic instructions become familiar, you begin to tune into some of the nuances of what makes a good loaf of banana bread, great. You become aware of how the ripeness of the bananas you use affects the outcome, or how a dash of cinnamon added to the batter delivers a wonderful accent, or exactly how long to bake it in your specific oven in order to get a perfectly brown exterior and a soft moist interior. If you changed all those variables every time you baked a loaf you'd never know from loaf to loaf why one ended up better than the other. The same holds true for walking (not running) this path. Give each new degree of change time to show itself and integrate into your overall sense of well-being before taking the next step on your journey.

The Importance of Hydration

Hydration is also a critical aspect of nutrition, foundational to maintaining health and ensuring that our bodies function optimally. Water makes up approximately 60% of the human body, and without sufficient water intake, the human body can only survive for a few days, which should be a fairly strong indication to the vital importance of maintaining proper hydration levels.

Water is integral to numerous bodily functions, including regulating body temperature through processes such as sweating and respiration. During physical activity or exposure to high temperatures, water helps dissipate excess heat, preventing overheating and ensuring that the body remains at a stable internal temperature. Proper hydration is also essential for digestion and nutrient absorption. Water aids in the breakdown of food, facilitating the movement of food through the digestive tract and assisting in the efficient transport of nutrients to cells. It helps produce digestive juices and supports the function of enzymes that are necessary for breaking down food into absorbable nutrients. Additionally, adequate water intake is crucial for preventing constipation, as it helps soften stool and promotes regular bowel movements, ensuring that waste is efficiently excreted from the body. Water plays a crucial role in maintaining joint health as well. Synovial fluid, which lubricates the joints, is primarily composed of water. Adequate hydration supports the maintenance of this fluid, reducing the risk of joint discomfort and stiffness.

Furthermore, water assists in detoxification by facilitating the removal of waste products through urine, sweat, and bowel movements. It supports the kidneys in filtering and excreting toxins, contributing to overall health.

Hydration also profoundly impacts cognitive function. The brain, being highly sensitive to changes in hydration status, relies on a consistent supply of water to perform optimally. Even mild dehydration can impair cognitive functions such as concentration, memory, and mood, leading to decreased mental performance and increased irritability. Studies have shown that as little as 1-2% dehydration can significantly affect cognitive abilities, resulting in slower reaction times, reduced alertness, and difficulties in focusing. This makes it evident how crucial regular water intake is for maintaining mental sharpness and overall cognitive health.

Daily Water Intake Formula

Daily Water Intake (in ounces) = Body Weight (in pounds) x **0.67**

For example, if you weigh 150 pounds, you would need approximately 100.5 ounces of water per day to meet your hydration needs. This formula provides a baseline for fluid intake but should be adjusted based on individual factors like physical activity, climate, and health conditions.

It's surprisingly easy to become dehydrated, especially when we're not actively paying attention to our water intake throughout the day. Factors such as physical activity, environmental conditions, and even daily tasks that divert attention can lead to insufficient water consumption. Often, by the time we feel thirsty, mild dehydration has already set in. Given the critical roles that water plays in the body—from digestion and detoxification to cognitive function and joint health—it's essential to stay properly hydrated throughout the day. Challenge yourself to get 1° better at drinking enough water every day. It's a simple habit that pays significant dividends in trying to establish an elevated daily experience by supporting the body's many vital functions.

Water Quality

High-quality water is an important part of the hydration equation and not all water, sadly, is the same. Consuming water that is free from contaminants such as heavy metals, chlorine, and other chemicals commonly found in tap water is crucial for maintaining overall wellness. To ensure water is maximally absorbed by the body, it is important to consume water that is mineral-rich, pH-balanced, and free from harmful contaminants. Using high-quality filtration systems can remove these impurities, ensuring that the water you drink is as absorbable as possible. Natural spring water is great because it contains beneficial minerals that are typically stripped away during the purification processes of other water sources.

For water to be maximally absorbed by the body, it needs to be in a state that the body can readily utilize. The key factors influencing water absorption include its mineral content, pH level, and the presence of any contaminants or particulates. One way to notice the quality of the water you are drinking is how often you need to pee... now, this can be indicative of a few things but one reason, if you are drinking the proper amount of water and find yourself having to pee all the time may be because your body isn't absorbing the water you are drinking as well as you could be—meaning it may be missing minerals or have a pH imbalance and more of it is passing through you than hydrating you. This is simply something to be aware of but still drink your water, it's the best beverage you can drink.

Mineral Content: Water that contains essential minerals, such as calcium, magnesium, and potassium, plays a crucial role in maintaining electrolyte balance. Electrolytes help regulate fluid movement across cell membranes, ensuring that water gets absorbed efficiently into cells. Hard water, which is rich in these minerals, can support hydration by providing a natural source of electrolytes. However, hard water's high mineral content can sometimes slow down absorption in sensitive individuals, and does have the potential to cause digestive discomfort should be considered. Conversely, soft water, which is lower in minerals, may be absorbed more quickly by the body, but its lack of naturally occurring electrolytes means it may not offer the same hydrating benefits as hard water. To ensure maximal hydration, a balance is necessary. Distilled water, which is free of all minerals, is not as hydrating as mineral-rich water because it does not contribute to the body's electrolyte balance. Drinking naturally mineralized water or water that has been remineralized—such as by adding hydrogen tablets or electrolyte supplements—can enhance the body's ability to absorb and utilize water effectively. I personally add a hydrogen tablet to my morning water to boost its mineral content and improve my daily hydration routine.

pH Level: The pH level of water can also impact its absorbability and plays an important role in determining water quality and its impact on the body. The pH scale, ranging from 0 to 14, measures how acidic or alkaline a substance is, with 7 being neutral. For water, a pH level of 6.5 to 8.5 is generally considered optimal for consumption. Water that is too acidic (below 6.5) can leach metals from pipes, which may lead to contamination with harmful substances like lead and copper.

Acidic water can also cause digestive discomfort and interfere with the body's natural pH balance. Conversely, highly alkaline water (above 8.5) can have an unpleasant taste and may cause mineral deposits, although some claim it can neutralize acid in the body. Maintaining a neutral or slightly alkaline pH in drinking water is important for optimal hydration and health. Water at this pH range supports cellular processes without causing irritation to the gut lining or contributing to health risks related to metal contamination or mineral imbalance.

Contaminants: Water that contains contaminants or particulates can also be less absorbable, as the body may need to expend additional energy to filter out impurities, potentially reducing the efficiency of hydration. Both public water supplies and bottled water can contain various particulates and contaminants that affect water quality and safety. Some of the most common particulates include:

Chlorine and Chloramines: Used as disinfectants in public water supplies to kill bacteria and other pathogens. While effective for sanitation, they can leave behind residues that may have an unpleasant taste and potential health impacts over long-term exposure.

Fluoride: Fluoride has long been touted for its dental benefits, but its presence in public water supplies raises concerns. Originally added to drinking water to reduce tooth decay, recent research has questioned its safety, pointing to potential risks including endocrine disruption, thyroid dysfunction, and impaired cognitive development. Chronic exposure, even at low levels, may accumulate in bones and tissues, posing long-term health concerns.

Heavy Metals: Lead, arsenic, and mercury are examples of heavy metals that can be found in public water supplies, often due to old plumbing infrastructure or industrial contamination. These metals are toxic and can cause serious health issues, particularly with prolonged exposure.

Microplastics: Tiny plastic particles have been detected in both public and bottled water. Microplastics can come from various sources, including degraded plastic waste and packaging materials. The long-term health effects of ingesting microplastics are still being studied, but their presence is a growing concern. Studies have shown that the average American now consumes a *credit card size worth of microplastics on an annual basis.* Let that sink in.

Pesticides and Herbicides: Agricultural runoff can introduce pesticides and herbicides into water supplies. These chemicals can persist in the environment and may contaminate drinking water, posing risks to human health.

Pharmaceutical Residues: Trace amounts of pharmaceuticals, such as antibiotics and hormones, have been found in water supplies, particularly where wastewater treatment plants discharge into water sources. These residues can enter the water supply through human waste or improper disposal of medications.

Nitrates: Commonly found in agricultural runoff, nitrates can contaminate water supplies, particularly in rural areas. High levels of nitrates in drinking water can be harmful, especially for infants and pregnant women.

Being aware of common particulates found in public and bottled water, such as chlorine, heavy metals, microplastics, pesticides, and pharmaceutical residues, can guide you in choosing the best filtration methods or water sources for optimal hydration and health. In practical terms, get your water tested (see *Additional Resources*) and then determine what kind of filtration system is most appropriate for the water you drink. While it may seem like a pain in the butt to 'test your water', it's an investment in your health and a small one time exercise to ensure you are flushing your system daily with the cleanest water available. And just don't drink water out of plastic bottles. It's bad for you and it's terrible for the environment.

Recommended Filtration Systems for High-Quality Water

Filtration System	Positives (+)	Downsides (-)
Berkey Water Filters	Excellent at removing a wide range of contaminants, including heavy metals, chlorine, and pathogens.	High upfront cost. Replacement filters are expensive.
Reverse Osmosis Systems	Highly effective at removing most contaminants, including fluoride and heavy metals.	Strips water of beneficial minerals; requires remineralization for pH balance.
Brita Pitchers	Affordable and easy to use; reduces chlorine, lead, and other common contaminants.	Limited filtration capacity; less effective at removing heavy metals and some chemicals.
ZeroWater Filters	Provides thorough filtration, reducing most dissolved solids and contaminants.	Can strip beneficial minerals; water may taste flat due to aggressive filtration.

Aquasana Whole House Systems	Comprehensive filtration for the entire home; removes chlorine, lead, and organic compounds.	Expensive installation and maintenance; not portable or convenient for renters.

These filtration systems vary in effectiveness based on the contaminants they can remove and whether they maintain or strip away beneficial minerals. Choosing the right system depends on individual needs, such as whether you prioritize portability, thorough filtration, or the retention of beneficial minerals for pH balance. Personally, I use a Berkey water filter and always carry my Yeti Insulated water bottle with me wherever I go.

Alcohol

On the opposite end of the spectrum from water is Alcohol, a diuretic. It causes your body to remove fluids from your blood through your renal system, which includes the kidneys, ureters, and bladder, at a much quicker rate than other liquids. Almost all of us at one time or another have enjoyed an adult beverage or two and I'm sure many of us have also enjoyed 'one too many'.

Alcohol is a pervasive part of many cultures around the world and has been for most of human civilization. And while its effects can feel great in the moment, it's worth understanding more about what's happening underneath the hood to better assess the pros and cons of knocking a few back.

When you consume alcohol, it binds to gamma-aminobutyric acid (GABA) receptors in the brain, increasing the inhibitory effects of GABA. This leads to the characteristic effects of alcohol, such as relaxation, reduced inhibition, and ultimately impaired motor function. At higher doses, alcohol's enhancement of GABA can lead to more profound sedation, loss of consciousness, and even memory blackouts. This amplification of GABA's inhibitory effects is similar to how anesthesia drugs function to induce unconsciousness, suppress pain, and immobilize the body during surgery. Unfortunately, alcohol consumption can have a wide range of harmful effects on the body, affecting multiple organs and systems. When alcohol is consumed, it is rapidly absorbed into the bloodstream through the stomach and small intestine. From there, it is transported to the liver, where the primary metabolism of alcohol takes place. The liver breaks down alcohol through a two-step process:

1. **Alcohol Dehydrogenase (ADH):** The enzyme alcohol dehydrogenase converts alcohol (ethanol) into acetaldehyde, a highly toxic and reactive substance. Acetaldehyde is much more harmful than ethanol itself and is a key factor in alcohol-related damage to the body.
2. **Aldehyde Dehydrogenase (ALDH):** The enzyme aldehyde dehydrogenase then converts acetaldehyde into acetate, a less harmful substance. Acetate is eventually broken down into carbon dioxide and water, which the body can eliminate.

Despite this detoxification process, acetaldehyde can accumulate in the body, especially if large amounts of alcohol are consumed in a short period. This accumulation can cause significant damage to tissues and organs.

Destructive Effects on the Body

When you consider the downsides of consuming alcohol—and that doesn't say anything about the empty calories it represents—it becomes fairly tough to make a case for drinking it on any kind of regular basis. Nothing about consumption of alcohol aligns with living an elevated life in the way we have defined it in TMM. Hopefully increased awareness about what consuming alcohol does to the body will make you think twice about making alcohol part of your everyday protocol.

Liver Damage: The liver is the primary site of alcohol metabolism, and chronic alcohol consumption can lead to liver diseases such as fatty liver, alcoholic hepatitis, and cirrhosis. The constant exposure to acetaldehyde and oxidative stress overwhelms the liver's ability to repair itself, leading to inflammation, scarring, and eventually, liver failure.

Brain and Nervous System: Alcohol is a central nervous system depressant. It impairs cognitive function, coordination, and decision-making. Over time, excessive alcohol use can lead to permanent brain damage, cognitive decline, and increased risk of neurodegenerative diseases like dementia.

Cardiovascular System: Alcohol can increase blood pressure and lead to cardiomyopathy (a condition where the heart muscle weakens), arrhythmias (irregular heartbeats), and an increased risk of stroke. Alcohol also contributes to the buildup of triglycerides in the blood, leading to the risk of heart disease.

PMS: Alcohol can exacerbate PMS (Premenstrual Syndrome) symptoms by altering hormone levels and disrupting mood-regulating neurotransmitters, such as serotonin. It can increase anxiety, irritability, and fatigue, and may also worsen physical symptoms like bloating and breast tenderness due to its impact on fluid retention and inflammation.

Digestive System: Chronic alcohol consumption can cause inflammation of the stomach lining (gastritis) and increase the risk of ulcers. It also disrupts the balance of gut microbiota, leading to digestive issues and an increased risk of gastrointestinal cancers.

Weight Gain and Muscle Growth: Alcohol is calorie-dense (7 calories per gram) and can contribute to weight gain, especially as it is often consumed alongside high-calorie foods. Moreover, alcohol metabolism takes precedence in the body, meaning that other nutrients (carbohydrates, fats, proteins) are more likely to be stored as fat when alcohol is present. Additionally, alcohol disrupts hormone balance, including testosterone and growth hormone, which are critical for muscle repair and growth. This disruption can impair muscle recovery and growth, making it harder to build and maintain muscle mass. In other words, drinking a beer after a hard workout can negate all the work you just put in to build muscle.

Sleep Disruption: While alcohol may initially make you feel drowsy, it actually disrupts sleep patterns. Alcohol reduces REM sleep, the most restorative phase of the sleep cycle, leading to poor sleep quality. This disruption can result in fatigue, impaired cognitive function, and a weakened immune system. Over time, poor sleep due to alcohol consumption can contribute to chronic sleep disorders and overall health decline.

Hangovers: A hangover is the unpleasant aftermath of excessive alcohol consumption and is caused by several interrelated factors, each contributing to the discomfort and distress that often follows drinking. One of the most severe causes is dehydration. As mentioned, alcohol is a diuretic that increases urine production, leading to significant fluid loss. This dehydration is responsible for many hangover symptoms, including severe headaches, dizziness, and a parched feeling in the mouth. Closely linked to dehydration is an electrolyte imbalance, as alcohol depletes essential electrolytes like sodium, potassium, and magnesium. This imbalance can result in muscle cramps, weakness, and overwhelming fatigue.

Homemade Electrolyte Drink Recipe

A simple and effective recipe for a homemade electrolyte drink using coconut water as the base, which is naturally rich in electrolytes.

Ingredients:
- 8oz (1 cup) coconut water
- 1/4 cup fresh fruit juice (orange juice is my fave)
- 1/4 teaspoon salt (sea or kosher)*

Total for 1 Serving (16 oz):
- **Calories:** 94
- **Potassium:** 725 mg
- **Sodium:** 1000 mg
- **Magnesium:** 65 mg
- **Calcium:** 71

*note on Himalayan Sea Salt – It has increasingly been found to be mined in China and contain heavy metals. AVOID. Use Diamond Crystal kosher salt or sea salt mined in the U.S.

Gastrointestinal distress is another major component of hangovers. Alcohol irritates the stomach lining and increases the production of stomach acid, leading to nausea, vomiting, and stomach pain. The toxic buildup of acetaldehyde contributes to the general malaise, headaches, and overall sense of being unwell that define a hangover. And alcohol causes fluctuations in blood sugar levels, which can lead to symptoms like fatigue, irritability, and shakiness. This disruption in blood sugar can make it difficult for the body to maintain stable energy levels, exacerbating the overall feeling of discomfort.

Alcohol-Related Diseases and Side Effects: Just as the benefits of healthy habits compound in your favor over time, detrimental behaviors can have the same kind of compounding effect in the opposite direction. And as with some many diseases, each individual is different and has a unique genetic makeup that protects or predisposes them to triggering it but regardless of your genetic code, chronic alcohol consumption is associated with a wide range of terrible diseases and side effects, including:

Liver Diseases: Fatty liver, alcoholic hepatitis, and cirrhosis are the most common alcohol-related liver diseases. These conditions can progress to liver failure, which is life-threatening.

Pancreatitis: Alcohol can cause inflammation of the pancreas, leading to pancreatitis, a painful and potentially dangerous condition.

Cancers: Alcohol consumption is a known risk factor for several types of cancer, including mouth, throat, esophagus, liver, breast, and colorectal cancer.

Immune System Suppression: Alcohol weakens the immune system, making the body more susceptible to infections and slowing recovery from illness and injury.

Mental Health Disorders: Alcohol is linked to an increased risk of mental health disorders, including depression, anxiety, and alcohol use disorder (AUD). Chronic alcohol use can exacerbate symptoms of these conditions and lead to a vicious cycle of dependency.

Gastrointestinal Issues: Chronic alcohol consumption can lead to a range of digestive issues, including gastritis, ulcers, and an increased risk of gastrointestinal cancers.

To be clear, there is nothing wrong with an occasional alcoholic drink. The fermentation process is truly a remarkable alchemical transformation humans have discovered and perfected. But culturally, alcohol is accepted and presented in a way that (deliberately) glosses over the clear and present dangers of regularly ingesting ethanol (poison) into our systems. The takeaway here is to be aware and intentional with alcohol consumption. As with food, both quality and quantity definitely matter.

Caffeine

Caffeine, like alcohol, is also a diuretic, meaning it increases urine production and can contribute to dehydration if water intake is not adequately maintained. Regular caffeine consumers often experience increased fluid loss, which places added strain on the kidneys, requiring them to work harder to filter waste. Over time, the cumulative effect of dehydration—especially when unaddressed—can impair the body's ability to maintain electrolyte balance, leading to fatigue, headaches, and diminished physical performance. Prolonged caffeine consumption also poses challenges to the digestive system, particularly the stomach. Caffeine stimulates the production of stomach acid, which can exacerbate conditions like acid reflux and gastritis. Over time, this heightened acid exposure may damage the stomach lining, increasing the risk of ulcers and discomfort. For individuals prone to acid reflux, caffeine's impact can be especially disruptive, as the relaxation of the lower esophageal sphincter allows stomach acid to backflow into the esophagus, causing burning sensations and potential long-term damage if untreated. Caffeine can also negatively influence the cardiovascular system by elevating heart rate and blood pressure, effects that, while temporary, can strain the heart over time if intake is excessive or habitual. Some individuals are more sensitive to these cardiovascular effects, experiencing heart palpitations or irregular rhythms after consuming even moderate amounts of caffeine.

When caffeine enters the bloodstream, it blocks the action of adenosine, a neurotransmitter that promotes relaxation and sleepiness. By doing so, caffeine stimulates the central nervous system, triggering the release of adrenaline from the adrenal glands. Adrenaline is the hormone responsible for the "fight-or-flight" response, which increases heart rate, blood pressure, and energy levels temporarily. Caffeine can elevate cortisol levels, especially in those of us who suffer from chronic stress. The response to caffeine varies from person to person depending on factors such as individual tolerance, sensitivity to caffeine, and habitual use but it's important to be aware of how caffeine affects the body. Given its diuretic and acid-stimulating properties, managing caffeine consumption is essential to maintaining digestive health, hydration, and overall well-being. Incorporating mindful consumption habits—like limiting intake to early in the day and balancing caffeine with ample water—can mitigate its negative effects while still allowing individuals to enjoy its stimulating benefits.

How To Eat Anything You Want... and still lose weight

The Law of Thermodynamics states that Energy cannot be created or destroyed. This is a law of the physical universe as we know it. This is not "opinion" and doesn't vary from person to person. So, if you are eating more calories than you are burning, regardless of the source of those calories you will put on mass somewhere on your body. By the same token, if you are burning more calories than you are consuming, even if those calories consist of pizza and beer, you will lose weight. If you aren't losing weight you aren't, by definition, in a deficit. In terms of actual numbers, a pound is roughly 3500 calories which means that in order to lose (or gain) a pound, you need to be in a deficit (or surplus) beyond your Total Daily Energy Expenditure (TDEE) by 3500 calories. So the reality is that you can eat whatever you want and still lose weight **but** in order to achieve a nutrient dense meal that gives you clean energy to burn throughout the day, maintains lean muscle, and doesn't cause inflammation or any number of other imbalances, the window for eating "anything you want" is actually pretty small. Having said that, once you are armed with the knowledge of how to plan your meals using the macros that bring you closer to your goals, you can make adjustments to your program to accommodate whatever it is you desire to eat.

Losing Body Fat and Building Muscle

This seems to be most people's holy grail. Getting lean while at the same time getting strong. Ultimately that means in order to lose body fat while preserving muscle, you need to be working hard enough (or exercising hard enough) so that your body recognizes that it needs to keep the muscle for the purposes of the stress it is consistently under, while at the same time keeping your body in a deficit so that it burns fat. Otherwise known as the razor's edge.

Muscle is a metabolically active tissue. This means that muscle needs fuel in order to survive. Without that fuel, it will "reduce itself" for the purpose of survival. If you are training hard and consistently, your body will preserve the muscle more so than if you reduced how often/hard you were training or became sedentary. Otherwise, when you reduce the calories, you will naturally and unequivocally lose muscle at a faster rate. Body fat is not metabolically active. This means that it does not require fuel to exist. On the contrary, it can be used as fuel. So the goal, in order to lose body fat while preserving muscle mass, would be to eat as much as you can while still remaining in a deficit to burn body fat. When you do this, you will preserve a greater percentage of muscle, while reducing body fat.

Let's circle back to the initial question. Are we able to build muscle while losing body fat?

The short answer is: Not really. For a brief period of time it may be possible as you are first starting out. Changing your eating habits while increasing your work output will have you both getting leaner and stronger. Unfortunately, you can't serve both masters. You can either build muscle or burn fat but not both at the same time. Eventually, you will reach a plateau at one end of the spectrum or the other at which point you will need to prioritize the makeup of your macros to favor the goal you desire more. If you want to lose weight it will come at the cost of strength gains. And if you want to build muscle, you are going to need to add mass. But, the more aware you become of your own body's capacity to adapt and the more dialed in you become to adhering to your macros on a daily basis, the better you will be able to 'ride the razor's edge', making small shifts (e.g., increasing protein, decreasing carbs) to continue to progress building muscle and losing fat. As with everything in the world of TMM, this is a slower, more gradual approach but one that reflects a deeper understanding and mastery of how your machine works. Another way to think about this is that looking 'shredded' or having 'muscle definition' is really just muscles being visible underneath a minimal layer of body fat. Body aesthetics are made in the kitchen, strength is built in the gym. This is completely a matter of personal preference here but in my opinion, ***it's easier (and more rewarding) to lose the weight first then hit the weights hard to build muscle and strength*** (if that's your goal).

Calculating Your Macros

Macros are where the rubber meets the road in terms of meal planning and developing a solid foundational understanding of what foods serve what purpose in fueling your body. Calculating your macros is not rocket science and once you've done it for a few weeks, it's probably something you can adjust on the fly in your head. In the *Additional Resources* is a link to an online macro calculator to make it easy for you to figure out your splits between protein, carbs, and fat. The weighing and measuring is your (important) task. As we learned earlier, 1g of protein and 1g of carbohydrates both equal 4 calories while a 1g of fat is 9 calories. To understand the calculation for yourself, first we get our total daily energy expenditure (TDEE) or caloric target based on our desired outcome over time (cut, build, or maintain). From there we figure out the calories of our protein intake (grams/lb of body weight). The calories of our fat intake (X% of TDEE) and then the amount of calories allocated to carbohydrates falls right into place (it's just what's left over). Our daily caloric target and our carbohydrate intake are really the big levers we play with to drive different results.

It should be noted that calories don't carry over from day to day. If you end the day in a deficit, when you wake up the next day, you're back at zero. You've either lost weight or gained mass in the time you've rested and recovered since your last meal the day before but don't try to cheat the system by overeating one day and undereating the next. While theoretically, this may net out, remember that meal timing, frequency, and consistency are what help teach the body to become an efficient metabolic machine. Having said that, I would encourage you to take note if you find yourself trying to 'game the system'.

If I give you a map that shows you the fastest way from point A to point B, you wouldn't decide to take a detour and disregard the map, especially if you are in unfamiliar territory, would you? If you are looking for detours, spend some time reflecting on what is behind those impulses to disregard or circumvent the plan that will unequivocally get you to your stated goal.

So if the goal is to...

Lose body fat - make sure you work out hard, prioritize protein, eat enough **while staying in a deficit**, and get plenty of recovery.

Losing Weight

Value	Formula	Example
Daily Caloric Load	Weight (lbs) x **10**	180 x 10 = **1800 calories**
Daily Protein Intake (g)	1g per pound	180 x 1 = **180g protein** (720 calories)
Daily Fat Intake (g)	37.5% of weight	180 x .375 = **75g fat** (675 calories)
Daily Carb Intake (g)	(Daily calories - (grams of protein*4) - (grams of fat*9))/4	1800-720-675=405/4=**101g carbs** (405 calories)

To put this in real world terms and within the 1° framework, spending one day in a 500 calorie deficit, you will lose about 64g of fat or about 2.3oz - distributed across your entire body, you probably won't see or feel much difference. Keep that deficit up however for 10 days and you will have lost 640 grams or 1.4 lbs of fat, and continue to stay focused on your goal for 30 days and that 64 grams lost will become 4.5lbs, continue for 3 months and your body will be completely transformed. Notice this has nothing to do with the kinds of calories, just the deficit. Nor does it have anything to do with your workout plan. When we combine the benefits of achieving a caloric deficit with high quality nutrition that provides clean burning energy supporting all the body's metabolic functions, then you start to feel and perform at the highest levels all day everyday, regardless of what activities you take on.

If the goal is to...

Build strength/size - make sure you workout hard, prioritize protein, eat enough **to build muscle without increasing body fat** and get plenty of recovery!

Building Muscle

Value	Formula	Example
Daily Caloric Load	Weight (lbs) x 15	180 x 15 = **2700 calories**
Daily Protein Intake (g)	1.1g per pound	180 x 1.1 = **207g protein** (828 calories)
Daily Fat Intake (g)	30% of weight	180 x .30 = **90g fat** (810 calories)
Daily Carb Intake (g)	(Daily calories - (grams of protein*4) - (grams of fat*9))/4	3060-720-607.5=472.5/4 =**266g carbs** (1062 calories)

Make sure you focus on progressive overload in your workouts, prioritize protein intake, consume a caloric surplus, and allow for adequate recovery. To put this in real-world terms and within the 1° framework, adding just 100 extra calories per day in a well-balanced diet will gradually support muscle growth. After one week, you might gain approximately 0.2 pounds of muscle, which won't be immediately noticeable. However, maintain that surplus for a month, and you'll have added around 0.8 pounds of muscle mass (1-2 lbs of muscle mass/month is a healthy target). Stay consistent for three months, and you'll see an increase of about 3 pounds of solid muscle, significantly improving your strength and physique. Again, this is just focusing on caloric intake and doesn't take into account the quality of your nutrition nor does it factor in the intensity of your workouts which unlike cutting, will have a significant impact on how much strength and size you are able to add. Regardless, when you ensure those extra calories come from nutrient-dense foods that provide essential amino acids and support muscle repair, your body will not only grow stronger but also recover more effectively, leading to more efficient gains and better performance in every workout.

If the goal is to stay right where you are...

Maintain your current fitness - make sure you exercise regularly, prioritize protein, eat enough *to support your level of physical activity* and get plenty of recovery!

Maintaining Fitness

Value	Formula	Example
Daily Caloric Load	Weight (lbs) x **12.5**	180 x 12.5 = **2250 calories**
Daily Protein Intake(g)	1g per pound	180 x 1 = **180g protein** (720 calories)
Daily Fat Intake (g)	37.5% of weight	180 x .375 = **94g fat**) (844 calories)
Daily Carb Intake (g)	(Daily calories - (grams of protein*4) - (grams of fat*9))/4	2340-720 -607.5=1012.5/4 =**172g carbs** (686 calories)

If the goal is to maintain your current fitness level, the key is consistency. Contrary to popular belief, metabolism doesn't just drop off suddenly; it's influenced by your activity level, muscle mass, and dietary habits. Continue to engage in regular workouts that challenge your body just enough to preserve your strength, endurance, and flexibility. Prioritize a balanced diet that meets your caloric needs without excess, ensuring you're getting a mix of macronutrients to fuel your activities and support recovery.

It is my fundamental belief that the minute we start sending the signals to our brain and body at a cellular level that we are 'too old', 'or that our best days are behind us' or let ourselves fall out of shape to the point that the effort to recover our fitness feels insurmountable then the body and our cells organize around those objectives. The systems that create energy, repair muscle and tissue, and combat senescence respond by slowing down...

but that's only because those are the signals you're sending, not because "your metabolism slows down". In real-world terms sticking to a routine where you consume just the right amount of calories to match your energy expenditure will keep your body in equilibrium. Over a week, you'll neither gain nor lose significant weight, and your muscle mass and performance will remain steady. Extend this consistency over a month, and you'll see that your strength, endurance, and overall fitness remain intact. Push this discipline across three months, and you'll find that you've successfully maintained your fitness level, and built a sustainable habit proving that with the right approach, your metabolism can and will remain robust because you've given it the signals that tell your body it still needs to produce. The key here is balance—continuing to nourish your body with high-quality foods and giving it the rest it needs ensures that you stay at your peak, without slipping backward or worrying unnecessarily about your metabolism letting you down.

Sources of Protein

As we've said multiple times over, the intention of this program is 'to meet you where you are', no matter where that is as a function of what we are recommending. When talking about proteins, there is probably not a bigger source of controversy or personal preference than in comparing animal versus plant based proteins. Without getting too far into the weeds of moral or ethical discussions, at TMM, suffice it to say we are strong proponents of humanely raised, ethically-sourced animal based proteins as the most complete and bioavailable source of nutrition one can find. Having said that, the nutritional goals we are setting out in this program can be accomplished for people on a plant based diet as well with a few important caveats which we will discuss below.

Animal Proteins

Animal-based proteins are considered complete proteins because they contain all nine essential amino acids in the proportions required by the human body. Essential amino acids are those that cannot be synthesized by the body and must be obtained from the diet. Examples include meat, fish, eggs, and dairy products, all of which provide a balanced and comprehensive amino acid profile necessary for protein synthesis and various physiological functions.

Animal proteins also have higher digestibility and bioavailability compared to plant proteins. Digestibility refers to how efficiently the body can break down and absorb the protein, while bioavailability indicates the proportion of the protein that can be utilized by the body. Animal proteins have higher digestibility scores and are more efficiently used by the body, leading to better muscle protein synthesis and overall protein utilization. Protein Digestibility-Corrected Amino Acid Score (PDCAAS) is a common method for evaluating protein quality, and animal-based proteins universally score higher on this scale compared to most plant-based proteins. This higher digestibility ensures that the body can more effectively utilize the protein consumed.

Egg White, Whey Protein, and Casein Protein all have a PDCAAS score of 1.00, indicating they provide all essential amino acids in adequate amounts and are highly digestible. Soy Protein has a PDCAAS of 0.91, making it a high-quality plant-based protein, though slightly less digestible or balanced in amino acid profile compared to animal proteins.

For reference, here's a chart comparing several animal and plant protein sources based on their Protein Digestibility-Corrected Amino Acid Score (PDCAAS).

Protein Source	Protein Type	PDCAAS Score
Egg White	Animal	1.00
Whey Protein	Animal	1.00
Casein Protein	Animal	1.00
Soy Protein	Plant	.91
Pea Protein	Plant	.69
Rice Protein	Plant	.47

Pea Protein and Rice Protein have lower PDCAAS scores (0.69 and 0.47, respectively), which reflects their lower digestibility and/or less complete amino acid profiles compared to the higher-scoring proteins.

Animal-based proteins also generally have a higher protein density per serving compared to plant-based proteins. This means that for a given serving size, animal-based sources provide more protein, making it easier to meet daily protein requirements without consuming excessive calories.

Serving Size Comparison for 20g Protein (Including Calories)

Protein Source	Type	Serving Size (oz) for 20g Protein	Calories (per 20g protein)	Notes
Chicken Breast	Animal	3.0 oz	~165 cal	Lean source with high protein
Salmon	Animal	4.0 oz	~220 cal	Rich in omega-3 fatty acids
Beef (ground)	Animal	4.4 oz	~330 cal	High-quality protein
Tofu (firm)	Plant	10.0 oz	~150 cal	Good all-around protein source
Lentils	Plant	11.0 oz	~310 cal	Protein and fiber
Quinoa	Plant	11.4 oz	~320 cal	

Animal-based proteins come with additional nutrients that complement their protein content. For example, many animal-based protein sources are rich in bioavailable forms of essential vitamins and minerals such as vitamin B12, heme iron, and zinc. These nutrients are crucial for various bodily functions, including red blood cell production, immune function, and overall metabolic processes as we've already discussed. Studies have also shown that animal-based proteins are generally more effective in promoting muscle mass and recovery compared to plant-based proteins. The higher content of essential amino acids, especially leucine, found in animal proteins plays a key role in stimulating muscle protein synthesis. There are, of course, many examples of athletes thriving on plant based diets. Just know that there is added complexity, preparation, and a lot more chewing to optimize your nutrition with a plant-based diet.

Protein Powders

Protein powders are a common way to boost your daily protein intake when trying to hit increased targets. In a pinch or on the road, protein powder can be a great way to keep the protein intake train going. However, we are going to recommend that you do your best to get your protein from whole food sources regardless of whether they are animal or plant based. After spending almost two years training at an elite powerlifting gym, it became abundantly clear to me that consuming protein powder on a daily basis caused some kind of gut stress to everyone who used it, and we were using 'the best of the best'. Beyond that, protein powders, especially plant-based ones, have been shown to have high levels of heavy metals (lead, cadmium, arsenic). And that does not qualify as high quality nutrition. Use protein powder in a pinch but not as a daily reliable source of protein.

Plant Proteins

To achieve high-quality nutrition on a plant-based diet while minimizing the impact of anti-nutrients, it's crucial to select and prepare foods thoughtfully. Just because they are technically edible, doesn't make them a good source of nutrition. In fact, many plants, due to Mother Nature's intelligent design, contain elements ('anti-nutrients') that deliberately make them hard to digest in an attempt to dissuade animals (humans included) from eating them. Anti-nutrients are naturally occurring compounds in plant foods that can interfere with nutrient absorption and overall health. Incorporating strategies to mitigate their effects can enhance the nutritional quality of your diet.

As pointed out earlier, an incomplete amino acid profile is one of the biggest issues with plant based proteins. To ensure a complete amino acid profile and sufficient protein intake, include a variety of plant-based proteins. Options such as tofu, quinoa, and lentils offer good digestibility and protein quality. However, some of these plant-based proteins can be high in phytic acid and lectins, so preparation methods are key. Reduce anti-nutrient levels in legumes and nuts through soaking, sprouting, and cooking. For example, soaking beans and lentils overnight and cooking them thoroughly can significantly lower their lectin and phytic acid content, making the protein and minerals more bioavailable. This adds time and complexity to your meal preparation but is critical for getting the most out of your plant based proteins.

Below is a chart detailing the amino acid profiles for major plant-based protein sources based on the latest available data. This chart provides information on the essential amino acids present in common plant-based protein sources, including their content per 100 grams. The highlighted numbers show where the protein source provides or exceeds the recommended daily amino acid intake

Amino Acid Profiles for Major Plant-Based Protein Sources

Amino Acid	Tofu (Firm)	Lentils	Quinoa	Chick peas	Hemp Seeds	rec daily intake
Histidine	.54g	.48g	.52g	.39g	.1g	.8g
Isoleucine	.16g	.73g	.83g	.59g	.5g	.1g
Leucine	.76g	.34g	.52g	.91g	.5g	.7g
Lysine	.29g	.99g	.90g	.73g	.4g	.9g
Methionine	.31g	.22g	.35g	.23g	.9g	.6g
Phenyl alanine	.16g	.04g	.96g	.73g	.4g	.2g
Threonine	.82g	.45g	.46g	.33g	.9g	.6g
Tryptophan	.22g	.13g	.16g	.09g	.4g	.3g
Valine	.13g	.68g	.78g	.54g	.4g	.0g

Food Combining

Food combining is a valuable strategy to achieve complete proteins, which contain all nine essential amino acids in the necessary proportions for the human body. The practice of food combining involves eating different plant-based protein sources together to create a complete protein profile, ensuring nutritional completeness, variety, and balance in the diet.

One effective combination is grains and legumes. For instance, rice and beans complement each other perfectly, rice is low in lysine but high in methionine, while beans are low in methionine but high in lysine. Together, they form a complete protein.

Hummus with whole grain bread is a classic example where chickpeas provide certain amino acids and whole grain bread provides others, completing the amino acid profile. Almond butter on whole wheat toast and lentil salad with sunflower seeds are also effective combinations. Grains and vegetables can also be combined for enhanced protein quality. An example is rice and broccoli, where the combination ensures a variety of amino acids and other nutrients. Other effective combinations include quinoa with stir-fried vegetables, millet with kale, legumes and bean chili with mixed vegetables, barley and lentils, and split pea soup with carrots and celery are all well balanced combinations.

Incorporating diverse foods throughout the day ensures that all essential amino acids are consumed, even if not in every meal. Utilizing a mix of legumes, grains, nuts, seeds, and vegetables helps cover different amino acid profiles. Given all the considerations and steps involved in creating a high quality plant-based diet, advanced meal preparation and planning are critical to your success.

Plant-Based Fats

When thinking about fats, Include healthy fats from sources generally low in anti-nutrients. Opt for avocados, nuts (such as almonds and walnuts), seeds (like chia and flax seeds), and oils like olive oil and coconut oil. These provide essential fatty acids and support overall health without introducing high levels of harmful compounds. You will want to make sure you are also getting enough Omega-3 Fatty Acids. While many plant based nutritionists talk about the benefits of plant-based omega-3 sources like flaxseeds, chia seeds, and walnuts, these are actually incomplete sources. Plant-based sources of omega-3 fatty acids, such as flaxseeds, chia seeds, hemp seeds, and walnuts, predominantly offer alpha-linolenic acid (ALA), which is a precursor to the more potent forms of omega-3s, eicosapentaenoic acid (EPA) and docosahexaenoic acid (DHA). While ALA is essential, it is less efficiently converted into EPA and DHA in the body. This conversion process is hindered by several factors, including the presence of omega-3 fatty acids in many processed foods, which compete with omega-3s for conversion enzymes. Consequently, individuals relying solely on plant-based sources may not achieve optimal levels of EPA and DHA, which are crucial for heart and brain health. For those seeking a more direct source of EPA and DHA, algal oil supplements are a viable option. Derived from algae, algal oil provides both EPA and DHA, bypassing the need for conversion from ALA.

While plant-based diets can be rich in essential nutrients, they often include various sources of fats that can impact a macro nutrient based eating plan. Many plant-based fats, such as those found in avocados, nuts, seeds, and oils, are high in calories. As you may recall, fats are calorie-dense, providing 9 calories per gram compared to 4 calories per gram for proteins and carbohydrates. This means that even small amounts of high-fat plant foods can significantly increase daily caloric intake and take up significant macro "real estate" in your daily planning, crowding out the other essentials - proteins and carbohydrates and limiting your options for getting other necessary vitamins and minerals.

Carbohydrates

There are obviously a lot of options when it comes to carbohydrates in a plant-based diet. However, it is important to know which plants actually contain anti-nutrients that can make it difficult on the body to get the nutritional benefits. Choose carbohydrates that provide sustained energy and are less affected by anti-nutrients. Sweet potatoes, butternut squash, and whole grain cereals offer good options. Quinoa, barley, and organic white jasmine rice are good whole grain choices, as they contain fewer harmful compounds compared to high-arsenic brown rice. Proper preparation methods like soaking are essential to further reduce anti-nutrient levels in these grains however. Incorporate a variety of vegetables, fruits, and legumes but be mindful of high-oxalate foods such as spinach and rhubarb. Opt for lower-oxalate alternatives like collard greens, bok choy, or bell peppers. These vegetables are rich in fiber and essential nutrients while being less likely to inhibit calcium absorption.

This is a good time to remind you why it's important to know where your food is coming from. Many of these plants (soybeans, oats, barley, wheat) are known to contain high levels of glyphosate, which, as we've discussed, is a highly toxic chemical you don't want to be consuming in large quantities (or at all if you can help it).

Addressing Micronutrient Needs

If you are going to follow a plant-based program, it's absolutely imperative that you address and plan for the micronutrient deficiencies inherent in a plant-based diet. This is just a universal fact of plant-based diets.

Vitamin B12: As Vitamin B12 is not naturally present in plant foods, consume fortified foods or supplements to prevent deficiency, which can lead to anemia and neurological issues.

Vitamin D: Obtain Vitamin D from fortified foods or supplements, especially if sun exposure is limited, to support bone health and immune function.

Omega-3 Fatty Acids (EPA and DHA): Omega-3 fatty acids are vital for brain and heart health. While ALA is found in plant sources like flaxseeds, conversion to EPA and DHA is inefficient, so algae-based supplements can help ensure adequate intake.

Iron: Plant-based iron (non-heme iron) is less bioavailable than heme iron from animal sources. To enhance absorption, consume iron-rich foods such as lentils, chickpeas, and pumpkin seeds with vitamin C-rich foods like citrus fruits or bell peppers. Be aware of phytic acid in grains and legumes that can inhibit iron absorption; soaking and sprouting can help reduce these effects.

Calcium: Choose calcium rich foods plant-based foods like almonds, chia seeds, figs, and calcium-set tofu. Leafy greens such as bok choy and collard greens are good calcium sources with lower oxalate content compared to spinach, which has high oxalate levels.

Selenium: Selenium is important for thyroid function and antioxidant defense, with its content in plant foods varying by soil quality. Including Brazil nuts in the diet can help ensure sufficient selenium intake.

Zinc: Include zinc-rich plant-based foods such as legumes, nuts, and seeds. Be cautious with high-phytate foods; soaking and sprouting can improve zinc bioavailability.

Hydration: Ensure proper hydration to support nutrient absorption and overall health. Drink ample water throughout the day, particularly when consuming high-fiber foods.

Key Nutritional Biomarkers

Biomarkers serve as critical tools for assessing and ensuring nutritional excellence. They provide measurable insights into how well the body is obtaining and utilizing nutrients, allowing for the optimization of diet and health. By monitoring specific biomarkers, you can identify potential deficiencies, excesses, and imbalances in your nutritional intake, facilitating proactive adjustments to achieve optimal health.

Key Biomarkers for Assessing Nutritional Excellence

Biomarker	Why It's Important	What to Track
Blood Glucose Levels	Indicator of carbohydrate metabolism and overall metabolic health.	Fasting blood glucose, Hemoglobin A1c (HbA1c)
Lipid Profile	Reflects fat metabolism and cardiovascular health.	Total cholesterol, LDL cholesterol, HDL cholesterol, triglycerides
Vitamin D Levels	Essential for bone health, immune function, and inflammation control.	25-hydroxyvitamin D (25(OH)D)
Hemoglobin and Hematocrit	Indicates iron status and overall oxygen-carrying capacity of the blood.	Hemoglobin levels, hematocrit percentage
Serum Ferritin	Reflects iron stores in the body and helps diagnose anemia.	Ferritin levels
Serum Folate and B12	Essential for DNA synthesis, red blood cell formation, and neurological function.	Serum folate, vitamin B12 levels
Calcium and Magnesium Levels	Crucial for bone health, muscle function, and numerous biochemical reactions.	Serum calcium, serum magnesium
Electrolytes	Important for hydration status and cellular function.	Sodium, potassium, chloride
C-Reactive Protein (CRP)	Marker of inflammation which can indicate dietary influences on chronic disease risk.	CRP levels

Omega-3 Index	Measures the amount of EPA and DHA in red blood cells, reflecting omega-3 fatty acid status.	Omega-3 index
Thyroid Function	Assesses overall metabolic rate and iodine status.	Thyroid-stimulating hormone (TSH), Free T3, Free T4

Explanation of Key Biomarkers

Blood Glucose Levels

Fasting blood glucose and HbA1c levels indicate how well the body manages carbohydrate intake and its ability to maintain stable blood sugar levels. Consistent readings within a healthy range suggest effective carbohydrate metabolism and overall metabolic health.

Lipid Profile

A comprehensive lipid profile, including total cholesterol, LDL, HDL, and triglycerides, provides insights into fat metabolism and cardiovascular health. Optimal lipid levels are indicative of a diet low in unhealthy fats and high in beneficial fats, such as those from fish, nuts, and seeds.

Vitamin D Levels

Vitamin D, measured as 25(OH)D, is vital for bone health, immune function, and reducing inflammation. Adequate levels indicate sufficient sun exposure and/or dietary intake, often through fortified foods or supplements.

Hemoglobin and Hematocrit

These biomarkers reflect the oxygen-carrying capacity of the blood and are indicative of iron status. Optimal levels suggest sufficient intake of iron-rich foods, such as leafy greens, legumes, and fortified cereals.

Serum Ferritin

Serum ferritin levels are a marker of iron storage in the body. Adequate ferritin levels indicate good iron status, preventing anemia and ensuring proper oxygen transport and energy levels.

Serum Folate and B12

These vitamins are crucial for DNA synthesis, red blood cell formation, and neurological function. Adequate levels of folate and B12 are necessary for overall cellular health and prevention of anemia and neurological issues.

Calcium and Magnesium Levels

Serum calcium and magnesium levels are essential for bone health, muscle function, and numerous biochemical reactions. Balanced levels indicate adequate dietary intake from sources like leafy greens, nuts, seeds, and fortified plant milks.

Electrolytes

Sodium, potassium, and chloride levels reflect hydration status and cellular function. Balanced electrolytes indicate proper fluid and nutrient intake, supporting overall cellular health.

C-Reactive Protein (CRP)

CRP is a marker of inflammation. Low CRP levels suggest a diet rich in anti-inflammatory foods such as fruits, vegetables, whole grains, and healthy fats.

Omega-3 Index

The omega-3 index measures the amount of EPA and DHA in red blood cells, indicating omega-3 fatty acid status. Higher levels suggest sufficient intake of omega-3-rich foods like flaxseeds, chia seeds, walnuts, and algae supplements.

Homocysteine

Elevated homocysteine levels can indicate deficiencies in B vitamins, particularly B6, B12, and folate. Maintaining low homocysteine levels suggests adequate intake of these essential nutrients.

Thyroid Function

Thyroid function tests, including TSH, Free T3, and Free T4, assess overall metabolic rate and iodine status. Healthy thyroid levels indicate sufficient iodine intake from foods like sea vegetables and iodized salt.

This is by no means a comprehensive list of biomarkers you can track but regular monitoring of these biomarkers can provide a solid baseline view of your nutritional status and help guide dietary adjustments to make sure your body is getting what it needs from your food intake.

Supplementation

Naturally we want to obtain the majority of our vitamins and nutrients from the whole foods we eat. That is the most optimal solution and definitely our goal in shifting to eating entirely high quality foods. Ensuring that you get sufficient quantities of key vitamins and micronutrients daily can be challenging, regardless of whether you follow an animal-based or plant-based diet as both animal-based and plant-based diets can have nutrient gaps. On top of that, modern food production practices, soil depletion, and the demands of busy lifestyles often mean that even a well-rounded diet might not provide all the essential nutrients your body needs to function optimally. Supplementation, when approached intentionally, can help fill in these gaps and support overall health by considering not only the nutrients themselves but also their bioavailability and how they work synergistically in the body. For example, while a diet rich in animal products typically provides ample protein, vitamin B12, and certain essential fats, it might be lower in fiber, antioxidants, and certain vitamins like vitamin C and folate. On the other hand, plant-based diets are often rich in fiber, vitamins, and antioxidants but as discussed, lack sufficient quantities of vitamin B12, iron, omega-3 fatty acids (EPA and DHA), and vitamin D. Additionally, factors such as individual health conditions, age, activity levels, and environmental stressors can increase the body's nutrient demands, making supplementation an essential consideration for everyone. These are recommendations based on experience and research but it's best to get your bloodwork done and consult with a healthcare provider before starting any new supplementation regimen to tailor it to your specific needs and circumstances.

Recommended Baseline Supplementation Stack

By considering the bioavailability of nutrients and how they work together in the body, you can create a supplementation stack that not only fills nutritional gaps but also enhances overall health. Pairing key vitamins and minerals like Vitamin D3 with K2, B12 with Folate, and Omega-3s with antioxidants ensures that your body can absorb and utilize these nutrients effectively, supporting your long-term well-being. Taking into account the bioavailability and synergistic relationships between nutrients, here's a recommended baseline supplementation stack:

Vitamin D3 (2000-5000 IU daily) **with Vitamin K2** (100-200 mcg daily): Vitamin D3 is crucial for bone health, immune function, and mood regulation. However, to ensure that calcium is properly utilized in the body and not deposited in arteries, it should be paired with vitamin K2. Vitamin K2 directs calcium to the bones where it's needed and away from the arteries, reducing the risk of calcification.

Vitamin B12 (1000 mcg daily) **with Folate** (400 mcg daily): Vitamin B12 is essential for nerve function, red blood cell production, and DNA synthesis. To maximize its effectiveness, it should be taken in conjunction with folate, another B-vitamin that works synergistically with B12 in methylation processes that are crucial for DNA repair and detoxification. Methylated forms of both (such as methylcobalamin for B12 and methylfolate for folate) are preferred for their superior bioavailability

Omega-3 Fatty Acids (EPA and DHA, 1000 mg daily) **with Vitamin E** (10-20 IU daily): Omega-3 fatty acids are vital for brain health, heart health, and reducing inflammation. To prevent oxidation of these delicate fats in the body, it's beneficial to take them with antioxidants like vitamin E. Look for fish oil supplements that include a small amount of vitamin E (typically around 10-20 IU) to protect the oil from oxidation.

Magnesium Glycinate or Malate (200-400 mg daily) **with Vitamin B6** (50-100 mg daily): Magnesium supports over 300 biochemical reactions in the body, including muscle and nerve function, blood sugar control, and blood pressure regulation. Pairing magnesium with vitamin B6 can enhance magnesium absorption and support nervous system function.

When choosing a vitamin B6 supplement, the two primary options are pyridoxine hydrochloride and PLP. Pyridoxine hydrochloride, a synthetic form, requires conversion by the body into PLP to become active. This conversion involves enzymatic steps that, in some individuals, may be less efficient due to genetic variations or certain health conditions. On the other hand, supplements containing PLP provide the active form directly, potentially offering better bioavailability and immediate utilization by the body.

Iron (18 mg daily for women, 8 mg daily for men) **with Vitamin C** (500 mg daily): Iron is necessary for oxygen transport in the blood, but its absorption can be enhanced by vitamin C. Vitamin C helps convert iron into a form that is more easily absorbed by the intestines. This is particularly important for non-heme iron (the type found in plant foods), which is less readily absorbed than heme iron from animal sources.

Zinc (15-30 mg daily) **with Copper** (1-2 mg daily): Zinc is important for immune function, wound healing, and DNA synthesis. However, zinc supplementation can interfere with copper absorption, leading to a deficiency over time. Therefore, it's wise to balance zinc intake with a small amount of copper.

Iodine (150 mcg daily) **with Selenium** (100-200 mcg daily): Iodine is essential for thyroid function, but its activity is closely related to selenium, which helps protect the thyroid from oxidative damage during the production of thyroid hormones. Ensuring adequate intake of both can support thyroid health.

Supplementation Stack for Hormonal Balance and PMS Relief

When it comes to female hormone health and managing PMS, the right supplements can provide critical support by targeting inflammation, stabilizing hormones, and replenishing essential nutrients that may be lacking. While these are covered above, we wanted to make sure to call out this stack specifically for menstrual support.

Zinc

Zinc is a powerhouse for hormone health. It helps regulate estrogen and progesterone levels, supports ovulatory health, and has anti-inflammatory properties that can reduce menstrual cramping. It's especially beneficial in the days leading up to your cycle, as it has been shown to inhibit prostaglandin production, which is responsible for much of the pain associated with periods. Including zinc-rich foods like pumpkin seeds and oysters can be a great first step, but for those with persistent PMS, a low-dose zinc supplement can provide added support.

Magnesium

Magnesium is often called the "calming mineral" for good reason—it's involved in over 300 biochemical reactions in the body, many of which play a role in muscle relaxation and nervous system regulation. This makes it especially useful for easing cramps, reducing tension headaches, and calming mood swings associated with PMS. Opt for magnesium glycinate for better absorption and to avoid digestive upset, and pair it with magnesium-rich foods like dark leafy greens and avocados.

Omega-3 Fatty Acids

Omega-3s, found in fatty fish like salmon or plant sources like flaxseeds, are crucial for reducing overall inflammation in the body. These healthy fats help lower the production of inflammatory prostaglandins, easing the severity of cramps and supporting a more balanced mood during the luteal phase. Studies have shown that omega-3 supplementation can significantly reduce the intensity of period pain and may even shorten the duration of symptoms.

Other Supplements Worth Considering

Creatine

Creatine is a naturally occurring compound found in muscle cells and is one of the most researched supplements for enhancing athletic performance. It helps produce adenosine triphosphate (ATP), the primary energy currency of the cell, particularly during short bursts of high-intensity exercise. Numerous studies have demonstrated that creatine supplementation can increase muscle mass, strength, and exercise performance. A meta-analysis published in the *Journal of the International Society of Sports Nutrition* found that creatine supplementation improved muscle strength by 8%, weightlifting performance by 14%, and sprint performance by up to 7%. Creatine may also have cognitive benefits. Research in *Psychopharmacology* suggests that creatine supplementation can enhance cognitive performance, particularly in tasks requiring short-term memory and quick decision-making, especially under stress or sleep deprivation.

Recommended Dosage: 3-5 grams per day. If building muscle is part of your objective, the most common protocol for creatine supplementation is to start with a loading phase of 20 grams per day (divided into 4 doses) for 5-7 days, followed by standard doses of 3-5 grams per day. An initial loading phase may help to increase total creatine stores at a faster rate than a lower dose, but the difference between a loading phase or just a regular dose of 3-5 grams will become negligible after one month of regular supplementation. Creatine can be taken with or without food, though absorption may be improved when taken with carbohydrates.

Psyllium Husk

Psyllium husk is a type of soluble fiber derived from the seeds of *Plantago ovata*. It is known for its ability to support digestive health by promoting regular bowel movements and relieving constipation. Studies show that psyllium husk can help manage cholesterol levels, particularly lowering LDL cholesterol, which is a risk factor for cardiovascular disease. A systematic review in the *American Journal of Clinical Nutrition* found that psyllium supplementation reduced LDL cholesterol levels by about 6% in people with mild to moderate hypercholesterolemia.

Research has shown that Psyllium can also aid in glycemic control by slowing down the absorption of sugars, making it beneficial for people with type 2 diabetes.

Recommended Dosage: A common dosage for psyllium husk is 5-10 grams (1-2 teaspoons) taken with water once or twice daily. It is essential to start with a smaller dose and gradually increase to allow the body to adjust. Make sure you are drinking plenty of water when taking psyllium (of course you are – we already talked about drinking enough water and you are on it!) to prevent digestive discomfort.

Collagen

Collagen is the most abundant protein in the body and plays a key role in maintaining the structural integrity of skin, hair, nails, joints, and connective tissues. Supplementation has been shown to improve skin elasticity and hydration, potentially reducing the appearance of wrinkles. A randomized controlled trial published in the *Journal of Cosmetic Dermatology* found that participants who took a collagen supplement daily for 12 weeks showed significant improvements in skin elasticity and hydration compared to those who took a placebo.

Supplemental collagen can benefit hair, teeth, and nails by providing essential amino acids that promote stronger, thicker hair, enhance scalp health, and support hair growth. For teeth, collagen aids in maintaining healthy gums, strengthening the jawbone, and providing a stable foundation that may protect against tooth damage and loss. When it comes to nails, collagen can improve growth rates, reduce brittleness, and increase resilience, leading to healthier and less fragile nails overall. By supporting the structure and strength of these tissues, collagen helps counteract the effects of aging and maintain vitality. A study in the *Journal of Arthritis Research & Therapy* reported that collagen supplementation decreased joint pain in athletes and individuals with osteoarthritis.

Recommended Dosage: The typical dosage for collagen supplements ranges from 5 to 15 grams per day. Collagen is often taken in powder form mixed with water or other beverages, and it can be consumed at any time of day.

Colostrum

Colostrum, the nutrient-dense first form of milk produced by mammals immediately after giving birth is rich in antibodies, growth factors, proteins, and various nutrients that support immune function, promote growth, and aid in tissue repair. Regular colostrum supplementation can enhance immune function by increasing immunoglobulin levels, which strengthens the body's defenses against infections. It also promotes gut health by supporting the integrity of the intestinal lining; studies have shown that colostrum can improve conditions like "leaky gut" in individuals with inflammatory bowel disease. Colostrum's growth factors and cytokines support skin health by promoting collagen production, improving hydration and elasticity, and potentially reducing signs of aging.

Recommended Dosage: a typical dosage of bovine colostrum is 20 to 60 grams per day, usually divided into smaller doses, such as 1 to 2 tablespoons (approximately 10 grams each) taken 1-3 times daily on an empty stomach to maximize absorption.

For what it's worth, I take or have taken all of these on a daily basis for quite some time and find them to be an integral part of sustaining my long term wellness.

Putting It All Together – Building Weekly Menu Plans

Level 1: Build the plan

- **Decide on your primary objective:** this will determine how you calculate your macros
  - Losing weight, building muscle or maintaining
- **Calculate your Macros:** now you have a plan.
- **Ask chatGPT:** to write you a few days worth of meal plans. Include your preferred protein sources and other ingredients or food combinations you like.
  - "Plan 5 days of meals, with 4 meals per day, where each day's macro totals are **exactly** xxg of protein, xxg of fat, and xxg of carbs. These totals must be met without exception. Ensure that each meal is within 5g of the target macros and that the daily totals are rigorously verified using the following conversions: 1g of protein = 4 calories, 1g of carbs = 4 calories, and 1g of fat = 9 calories.
  - Use the following guidelines:
    - Ensure the most calorie-dense meals are earlier in the day.
    - Do not repeat a meal more than three times across the 5 days.
    - Specify all ingredients in grams, and provide the macronutrient and caloric totals for each meal as well as for the entire day.
- **Recognize the Signs of Dehydration:** Be aware of signs such as fatigue, headaches, and joint pain, and start by increasing water intake rather than taking medications to treat symptoms.

A note on using ChatGPT: Although the prompt is very clear about the target numbers, do an occasional double check just to make sure the math is correct. I've had it give me values that don't add up, simply to give me a response it thinks I am looking for..

Level 2: Execute the Plan

- **Drink Adequate Water Daily:** This is actually harder than it sounds. Aim to drink at least *half your body weight* in ounces (e.g. 160lbs = 80oz) of water each day to maintain optimal hydration levels. If you are exercising, you will want to drink 10-20% more water on top of this number during and after your exercise session. Or use the hydration formula - body weight x .67oz per day.
- **Get a food scale:** You can't do this effectively without a scale. Eventually you'll get pretty good at eyeballing but regularly spot check your quantities, especially if you've stopped achieving results. Nothing fancy needed, links in *Additional Resources*
- **Prep your meals for the week:** Remember, this is about fuel, not fine dining. Being able to take the ingredients on your meal plan, heat them up and go will be critical to maintaining adherence. It will also facilitate assembling meals 'to go' when you're going to be on the move.
- **Stick to the plan:** 80% adherence to the plan is effectively 0% adherence to the plan. Consistency is the key here. This will be the most difficult part of the exercise because it requires a fundamental paradigm shift in the way you think about and consume food. Don't expect to nail it out of the gate. Remember:
    You can't be mad about not getting the results you want for work you didn't put in.
    - Use ChatGPT to your advantage. If you know you are going to go out and have margaritas or pizza or whatever, ask Chat GPT to recalculate your macros for that day to include whatever off plan items you are going to enjoy. While it might not be perfect, you can mitigate some of your off-plan shenanigans with a little prior planning.
- **Establish a Baseline:** Get your bloodwork done at least 1x/year but ideally more like 2-3x/year.
- **Create a Daily Supplement Stack:** based on your bloodwork, look to supplement your high quality diet with the vitamins and minerals where you are deficient.

Level 3: Strict Adherence to the Plan

- **100% Adherence:** Don't miss any meals - don't miss timing, don't miss your macro targets, drink enough water.
- **Revisit and Revise:** As you achieve or get close to your objectives, you will set new goals and new goals will require a new plan. The more exacting you become, the more specific your plan will need to be and you may want to revisit this on a weekly basis, consistently adjusting another degree.
- **Eliminate Alcohol:** There is nothing elevating about alcohol. It is, strictly speaking, poison. You don't need it and it's not making you better.
- **Eat Hydrating Foods:** Incorporate more water-rich fruits into your diet (e.g., watermelon, cucumber, strawberry, chia seeds, peaches) to boost hydration and provide essential nutrients.

Nutrition - subscribepage.io/Nutritionresources

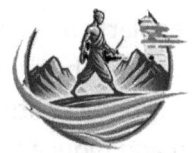

EXERCISE

MOVEMENT ALONG THE PATH

Regular physical activity enhances your overall health 'resume', cultivates resilience and strengthens a sense of vitality that permeates every area of life. Scientific research consistently demonstrates that an active lifestyle is one of the most powerful ways to improve both the quality of life and lifespan. Several large-scale studies demonstrate that even moderate amounts of exercise (20 mins per day) can significantly reduce all-cause mortality. Similarly, research shows that people who engage in regular physical activity live, on average, 3-4 years longer than their sedentary counterparts. Beyond simply extending lifespan or more importantly, "healthspan", exercise enhances the quality of life by improving functional mobility, energy levels, mood, and resilience to stress—aligning directly with The Modern Monk's objective of living a vibrant and fulfilling life. Put another way, there is no reason that as we get older our bodies, our meat-suits, should become prisons that limit our experience. Like the animals in the wild, we want to and should be functioning at a high level right up to our last breath. And exercise is one of the fundamental ways to ensure that level of performance and resilience.

When we exercise regularly, a cascade of beneficial chemical reactions occurs within the body. Exercise stimulates the release of endorphins, the body's natural "feel-good" chemicals, which help reduce pain and induce feelings of euphoria, often referred to as the "runner's high." This boost in mood helps manage stress and promotes mental well-being. Exercise also increases levels of brain-derived neurotrophic factor (BDNF), a protein that supports the growth and survival of neurons in the brain. Elevated BDNF levels enhance cognitive function, memory, and neuroplasticity, making exercise a powerful tool in maintaining brain health and lowering the risk of cognitive decline. Additionally, exercise improves insulin sensitivity (the opposite of the dreaded insulin resistance) by increasing the muscles' ability to take up glucose from the bloodstream, which is critical for preventing type 2 diabetes and maintaining stable energy levels. Regular physical activity also triggers anti-inflammatory effects by releasing cytokines and enhancing immune function, which helps protect against illness and age-related decline. And if that wasn't enough, exercise stimulates the production of new mitochondria and improves their function, leading to increased energy production, reduced oxidative stress, and slowed cellular aging.

Defining Exercise

Exercise can be broadly defined as any physical activity that challenges the body to move and exert effort, with benefits available across a wide range of activities—from walking, yoga, and calisthenics to strength training, martial arts, high-intensity interval training (HIIT), and sports. This broad definition allows people at any fitness level to find a form of movement that fits their lifestyle and aligns with their goals. Whether someone is taking their first steps toward fitness or pursuing mastery in a specific discipline, exercise offers a universal path to better

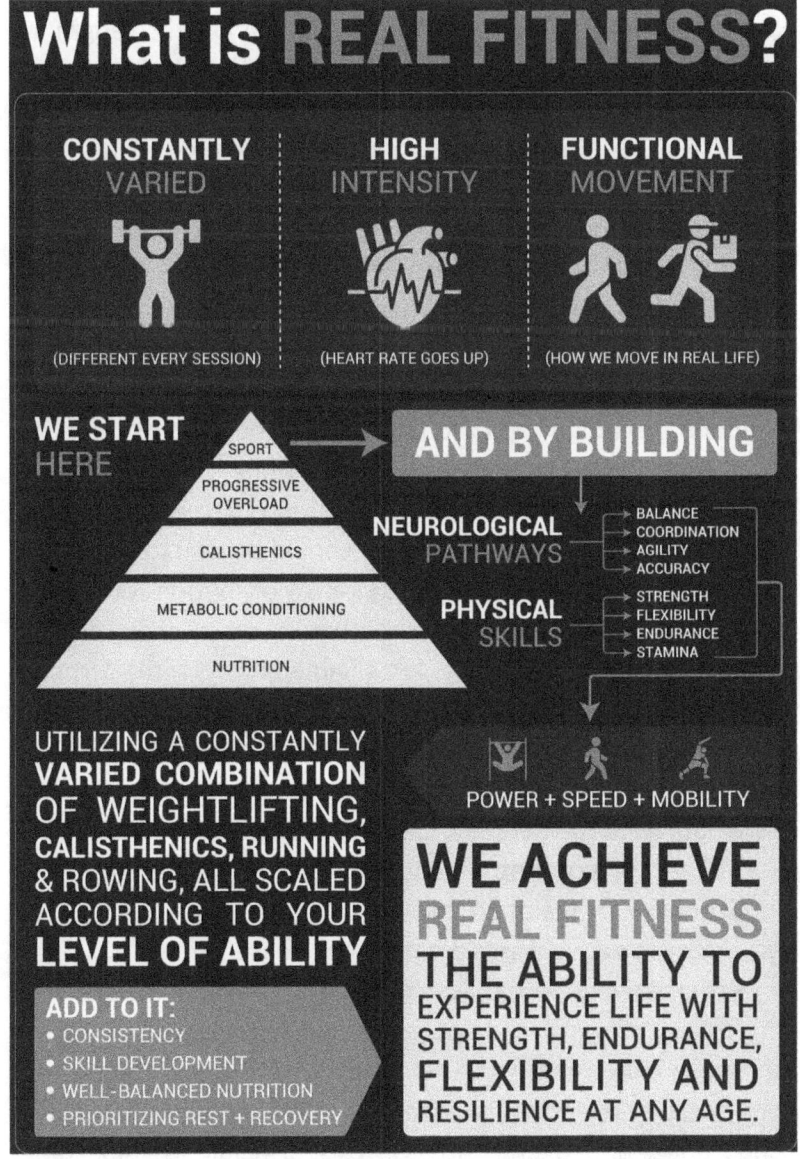

health and well-being. Within this broad spectrum, certain foundational principles stand out for their unique contribution to longevity and functional health—specifically, functional mobility, progressive overload, and interval training.

Functional mobility is the cornerstone of a long, active life, as it enhances range of motion, stability, and strength in ways that directly translate to everyday activities. Functional exercises mimic natural, real-world movement patterns like squatting, bending, reaching, and lifting, helping to prevent injury, improve posture, and maintain independence as we age. It absolutely breaks my heart to see older people hunched over like question marks, no longer able to straighten their backs and stand upright, especially when it's often so easily preventable.

Calisthenics—bodyweight exercises like push-ups, pull-ups, squats, and planks—are particularly effective for building functional strength and mobility. These movements develop coordination, balance, and stability while also improving flexibility and range of motion. And it stands to reason that this is an excellent way to exercise—we should be able to move our own body weight through a wide range of motion for a very long time. The accessibility of calisthenics, which require little to no equipment, makes it a sustainable and versatile form of exercise that can be adapted to all fitness levels. More and more frequently I hear people my age or even younger bow out of activities like skiing, hiking, music festivals, group sports or whatever because they 'can't move like they used to'. By regularly incorporating functional exercises and calisthenics, individuals can maintain the physical capability needed to navigate life's adventures demands with ease.

Progressive overload is another key principle, the gradual increase of stress placed on the body during exercise. Whether through increasing weights, reps, intensity, or duration, progressive overload is essential for improving strength, endurance, and overall fitness. This principle is important because the body adapts to stress over time, requiring continual progression to trigger further gains. Within The Modern Monk framework, progressive overload is not just a physical practice but also a metaphor for life: small, consistent challenges lead to growth and transformation. Interval training, particularly high-intensity interval training (HIIT), is highly effective for improving cardiovascular fitness, metabolic health, and fat loss. And for me personally, CrossFit has been the synthesis of all of these principles wrapped into one that has been a blessing for helping me get into the best shape of my life, one step at a time.

Shugyo (修行)

Shugyo refers to dedicated training and self-cultivation, often used in the context of martial arts, Zen practice, or other demanding endeavors. The kanji characters represent the idea of "austere practice" or "rigorous training." For the Modern Monk, Shugyo is the dedication to practices that push one beyond comfort zones in pursuit of mastery and deeper understanding. It involves embracing discomfort, commitment, and focused effort to sharpen the mind, strengthen the body, and cultivate resilience. Shugyo embodies the ethos of committing to challenging endeavors that forge character and unlock higher levels of capability and awareness.

Walking, running, martial arts, tennis, CrossFit, calisthenics, it doesn't matter what flavor suits you, by remaining active and understanding the profound biochemical changes that occur during exercise, anyone can create a custom regimen to suit them that supports longevity, vitality, and overall well-being. As science shows conclusively, the benefits of exercise extend beyond lifespan to deeply enhance the quality of life—a core goal for anyone on the path to living as a Modern Monk.

Forms of Exercise

Each form of exercise offers unique benefits that can be tailored to individual goals, whether they relate to improving body composition, building muscle, or optimizing metabolism. Below is an analysis of eight forms of exercise—walking, running, interval training, calisthenics, CrossFit, sports, yoga, and martial arts (specifically Brazilian Jiu-Jitsu)—along with the minimum recommended dose per week to yield positive results. But don't feel limited to this list by any means and don't feel like you have to stick to one type of exercise. There are a million different ways to stay active. The body thrives on variety and stagnates on repetition (it's a pattern recognition machine) so picking a couple of different ways to exercise during the week is a great way to keep things fresh and exciting while also working on different objectives. What is most important is that you are consistent in the activity you choose and in order to be consistent you need to be doing something you want to be doing.

Walking

Walking is one of the most accessible and sustainable forms of exercise, suitable for all fitness levels. It is particularly beneficial for longevity, cardiovascular health, and maintaining a healthy metabolism. Walking helps manage body weight, reduces the risk of chronic diseases like heart disease and diabetes, and improves mental health by reducing stress and anxiety. The widely popular goal of achieving 10,000 steps per day has become synonymous with maintaining an active lifestyle. While the origins of the 10,000-step guideline can be traced back to a marketing campaign for a Japanese pedometer in the 1960s, research in recent years has validated the benefits of reaching this threshold for health and well-being. According to the World Health Organization (WHO), adults should engage in at least 150 minutes of moderate-intensity activity or 75 minutes of vigorous-intensity activity per week. Walking 10,000 steps, which equates to approximately 5 miles, meets or exceeds this recommendation for many people. The goal serves as a simple, measurable way to promote physical activity, which is essential for cardiovascular health, weight management, mental health, and longevity.

Minimum Recommended Dose: 150 minutes per week (30 minutes, 5 times per week). *Benefits:* Improved cardiovascular health, weight management, reduced risk of chronic diseases, enhanced mental well-being.

Running

Running offers a more intense cardiovascular workout than walking and is highly effective for improving body composition, boosting metabolism, and supporting heart health. Running enhances aerobic capacity and promotes efficient calorie burning. A study published in *JAMA Internal Medicine* found that running just 5-10 minutes a day at a moderate pace is associated with a significantly lower risk of death from all causes, particularly cardiovascular disease. Running also activates large muscle groups (quads), promoting fat loss while preserving lean muscle mass.

Minimum Recommended Dose: 75 minutes per week (25 minutes, 3 times per week) at a moderate to vigorous intensity. *Benefits:* Enhanced cardiovascular fitness, improved body composition, increased bone density, higher calorie expenditure.

Interval Training

Interval training, particularly high-intensity interval training (HIIT), alternates between periods of intense effort and short recovery times. HIIT is extremely efficient, offering maximum benefits in a short time frame. HIIT training has been shown to improve both aerobic and anaerobic fitness, enhance metabolism, and promote fat loss while retaining muscle mass. HIIT has also been shown to improve insulin sensitivity, making it effective for metabolic health and reducing the risk of type 2 diabetes.

Minimum Recommended Dose: 60 minutes per week (20 minutes, 3 times per week). *Benefits:* Improved cardiovascular and metabolic health, fat loss, enhanced muscle retention, better insulin sensitivity.

Calisthenics

Calisthenics involves bodyweight exercises like push-ups, pull-ups, squats, and planks. This form of exercise is highly effective for building functional strength, improving mobility, and enhancing muscle endurance. Calisthenics can be done anywhere, requires no equipment, and is scalable for all fitness levels. Research in the *Journal of Strength and Conditioning Research* shows that calisthenics is effective for improving muscle mass, strength, and functional performance. It also promotes joint health and stability, reducing the risk of injury.

Minimum Recommended Dose: 90 minutes per week (30 minutes, 3 times per week).
Benefits: Functional strength, improved mobility, muscle endurance, enhanced joint stability.

CrossFit

CrossFit is a high-intensity, varied workout regimen that combines elements of weightlifting, calisthenics, and cardiovascular exercises. According to research in the *Journal of Strength and Conditioning Research* participants in CrossFit programs show significant improvements in VO2 max (a marker of aerobic capacity), muscle strength, and body fat reduction. CrossFit's community aspect also provides motivation and accountability, which can help with consistency. This is far and away my preferred method of exercise.

Minimum Recommended Dose: 90-120 minutes per week (3 sessions of 30-40 minutes). Benefits: Improved overall fitness, muscle development, fat loss, enhanced metabolic rate.

Sports

Engaging in sports, whether recreationally or competitively, provides a full-body workout that improves cardiovascular health, agility, coordination, and muscle strength. Sports like tennis, soccer, and basketball combine aerobic and anaerobic exercise, making them effective for both cardiovascular fitness and muscle endurance. The dynamic nature of sports also keeps exercise enjoyable, which is critical for long-term adherence.

Minimum Recommended Dose: 90 minutes per week (one or two sessions).
Benefits: Enhanced cardiovascular fitness, agility, coordination, muscle strength, and mental well-being.

Yoga

Yoga offers a unique combination of physical exercise, mental relaxation, and flexibility training. It improves functional mobility, balance, and core strength while promoting mental well-being through mindfulness and breath control, reducing stress, improving heart health, and enhancing overall quality of life. Yoga is also particularly beneficial for joint health and reducing the risk of injury.

Minimum Recommended Dose: 60-90 minutes per week (two sessions of 30-45 minutes).
Benefits: Improved flexibility, balance, joint health, mental clarity, and stress reduction.

Martial Arts (Brazilian Jiu-Jitsu)

Brazilian Jiu-Jitsu (BJJ) is a form of martial arts that combines grappling and ground-fighting techniques, offering both cardiovascular and muscular benefits. BJJ is effective for building functional strength, endurance, and flexibility. It also improves problem-solving skills and mental toughness due to its strategic and dynamic nature. BJJ training enhances aerobic and anaerobic capacity, while also promoting fat loss and muscle growth. Additionally, BJJ develops core stability and flexibility, which are crucial for overall functional fitness.

Minimum Recommended Dose: 90 minutes per week (two sessions of 45 minutes). *Benefits:* Enhanced functional strength, cardiovascular fitness, mental toughness, flexibility, and stress management.

Each form of exercise offers unique benefits that cater to different aspects of health, longevity, and fitness. Walking provides a foundation for cardiovascular health and is a sustainable lifelong habit. Running is ideal for calorie burning and cardiovascular endurance, while interval training offers time-efficient improvements in metabolic health and fat loss. Calisthenics and CrossFit build functional strength and comprehensive fitness, while sports add an element of enjoyment to physical activity. Yoga and Brazilian Jiu-Jitsu contribute to physical and mental well-being, with yoga emphasizing flexibility and mindfulness, and BJJ offering dynamic full-body conditioning.

Incorporating a mix of these activities, even at minimal recommended doses, can lead to significant improvements in lifespan, body composition, muscle development, and metabolism, setting the foundation for a healthier and more fulfilling life.

One thing to keep in mind, just as it is important to continually check-in with ourselves about how our meditation practice is feeling, about what foods make us feel best and how our weight is tracking to our goals, tracking progress is equally important with exercise. In order to determine if we are having success in training, we need to know where we started. Not only is this important for stimulating continuous growth, but there is real benefit to being able to look back and realize just how far you've come, whether it be how long it takes you to run a mile or the number of pull-ups you can do or what your maximum deadlift is. If we are consistent with our training in any discipline, progress is inevitable but when approached slowly and methodically, it can be deceptive just how far we've come because there's always another challenge ahead. So make sure to keep track of your workouts, even just in a notes app on your phone to give you a reference for how your hard work has paid off or to highlight where you might want to focus your effort to improve.

Recovery

Recovery is the often overlooked and underutilized, yet critical, element of any successful training program. It is easy to get caught up in the thinking that 'more training' directly correlates to 'more results' but realistically, it's the exact opposite. More/over training results in injury and injury prevents training from occurring at all. While training stresses the body to stimulate adaptation, it is during recovery that these adaptations occur. Recovery becomes even more essential as we age, when the body's ability to bounce back from physical exertion gradually diminishes. Scientific research consistently shows that adequate recovery is necessary for muscle growth, injury prevention, and sustained performance. As we get older, our bodies require more time to recover from exercise due to reduced muscle protein synthesis, slower tissue repair, and declining hormonal responses. Neglecting recovery can lead to burnout, overtraining, and injuries that can derail even the most basic training programs. Injury, especially as we age, is not just a temporary setback; it can have long-lasting effects on motivation and the ability to train consistently, which is vital for longevity and overall health. Having to 'climb the mountain' again after significant time off due to injury is one of the hardest, least enjoyable obstacles to have to overcome. So best to get your rest and not have to face that mountain at all.

Recovery is more than just physical; it's an opportunity to cultivate deeper body awareness and listen to the signals that the body sends. Joint soreness, fatigue, and even mood changes are all ways the body communicates its need for rest and regeneration. Being attuned to these signals and responding accordingly is a practice in self-awareness that aligns with The Modern Monk framework. The body's feedback loops are critical; ignoring them often leads to setbacks, while honoring them can sustain your continued progress over the long term.

Essential Recovery Protocols

To maintain a consistent training schedule and avoid injury, it's important to engage in scientifically-backed recovery protocols. Here are some of the most effective strategies:

Sleep

Once again, we are talking about sleep. Sleep is arguably the most important recovery tool in the arsenal. During deep sleep stages, the body releases growth hormone, which is essential for tissue repair and muscle growth. For optimal recovery, 7-9 hours of sleep per night is generally recommended, though individual needs may vary. Establishing a consistent sleep schedule and creating an environment conducive to quality sleep—cool, dark, and free from electronics—will enhance recovery outcomes.

Minimum Effective Dose: 7-9 hours of sleep per night, prioritizing deep and REM sleep stages.

Cold Plunge

Cold plunges (or cold water immersion) have gained popularity due to their ability to reduce muscle soreness and inflammation. The cold constricts blood vessels, which helps flush out waste products like lactic acid, while reducing swelling and muscle damage. A meta-analysis in the *Journal of Sports Science and Medicine* found that cold water immersion significantly reduces delayed onset muscle soreness (DOMS) and enhances recovery, particularly after high-intensity exercise.

However, timing is key when combining cold plunges with strength training. Post-workout cold plunges can blunt the body's adaptive response, which is crucial for muscle growth. To avoid this, it's recommended to wait at least 4-6 hours after strength training before using cold immersion, or better yet, save cold plunges for rest days. When used strategically, cold therapy enhances recovery without interfering with muscle adaptation. I can't recommend this protocol enough. It's life changing.

Minimum Effective Dose: 10-15 minutes in water between 45-59°F (10-15°C), spread over 3-4 sessions per week.

Sauna

Heat exposure via saunas promotes recovery by increasing circulation and helping the body eliminate toxins. Regular sauna use is associated with improved cardiovascular health, reduced muscle soreness, and increased longevity. The heat stimulates the production of heat shock proteins, which aid in muscle repair and reduce oxidative stress. Sauna sessions also support relaxation, improving sleep quality and mental recovery.

Minimum Effective Dose: 15-30 minutes in a sauna at 176-194°F (80-90°C), 2-4 times per week.

Cold Plunge and Sauna Combination: Alternating between cold plunges and hot saunas creates a powerful contrast therapy that promotes blood circulation and reduces muscle fatigue. A typical protocol involves 10-15 minutes in a sauna followed by 2-5 minutes in a cold plunge, repeating this cycle 2-3 times. This contrast between heat and cold stimulates the autonomic nervous system and enhances recovery by alternating between vasodilation (in the sauna) and vasoconstriction (in the cold plunge), flushing out metabolic waste and reducing inflammation. Remember to always end on cold and allow your body to bring its temperature back up naturally.

Red Light Therapy

Red light therapy (also known as low-level laser therapy) uses specific wavelengths of red and near-infrared light to penetrate the skin and promote cellular regeneration. A study in *The American Journal of Sports Medicine* found that red light therapy accelerates muscle recovery by enhancing mitochondrial function and reducing oxidative stress. It has also been shown to improve circulation, reduce inflammation, and enhance collagen production, which aids in muscle and joint repair.

Minimum Effective Dose: 10-20 minutes per session, 3-5 times per week, using a device emitting wavelengths between 600-850 nm.

Peptides

Peptides, specifically growth hormone-releasing peptides (GHRPs) and BPC-157, are increasingly used to accelerate recovery by enhancing tissue repair, reducing inflammation, and improving joint health. Some of the most well-documented GHRPs include:

CJC-1295: A growth hormone-releasing hormone (GHRH) analog, CJC-1295 increases growth hormone and IGF-1 levels, promoting tissue repair and muscle growth. It is often combined with Ipamorelin for synergistic effects.

Ipamorelin: A GHRP that stimulates the release of growth hormone without the associated spikes in cortisol or prolactin, making it ideal for muscle recovery and fat loss.

BPC-157: A synthetic peptide derived from a protective gastric protein, BPC-157 accelerates healing in tendons, ligaments, and muscles. It has been shown in studies published in *Gut* and *Journal of Orthopaedic Surgery and Research* to promote tissue regeneration and reduce inflammation, making it particularly effective for injury recovery.

These peptides work at a cellular level to stimulate growth factors that expedite recovery and improve overall muscle and joint health.

Minimum Effective Dose: Dosing protocols vary based on the peptide, but BPC-157 is commonly administered at 200-500 mcg daily, while CJC-1295 and Ipamorelin are often taken at doses of 100-200 mcg each, typically before bedtime.

Peptides vs. Steroids: What's the Difference?

Peptides and steroids are both performance-enhancing compounds, but they differ significantly in their mechanisms of action, and thus in their effect on the body, and potential side effects. Understanding these differences is key for those considering their use for recovery, muscle growth, or overall health.

Peptides

Peptides are short chains of amino acids that act as signaling molecules within the body. They play a crucial role in regulating various physiological processes, including tissue repair, immune function, and hormone production. In the context of performance and recovery, the most commonly used peptides are growth hormone-releasing peptides (GHRPs), such as CJC-1295, Ipamorelin, and BPC-157.

These peptides work by stimulating the body's natural production of growth hormone or by promoting the healing and regeneration of tissues. For example, GHRPs trigger the release of growth hormone from the pituitary gland, leading to increases in muscle growth, fat loss, and recovery. BPC-157, on the other hand, is involved in healing soft tissues like tendons, ligaments, and muscles by promoting angiogenesis (the formation of new blood vessels) and reducing inflammation.

Steroids

Anabolic steroids are synthetic derivatives of testosterone, the male sex hormone. They are primarily used to enhance muscle growth, strength, and endurance by directly increasing protein synthesis and nitrogen retention in muscle cells. Steroids are highly effective for building muscle and improving performance, but they come with significant risks and side effects, especially when used improperly or without medical supervision.

Steroids exert powerful effects on the entire endocrine system, leading to a wide range of potential side effects. Common side effects of steroid use include liver damage, cardiovascular issues (like increased risk of heart attack or stroke), hormone imbalances, and psychiatric effects like aggression or mood swings. In men, prolonged steroid use can cause testicular shrinkage, reduced sperm count, and gynecomastia (enlargement of breast tissue). In women, it can lead to virilization effects, such as deepening of the voice and facial hair growth.

Peptides have fewer to no side effects compared to anabolic steroids for several reasons:

Targeted Action: Peptides work by mimicking natural processes in the body rather than introducing foreign hormones. For instance, GHRPs stimulate the body's own production of growth hormone rather than directly supplying an exogenous hormone like steroids do. This results in a more regulated and physiologically normal increase in hormone levels, reducing the risk of severe side effects.

Selective Pathways: Peptides are designed to target specific pathways, such as tissue repair or growth hormone release, without affecting other hormonal systems. Steroids, on the other hand, can disrupt the entire endocrine system, leading to a cascade of unintended effects.

Fewer Hormonal Disruptions: Peptides generally do not cause the drastic hormonal imbalances seen with steroid use. For example, peptides that stimulate growth hormone do not interfere with testosterone production or cause estrogen-related side effects, making them safer for long-term use.

Lower Toxicity: Peptides are typically composed of naturally occurring amino acids, which means they are broken down and eliminated by the body more easily than synthetic steroids, which can be toxic, especially to the liver and cardiovascular system.

To be clear, **we are not in favor of taking steroids to enhance performance.** The incremental addition of exogenous (external) hormones into the system has been shown to have significant negative effects on the body. Peptides on the other hand, trigger the signaling mechanisms within the body to facilitate natural hormone production allowing the body to use its own systems and pathways to function as intended.

The Importance of Quality

The quality of peptides is crucial for both efficacy and safety. Unfortunately, the market is flooded with low-quality or counterfeit peptides, especially when sourced from unregulated online vendors. To ensure you're purchasing from a reliable peptide source, there are several key factors to consider. First, prioritize suppliers that offer third-party lab results verifying the purity and concentration of their products. Certificates of analysis (COAs) are essential for confirming that the peptides are free from contaminants and meet quality standards. Additionally, researching the reputation of the supplier is critical. Trusted sources will have positive reviews from verified customers and a proven track record of delivering consistent, high-quality products. Whenever possible, purchase peptides from suppliers operating within regulated markets, such as licensed compounding pharmacies or medical professionals who specialize in peptide therapy, as these sources are more likely to follow strict quality control measures. It's also important to avoid common pitfalls when buying peptides. Be cautious of products sold at unusually low prices, as these are often diluted or counterfeit. Similarly, steer clear of peptides that are marketed with exaggerated claims or lack clear information on dosage and usage. Taking these precautions can help ensure that you're getting effective and safe peptides that support your health and wellness goals.

Additional Recovery Protocols

Active Recovery: Low-intensity activities like walking, swimming, or gentle cycling can promote blood flow, helping to flush out metabolic waste while reducing stiffness and soreness. A study in *Sports Medicine* highlights that active recovery enhances circulation and accelerates the removal of lactate and other waste products.

Massage and Myofascial Release: Techniques like foam rolling and sports massage break up adhesions in muscle tissue, increase blood flow, and reduce muscle tension. Research in the *Journal of Athletic Training* shows that myofascial release can reduce DOMS and improve range of motion.

Nutrition and Hydration: Proper nutrition, including sufficient protein intake and micronutrients like magnesium and omega-3s, are vital for muscle repair and reducing inflammation. Staying hydrated ensures optimal circulation and helps deliver nutrients to recovering tissues.

Just as sleep is critical for ensuring the quality of our waking hours, recovery is just as important as training for ensuring our ability to stay at the top of our game. As we age, the need for deliberate recovery protocols becomes even more critical to maintain consistent progress and avoid setbacks from injury. By integrating sleep, cold plunges, sauna sessions, peptides, red light therapy as recovery strategies, we support the body's natural repair processes, enhance performance, and ultimately achieve long-term health and longevity. Just as we listen to our bodies during training, tuning into recovery signals and responding appropriately ensures that we can continue to train, grow, and live with vitality for years to come.

Masturbation (males only)

> "The reabsorption of semen by the blood is the strongest nourishment and, perhaps more than any other factor, it prompts the stimulus of power, the unrest of all forces toward the overcoming of resistances, the thirst for contradiction and resistance. The feeling of power has so far mounted highest in abstinent priests and hermits (for example, among the Brahmins)."
>
> — Frederic Nietzsche

The idea that males can benefit from abstaining from masturbation, often referred to as *sexual transmutation* or *semen retention*, has roots in both ancient practices and modern discussions about optimizing energy, focus, and vitality. The notion that the body reabsorbs the energy conserved from sexual abstinence is grounded in the belief that nutrients and hormones associated with ejaculation are repurposed for other vital functions. For instance, semen contains high levels of zinc, an essential mineral for immune function, cognitive health, and muscle repair. By retaining semen, it is believed that the body can redirect these resources toward physical and mental performance.

The energy itself is viewed as a form of *Qi* (life force) in traditional Chinese medicine or *prana* in yoga. Through practices like meditation, deep breathing, and focused intention, this energy can be transmuted into creativity, physical power, and heightened awareness. Abstaining from masturbation is believed to offer several potential benefits, particularly in the areas of energy conservation, mental clarity, confidence, and spiritual growth. One of the primary benefits is increased energy and vitality. Ejaculation involves a significant expenditure of energy, depleting stores of nutrients like zinc, magnesium, and other essentials. Proponents argue that by abstaining, the body reabsorbs this energy and redirects it toward other functions such as muscle growth, cognitive performance, and overall stamina. The principle is based on the idea that sexual energy is one of the most potent forms of energy, and retaining it can lead to heightened vitality.

Abstaining from masturbation is also associated with enhanced mental clarity and focus. Some studies and anecdotal reports suggest that frequent ejaculation can lead to feelings of lethargy, brain fog, and reduced motivation. By preventing these energy dips, abstaining is thought to improve mental sharpness, discipline, and focus, possibly due to conserving neurotransmitters like dopamine, which plays a key role in motivation and reward pathways.

In spiritual practices like Taoism and certain forms of yoga, sexual energy is considered a powerful force that, when harnessed, can be transmuted into higher states of consciousness, creativity, and personal development. By redirecting sexual energy away from immediate gratification, practitioners believe they can achieve deeper emotional balance, spiritual insight, and personal growth.

Ejaculation Frequency

In Taoist practice, there is a formula used to determine the optimal frequency of ejaculation based on a man's age. The formula is: (age in years - 7) ÷ 4, which gives the number of days a man should wait between releases to maintain optimal health and energy levels. For example, a 40-year-old man would calculate as: (40 - 7) ÷ 4 = 8.25, meaning he should ideally wait about 8 days between ejaculations. This formula is based on the belief that frequent ejaculation depletes vital energy, which can be better conserved and redirected toward enhancing longevity and overall vitality.

Note: This includes coitus to completion. There is no moratorium on sex itself, only the finishing.

While scientific evidence supporting all aspects of these claims is limited, the practice of semen retention has been celebrated in various cultures for centuries (much like meditation) and as science continues to validate energetic principles identified by long standing spiritual traditions (also like meditation) I believe there is merit in at least experimenting with a protocol like this one. There is no downside to trying it out and seeing for yourself if there is a difference in how you feel.

Putting it All Together – Staying Active

Level 1: Get in the game
- **Get your 10000 steps:** start with 10000 steps a week and then build from there. 10000 steps 3x/week and so on until you are hitting your target 5 days a week. If it seems like a lot, break it up into three 30min sessions in a day (7am/1pm/6pm).
- **Add some bodyweight exercise:** Create a routine that includes some movement of the body through functional positions (e.g., push-up, pull-up, squat, planks, etc)
  - Calisthenics: can be done anywhere, requires no equipment, and is scalable for all fitness levels
  - Yoga: Great full body movement sequences with plenty of scaling options for all levels of practitioner. Look for hatha or vinyasa flow classes
- **Recovery:** Build 1-2 rest days into your weekly routine.

Level 2: Up your game
- **Progressive Overload Activities:** Whether through increasing weights, reps, intensity, or duration, progressive overload is essential for improving strength, endurance, and overall fitness. Don't think you need to do this on your own. Programs like Orange Theory or 9Round Fitness are great ways to get started without having to know anything about training yourself.
  - Interval training
  - Weight lifting
  - Running
  - Pilates

- **Recovery:** In addition to programmed days of rest, add some targeted recovery to sooth muscles and reduce inflammation.
  - Cold Plunge or Sauna: start with one (cold plunge can be done in the bathtub if need be) and build up to incorporating both in your weekly routine.
  - Regular sports massage: Finding a quality practitioner is key here as this can be an expensive addition. Ask for recommendations at your gym. Use a foam roller and/or a lacrosse ball as an effective low cost alternative.

Level 3: Play an actual Game

- **Join Organized Athletics:** There are numerous benefits to joining group sports from the power of community to the presence of a coach that can greatly enhance your capabilities and your dedication to practice.

  - CrossFit/Hyrox: my current personal favorite. It combines strength, mobility, intensity, competition, coaching and community in 1hr sessions that are coached and led.

  - Sports: Do what you love. Soccer, Tennis, Cycling, Running, Crew. I'd recommend avoiding the more 'weekend warrior' type sports like softball or pick-up basketball where injuries tend to abound.

  - Martial Arts: The ultimate TMM practice. A slow, consistent, dedicated path to mastery of body and mind.

- **Recovery:** Train hard, recover hard. Inevitably something is going to get tweaked, twisted, or torn. You don't want to be out of action for too long and science is beginning to provide ways to speed your natural healing processes.
    - Peptides: this is your secret recovery (and muscle building weapon). Period. Find a quality clean source.
- **Masturbation protocol:** This is maximum TMM. Allow yourself to become 1° clearer, more focused and alive by holding back per the Taoist formula. When you then experience "release" (especially manual), tune-in to how your body feels afterwards. There is an unmistakable feeling of 'emptiness' that is pretty fascinating.

Exercise - subscribepage.io/exerciseresources

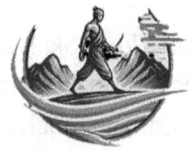

NEUROPLASTICITY
TIME TO TRAIN THE BRAIN

A healthy, well-functioning brain is essential for longevity, health span, and maximizing our life experiences. It's the central organ that governs not only our thoughts and emotions but also every function of our body. We've spent the majority of our time focused on elevating the physical function of the body but now we are turning our attention to the motor that runs the entire machine. As we strive to live an elevated life, the importance of maintaining optimal brain function becomes paramount. It is through the brain that we interpret our world, form memories, and make decisions that shape the future. The ability to remain adaptable, learn new skills, and engage with novel experiences is fundamentally linked to the brain's capacity to adapt and reorganize itself—its neuroplasticity. By actively nurturing our brain health, we can slow the effects of aging, enhance our cognitive abilities, and ensure that we continue to live with purpose and engagement, fully experiencing each moment and extending our health span well into later years. In the context of longevity and health, the brain is not just another organ—it is the motor that runs the entire machine, and its care and optimization are foundational to a life well-lived.

These two sections, *Building Skills* and *Cultivating Experiences* are fundamentally rooted in the idea that our brains are incredible pattern recognition machines. They process massive amounts of inputs all day every day—sights, sounds, smells, tastes, and tactile sensations to make split second decisions on how best to keep us alive in any given moment based on the pattern recognition of prior experiences. As we go through life, especially in today's society, it's extremely easy to let ourselves fall into a repetitive pattern of performing the same actions at the same time in the same places with the same people, day in and day out. And because the brain is so good at recognizing patterns, if these day in and day out patterns persist long enough, life begins to operate on 'auto-pilot'—our unconscious and programmed responses run our lives, and the brain checks out because it knows or can predict with a high degree of certainty what's coming next.

When this happens, our experience of time speeds up and begins to slip away. Weeks become months, months become years, and before we know it, a decade has disappeared.

This theory related to time perception is known as the *contextual-change model*, which suggests that our perception of time is based on the amount of information processed by the brain. This is why time seems to "slow down" during periods of learning or intense experiences (new stimuli) but appears to "speed up" during routine activities when new information is not being processed. When the brain encounters new stimuli or engages in novel activities, it requires more processing power, leading to a more detailed memory encoding and a perception that time is dense and slow moving. Conversely, when experiences are repetitive or familiar, the brain processes them more quickly, leading to less detailed memory encoding (because nothing is really different). Think about the last time you drove home from work or to pick up the kids, if you can remember anything about it at all. More than likely, it happened in a flash and unless something extraordinary happened along the way, that segment of time in your life basically vanished. On the other end of the spectrum, think back to a vacation you spent in a new place. The first few days seem to stretch out forever while the last few (once your brain has become acclimated) feel like they fly right by. Research indicates that the brain's experience of time is not linear but instead fragmented into discrete moments that are processed and stitched together by different neural circuits. This process depends on attention, the level of novelty, and emotional engagement, all of which contribute to how we subjectively experience the flow of time.

Nerves, reflexes, and memory, just like muscles, atrophy from lack of use. As we get older, it seems our culture has institutionalized 'resting on our laurels' or 'easing on down the road'. However, in making a conscious effort to continuously exercise brain functions by learning new skills or cultivating new and unfamiliar experiences, we keep the brain actively processing for new patterns and new connections. Our memories then are constantly filled with new details to sort and compare and our reflexes are continuously engaged in navigating unfamiliar territory—new neural pathways are formed and strengthened. When we engage in activities that demand high levels of attention and focus, neuromodulators like acetylcholine and dopamine are released, increasing the brain's alertness and ability to form new connections. This heightened state of focus can make time feel drawn out because the brain is encoding more detailed information. Time then appears to slow down rather than slip away. Our newly developed interests, skills, and expertise bring us into contact with new and interesting people we might not otherwise have had the pleasure of meeting or forming connections with and the circle of our life experience grows rather than consolidates.

For TMM, this is another cornerstone practice for living an elevated life.

Building Skills

Skill acquisition plays a vital role in shaping a fulfilling and adaptive life. Whether the goal is personal growth, professional success, or enriching life experiences, the ability to learn new skills is essential. In modern self-improvement philosophies that emphasize continuous growth, adaptability, and purpose, skill acquisition becomes a key component in creating a life that feels both meaningful and rewarding. In the context of leading an elevated life, learning new skills serves as both a tool for growth and a source of fulfillment. The process of acquiring new abilities not only helps in achieving specific goals but also strengthens the overall capacity to face new challenges with confidence and curiosity. It's a practice that enhances resilience, curiosity, and adaptability, which are crucial qualities for navigating life's uncertainties. Engaging with new challenges opens opportunities for growth in ways that not only build confidence but they provide new and exciting stimuli to the brain, forcing it to stay alert, active, and engaged in finding new patterns and building new neural pathways to support the demands of whatever skill you are developing.

The Science Behind Learning New Skills

The process of learning is driven by neuroplasticity, the brain's ability to reorganize itself by forming new neural connections. When acquiring a new skill, the brain's prefrontal cortex is initially engaged, focusing on the task at hand with intense concentration. With practice, these skills transition to being more automatic, utilizing different brain regions such as the basal ganglia and motor cortex. This shift from conscious effort to unconscious proficiency allows for smoother and more efficient execution.

One key to triggering neuroplasticity is engaging in focused practice, often requiring a state of heightened alertness or even mild stress. This focused state creates a window where the brain is primed to learn and form new connections. However, this is just one part of the process. The true consolidation of these new skills occurs during rest and sleep, particularly in deep sleep stages (here we are, back to sleep again—full circle). During this time, the brain reviews and strengthens the neural pathways, making the learned skill more permanent. While neuroplasticity tends to decline with age, this can be offset by a concerted effort to learn new skills. But as we've discussed, practice should be a pleasure not a discipline so when thinking about what new skill to learn, focus on something that you find fascinating and thoroughly interesting. Do it for you, not because you think it sounds cool or you'll find yourself quickly unmotivated to keep going.

One of the great things about the internet age and YouTube in particular is that you can find instructional videos on almost anything to almost any degree of mastery. While there is some romance in going on a quest to find a mentor, the reality is that many are just a few keystrokes away. Your success, like everything in this program, is going to happen through small and steady progress. Breaking down complex skills into smaller, manageable components and practicing them in a focused manner is essential. Regular, consistent practice helps reinforce learning and makes it easier for the brain to form lasting connections. And high-quality sleep is essential for hard coding your practice into the nervous system. During deep sleep, the brain consolidates the learning, ensuring that the practiced skill becomes a lasting part of one's repertoire. Consistent rest and relaxation are, therefore, as important as the practice itself. As I've begun to learn to play the piano, I make it a point to practice before I go to bed at night and what I've found is that when I get stuck on making a finger shape to hit a specific chord or I can't quite nail a rhythm pattern, while I'm sleeping, my brain works on the problem and the next time I practice, I'm suddenly able to play something I struggled with just 24 hours prior. It's amazing to experience and quality sleep is crucial in activating that process.

By understanding the mechanics of how the brain acquires and retains new skills, one can adopt methods that maximize their learning potential throughout life. Whether aiming to master a new language, improve a physical skill, or develop professional expertise, the combination of deliberate practice, mindfulness, and quality rest leads to more effective skill acquisition.

The Power of Habits

At its core, learning a new skill is about consistent practice and gradual improvement. Habits are what drive this consistency. When a task becomes habitual, it requires less mental energy to perform, allowing you to focus on refining the skill itself. This is where the concept of starting small comes into play. By identifying the key habits that support your skill goals, you can create a clear and achievable pathway to mastery.

> "We are what we repeatedly do. Excellence, then, is not an act, but a habit."
>
> - Aristotle

For example, cultivating gratitude—a skill that can enhance mental well-being—might begin with the simple habit of writing down three things you're grateful for each day. Over time, this daily reflection builds a mindset of appreciation and mindfulness. Similarly, if you want to learn how to hunt, breaking that goal into smaller habits like regular target practice or camping trips develops foundational skills that build toward the larger goal. Another example might involve learning to play a musical instrument. Starting with the small habit of dedicating just 10 minutes each day to practicing scales or finger exercises can, over time, build muscle memory and technique, eventually allowing for more complex compositions and improvisation. Or consider the process of learning a new language: beginning with the daily habit of memorizing just five new words and using them in sentences helps build vocabulary steadily, creating a solid foundation for fluency.

One of the most effective ways to systematically build skills is by adopting a quarterly habit development protocol. This approach helps break down complex goals into manageable steps, allowing consistent progress over time. Whether you are developing a creative skill like painting, a technical skill like coding, or a physical skill like running a marathon, this method encourages small but steady changes that accumulate into significant progress.

Identify a Skill Goal: Begin by defining a specific skill you wish to acquire over the next year, such as becoming conversationally fluent in a new language or proficient in playing an instrument like the guitar. Break the skill down into smaller components that can be developed sequentially, like vocabulary acquisition and grammar practice for a language, or finger dexterity and chord transitions for an instrument.

Set a Quarterly Habit: For the first quarter, choose a habit that directly supports your overall goal. If learning a language, your initial habit could be dedicating 15 minutes each morning to using a language app like Babbel or Pimsleur to practice basic phrases and vocabulary. For an instrument, the habit might be practicing scales or chord transitions for 10 minutes daily. The key is to keep the habit simple and sustainable, focusing on consistency rather than volume.

Track and Adjust: Throughout the quarter, monitor your progress. Track your habit daily and assess whether it's helping you build the foundational skills you need. For language learning, this could mean reviewing your ability to recall common phrases or understanding basic conversations. For an instrument, it could be tracking improvements in muscle memory and smoothness of transitions. Adjust the habit if needed—such as increasing practice time or shifting focus—while ensuring it remains aligned with your goals.

Build on the Habit: At the end of the quarter, evaluate your progress and layer on a new habit that builds upon what you've already established. After three months of practicing vocabulary and basic phrases, you might introduce a weekly session focused on conversation practice with a language partner. If learning an instrument, you could start incorporating more complex exercises, like playing simple songs or practicing rhythm and timing.

Rinse and Repeat: Continue this cycle each quarter, gradually increasing the complexity and depth of your habits as your skills improve. Over the course of a year, these incremental steps can lead to substantial progress, whether it's holding a conversation in your new language or confidently performing a piece on your instrument.

Aligning Goals and Desires

Habits form more easily when they align with a deep desire or intrinsic motivation. The fallacy of discipline suggests that sheer willpower alone is not a sustainable strategy for building habits. Instead, when you genuinely desire to learn a skill, the process of habit formation becomes more natural and enjoyable. This alignment minimizes resistance, making it easier to stay consistent.

Ikigai (生き甲斐)

Ikigai is a Japanese concept that translates to "reason for being" or "a reason to wake up in the morning." It is often depicated as the intersection between what you love, what you are good at, what the world needs, and what you can be paid for. For TMM, Ikigai represents finding alignment between purpose, passion, and daily life. It is the pursuit of meaningful living by understanding and embracing one's unique path, leading to a life of fulfillment and contribution. Pursuing your passions will motivate you to bring something new and authentic into the world, automatically making the world a better place for it.

Spend some time contemplating what it is that you desire most to achieve. For some, this may be something that you've been putting off a long time and for others it may be diving deep on a new obsession. No matter how the inspiration comes to you, think about learning this new skill not as a hobby but as a natural extension of who you are as a person or who you'd like to become.

The path to skill acquisition is not about massive leaps but rather small, consistent steps. By focusing on habit formation and gradually building up to more complex practices, you create a sustainable learning process that leads to long-term success. Whether it's learning gratitude, honing a craft, or mastering a new discipline, habits are the foundation upon which true skill is built. By adopting a quarterly protocol and aligning habits with your desires, you create an approach that not only builds skills but also enhances your overall life satisfaction and fulfillment by giving you something new and novel to look forward to each day and breaking a repetitive daily pattern.

Winning Habits

Within the TMM framework, there is another way to think about forming new habits that reflects the power of small 1° shifts. Rather than nesting new habits solely within skill acquisition, base them in becoming a better version of yourself. In other words, quarterly, give yourself the task of acquiring a winning habit. These habits aren't necessarily monumental changes but are consistent actions that align with the person you aspire to be. For example, committing to not being late anymore can lead to greater respect for your time and that of others, improving both your personal and professional relationships. Calling friends on their birthdays fosters deeper connections and nurtures the bonds that bring meaning and support into your life. Training yourself to find something positive in any situation helps rewire your mindset toward gratitude and appreciation even in challenging circumstances. By focusing on small, intentional habits that reflect your core values and desired identity, you gradually build a foundation for transformation. Over time, these incremental changes accumulate, leading to significant growth, all while reinforcing the belief that you are constantly moving toward a better version of yourself.

Cultivating Experiences

Neuroscience teaches us that our perception of time is shaped by novelty, emotional engagement, and the cognitive effort required to process new experiences. When we engage in the same routines day after day, time seems to slip by quickly because the brain isn't encoding new, detailed information. However, when we experience something novel, the brain works harder to process the new environment, challenges, and emotions, leading to richer, more vivid memories and the sense that time is expanding. These memories become touchstones that define our lives, marking significant periods and unique experiences. But, life moves pretty fast and without intentional commitment, our habitual patterns leave us with less time to do something new or exciting.

Instead of letting time disappear, make a concerted effort to plan short but unique experiences for you, your family and/or with friends every few months. The world is an incredibly interesting and diverse place with countless opportunities to explore, see something new, build your knowledge base, and expand your comfort zone. Making this a habitual practice not only enriches your life with diverse experiences but also creates a pattern of living that stretches your perception of time and enhances life satisfaction. If you were to engage in this practice of planning a mini-adventure every 2 months consistently, for the next 40 years, you would be on pace to accumulate 240 unique adventures—each representing a distinct chapter in your life story. These adventures, whether it's exploring a new city, discovering a cultural landmark, taking a seminar from a renowned teacher, or embarking on an outdoor expedition to a location you've never been to, would stand out against the backdrop of daily routine, offering moments of growth, discovery, and fulfillment. But don't do it alone! Engage your friends and your family in these adventures and side-quests in life. Perhaps the only thing more satisfying than experiencing something new and exciting is sharing it with someone you love.

At the pinnacle of the Modern Monk process, we introduce a concept that singularly embodies the ethos and intent of what it means to continuously walk the path towards living an elevated life.

Specifically, this is the concept of a *Misogi*—a once-a-year commitment to achieving something that stretches your limits and alters the course of your life by more than 1°. In traditional Japanese culture, *Misogi* involves ritual purification, but in the Modern Monk context, it can be reimagined as a transformative challenge that stands out as the defining event of your year. This could be quitting a destructive habit like smoking, accomplishing a significant personal goal like writing a book or starting a business. The key is that this Misogi is daunting, perhaps audacious, and requires serious commitment to achieve. This is the type of "boundary stretching" that brings about profound personal change and positions you to accomplish things you might have only dreamt about.

Misogi (禊)

Misogi is a traditional Japanese Shinto practice of purification, typically ivolving a cold-water ritual. It symbolizes cleansing oneself of impurities, both physical and spiritual. In the context of the Modern Monk, Misogi represents the idea of setting audacious goals for oneself that renew and refresh the mind, body, and spirit in their pursuit. The essence of Misogi is to strip away the distractions, doubts, and negativity accumulated in daily life, allowing one to emerge revitalized and focused. It's a commitment to constant self-evolution and growth, embodying resilience and a connection to something deeper within.

Beyond the benefits that you get from the sense of accomplishment in expanding your horizons and enriching your life experience once you have completed your Misogi, there is also significant value in the planning process of determining your mini-adventures and ultimately your annual Misogi. These plans and intentions become the foundations around which the rest of your life develops. In 2024, my Misogi was to finish my first feature-length film. Much of that year was consumed with this process but by the time you read this, the film will be released into the world and it will be one of the great accomplishments in my life to date—and something I never would have considered possible at this point in my life without this concept. I had to sacrifice to make it happen, but I committed to the dream and in retrospect, it was completely worth it.

The value of creating a Misogi each year lies in its ability to anchor your life around a singular, memorable achievement. Neuroscience supports the idea that events which demand focused attention, effort, and emotional investment create more lasting and impactful memories. You might forget the routine tasks of a given year, but you won't forget the pursuit of the Misogi that pushed you to attempt something you didn't think was possible and left you a different person for having accomplished it or for even having tried. These Misogi challenges serve as milestones that not only define your year but also contribute to your ongoing growth and evolution, creating a legacy of personal transformation. Don't let life pass by without giving yourself a chance to do something (many things) extraordinary. Climbing Mt. Fuji, complete an Iron Man triathlon, visit every continent, bag multiple 14000 ft peaks, publish a book of your photography, see the Aurora Borealis in person. Whatever you decide to take on, make it audacious, make it unique, make it memorable. At Google X, the secret Silicon Valley innovation lab, they believe that if you take a moonshot and you miss, you will still end up a lot farther along than you would have if you kept within the boundaries of conventional thinking.

moon·shot
/ˈmoōnˌSHät/
noun

1. **(Informal):** A highly ambitious and innovative project or idea, a plan or aim to do something that seems almost impossible.

Combining the practice of regular mini-adventures with an annual Misogi ensures that your life is not only filled with meaningful and memorable moments but that your development as a human being continues to expand year after year. Over time, these experiences build a rich tapestry of growth, adventure, and resilience, allowing you to live intentionally, fully engaged with the world, while at the same time evolving into the best version of yourself.

Putting it all together – Charting the Path

Whether you realize it or not, by the time you have gotten this far in the program, creating new winning habits and acquiring new skills is exactly what you have been doing from the beginning. Developing quality sleep habits, practicing meditation, eating to a plan, getting enough hydration, These are all examples of building new skills and habits that didn't previously exist in the quiver of your experience. As you consider the options in traversing this part of the path, don't get overwhelmed. You don't need to add even more to your plate. Consider focusing on building the winning habits outlined to this point. Once those are solidified in your new way of being, then move on to create new habits and acquire new skills beyond the scope of this framework.

Level 1 – Set Sail
- Pick one (1) winning habit to develop this quarter
- Plan one (1) mini-adventure to go on this quarter

Level 2 - Aim for the Horizon

- Pick a new skill to acquire
  - Develop a habit related to acquiring that skill
- Develop one (1) new winning habit each quarter this year
- Plan three (3) mini-adventures to undertake this year

Level 3 - Discover Uncharted Territory

- Identify your Misogi for this year
- plan six (6) min-adventures for this year
- Develop four (4) winning habits this year
- Acquire a new skill
  - Break the skill into habits
  - Track and adjust your progress quarterly

Neuroplasticity - subscribepage.io/Resources

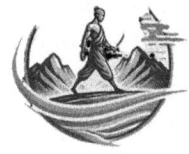

BONUS MATERIAL

WALKING THE INNER PATH

To truly walk the path to an elevated life, at some point, we inevitably need to address and heal our deepest traumas and uncover the unconscious cultural programming that influences our daily decisions and behaviors. This internal work enables us to break free from repetitive patterns that limit our potential and restrict our experience of life.

The Importance of Healing Trauma for an Elevated Life

We all carry limited beliefs, traumas and other perspectives that, whether we are conscious of them or not, impact how we show up in the world and more specifically, how we view ourselves in the context of the larger world around us. And oftentimes, these limiting beliefs are at the core of why we aren't making the best choices to support our health and well-being. As this program is presented, there are many opportunities and practices to cultivate a greater self-awareness and clear directions about how to move forward. But sometimes, even that is not enough. Sometimes, we need extra help to navigate our inner landscape. Engaging in internal work through these non-traditional modalities is not just about healing past wounds; it's about creating the mental and emotional space necessary for living an elevated life. Science increasingly validates the real and lasting effects of these substances on brain chemistry and emotional health, confirming their potential to facilitate profound transformation. By allowing individuals to access and process deeply buried trauma and uncover unconscious programming, these modalities enable a shift from reactive, patterned behavior to conscious, intentional living. This transformation is crucial for expanding one's experience of life, fostering deeper connections, and realizing one's full potential —I know they have been crucial in my own development and process of healing. I wouldn't include them here if I didn't believe they can be extremely useful in walking the path to self-realization.

However, it is vital that these powerful tools be used responsibly, under the supervision of licensed professionals who can ensure a safe and supportive environment.

Healing Trauma Through Non-Traditional Modalities

Non-traditional healing modalities like plant medicines and psychoactive compounds—Ayahuasca/DMT, Psilocybin, MDMA, and Ketamine—offer profound opportunities to explore the unconscious mind, release trauma, and rewire the brain for new ways of thinking and being. Modern science continues to explore and validate how these substances produce real and lasting effects on brain chemistry and emotional health, offering a path to more profound self-awareness, healing, and transformation. The intent here is not to prescribe or suggest protocols for these compounds, but rather to introduce them as an invitation for further discovery if one or more feel like they could be of help to you. I have personally worked with all of these modalities over the course of the last decade or more and have found each one to be its own blessing with its own healing gifts to offer.

IMPORTANT: these substances are being discussed for therapeutic use only; their powerful effects should only be explored under the guidance and supervision of licensed professionals who can ensure the proper dosages, purity of ingredients while also establishing the necessary "set and setting" for safe and effective healing.

"Set and Setting" in Psychedelic Therapy

"Set and setting" are the cornerstones of effective internal work. The terms describe the internal and external conditions that profoundly influence the outcome of experiences with psychoactive substances like Ayahuasca, Psilocybin, MDMA, and Ketamine. These concepts are critical for doing deep and effective internal work with these compounds, as they shape the psychological, emotional, and physiological responses individuals have during their sessions. Understanding and carefully managing "set and setting" is paramount for maximizing the therapeutic potential of these substances and ensuring a safe, transformative experience.

"Set" refers to the individual's mindset, which includes their mood, expectations, and psychological state before embarking on a psychedelic experience. A person's mindset is shaped by their personality, mental health, intentions, and the preparation they undertake before the session. For example, if someone approaches the experience with openness, curiosity, and a willingness to explore their inner world, they are more likely to gain meaningful insights and achieve emotional breakthroughs. Conversely, entering with fear, anxiety, or skepticism can increase the likelihood of a challenging or adverse experience. A study published in *The Journal of Psychopharmacology* emphasizes the importance of proper preparation and psychological readiness to optimize outcomes with psychedelic-assisted therapy, noting that individuals who were well-prepared had fewer adverse reactions and more positive, transformative experiences. An important distinction here is not that you have "no issues"—to the contrary, this work is about uncovering and resolving difficult situations and memories—but that you approach the work with intention and an openness to what you can discover about yourself.

"Setting" refers to the physical and social environment in which the experience takes place. This includes the location, sounds, smells, lighting, and the presence of other people, such as therapists or guides. The setting should foster safety, comfort, and trust, which is crucial for enabling deep emotional work. For instance, sessions are typically conducted in calm, quiet environments where the individual feels secure, reducing the likelihood of distractions or stressors that could trigger anxiety or panic. Research in *Frontiers in Psychology* highlights that a carefully controlled environment can significantly impact the therapeutic effectiveness of psychedelics, with participants reporting greater feelings of safety and a willingness to explore difficult emotions in settings designed to support introspection.

The synergy between "set and setting" is essential for effective healing. When both are carefully managed, they create a supportive space that allows the participant to confront trauma, uncover unconscious programming, and process difficult emotions without becoming overwhelmed. For example, MDMA-assisted therapy for PTSD relies heavily on a safe, controlled setting where a therapist provides guidance and support, facilitating the patient's ability to process traumatic memories without the intense fear response that typically accompanies them. A study published in *The Lancet*

Psychiatry found that the therapeutic setting, including the therapist's presence and emotional support, was crucial for the effectiveness of MDMA in treating PTSD, as it allowed patients to engage with their trauma in a new, more constructive way.

Moreover, the "set and setting" concept extends beyond just reducing risks—it enhances the profound, positive potential of these substances. For example, with psilocybin therapy, an open, prepared mindset combined with a nurturing, secure environment can facilitate a state of "ego dissolution," where individuals experience a profound sense of interconnectedness and unity, often leading to deep insights about their lives and purpose. As research in *The Journal of Psychopharmacology* suggests, these profound experiences can help reframe deeply ingrained negative beliefs, promoting lasting behavioral change and emotional healing. "Set and setting" are not just helpful; they are absolutely paramount for deep and effective internal work with these powerful compounds. They create the optimal safe conditions necessary for accessing the unconscious mind, processing trauma, and rewiring the brain for healthier patterns. Properly managing these factors, always under the guidance of licensed professionals, maximizes the therapeutic potential of these substances and helps ensure that the experience is safe, meaningful, and truly transformative.

Ayahuasca/DMT

Ayahuasca is a traditional Amazonian plant medicine with a rich history dating back hundreds, if not thousands, of years. It has been used by indigenous tribes in the Amazon basin for spiritual, medicinal, and shamanic purposes. The word "Ayahuasca" comes from the Quechua language, where "Aya" means spirit or soul, and "Huasca" means vine or rope—often translated as the "vine of the soul." The origins of Ayahuasca are deeply rooted in the cultural and spiritual practices of various indigenous groups in countries like Peru, Brazil, Colombia, and Ecuador, where it is considered a sacred tool for healing, divination, and communication with the spiritual realm.

Ayahuasca is typically made from two primary plant components: the *Banisteriopsis caapi* vine and the leaves of the *Psychotria viridis* shrub. The *Banisteriopsis caapi* vine (the 'jagube') contains potent monoamine oxidase inhibitors (MAOIs) called harmine, harmaline, and tetrahydroharmine. These compounds prevent the breakdown of the psychoactive compound DMT (dimethyltryptamine) found in the leaves of the *Psychotria viridis (the 'reina')*. DMT is a powerful hallucinogenic substance that is otherwise quickly metabolized by the body's enzymes, rendering it inactive when ingested orally. The combination of these two plants however, allows DMT to enter the bloodstream and cross the blood-brain barrier, inducing the intense, visionary experiences associated with Ayahuasca.

The preparation of Ayahuasca is a meticulous and time-consuming process often carried out by an experienced shaman, or ayahuasquero. The *Banisteriopsis caapi* vine is harvested, cleaned, and then pounded to expose its inner fibers. The *Psychotria viridis* leaves are usually picked fresh. Both components are boiled together in water for several hours, sometimes even days, until a thick, dark, and bitter liquid is produced. The process may involve multiple boiling and straining cycles to concentrate the brew. The preparation method varies among different indigenous groups and ayahuasqueros, with some adding additional plants to alter or enhance the brew's effects.

A typical Ayahuasca "journey" takes place in a ceremonial context, guided by a shaman or facilitator with extensive experience in the practice. Participants usually gather in a quiet, dimly lit environment—often a maloca (a traditional Amazonian ceremonial hut) or a dedicated ceremonial space. Ayahuasca ceremonies are typically conducted in a communal setting, which fosters a sense of shared experience and collective healing. The communal aspect helps participants feel supported and connected, which can amplify the healing effects. Studies have shown that social support is a critical component of psychological well-being, and participating in Ayahuasca ceremonies can provide a profound sense of community and belonging. The ceremony begins with rituals, prayers, or chants to set intentions and create a sacred atmosphere. The shaman, who has prepared the brew, serves Ayahuasca in small cups to each participant. The effects of Ayahuasca generally begin 20 to 60 minutes after ingestion and can last between four to eight hours, depending on the dosage, the individual's sensitivity, and other factors. The experience, known as a "journey," is characterized by intense visions, emotions, and physical sensations. Participants may encounter vivid, colorful imagery, profound emotional insights, and deep psychological introspection. It is common for people to experience both challenging and euphoric moments during the journey, which are often described as confronting personal fears, traumas, or unresolved emotions. Physical responses, such as purging (vomiting or diarrhea), are also typical and are considered a form of cleansing, both physically and spiritually.

Throughout the experience, the shaman or ayahuasquero plays a crucial role by guiding participants with sacred songs known as icaros, which are believed to help navigate the visionary state and facilitate healing. The setting is carefully controlled to maintain a sense of safety and support, allowing participants to surrender fully to the process.

The psychoactive properties of DMT, facilitated by the MAOIs in the *Banisteriopsis caapi* vine, create an altered state of consciousness where individuals can access parts of the mind that are usually inaccessible. This allows participants to confront deep-seated traumas, unconscious fears, and suppressed emotions that often drive negative behaviors or thought patterns. A study in the *Journal of Psychopharmacology* demonstrated that Ayahuasca could reduce symptoms of depression and anxiety by promoting psychological flexibility and enhancing mindfulness.

Ayahuasca has also been shown to affect brain function by promoting neuroplasticity—the brain's ability to reorganize itself by forming new neural connections. This process can help "reset" dysfunctional neural circuits associated with mood disorders, depression, and PTSD. Research in *Frontiers in Pharmacology* suggests that Ayahuasca may increase levels of brain-derived neurotrophic factor (BDNF), a protein that supports neuron growth and survival, contributing to long-term emotional and cognitive health.

Many participants report experiencing profound spiritual insights, a sense of interconnectedness with all life, and a deeper understanding of their place in the universe. These experiences can facilitate a sense of peace, acceptance, and meaning. According to a study published in *Transcultural Psychiatry*, Ayahuasca use was associated with higher scores on measures of "spirituality" and "personal development," which correlated with improved mental health outcomes. The purging effect that often accompanies Ayahuasca use is viewed as a form of physical and energetic cleansing and differs significantly from what we think of as vomiting when we are sick. In traditional Amazonian cultures, this is seen as a way to rid the body of negative energies, emotions, or toxins, contributing to a sense of renewal and revitalization. The physical detoxification aspect is not yet fully understood in Western medicine but is considered a crucial part of the healing process within indigenous practices but I can attest from extensive personal experience how sentient this medicine can be in not only finding areas that need healing but in guiding the experience to lead to deeper understanding and ultimately healing in ways I would never have imagined.

Ayahuasca's powerful healing potential lies in its ability to facilitate access to the unconscious mind, promote neuroplasticity, provide spiritual insights, and support both individual and communal healing processes. However, it is essential to approach this medicine with respect, proper preparation, and under the guidance of experienced shamans or facilitators who understand its complexities. As scientific research continues to explore and validate the therapeutic benefits of Ayahuasca, it remains a vital and transformative tool for those seeking deep emotional and spiritual healing.

Psilocybin

Psilocybin, the active compound found in certain species of "magic mushrooms," is gaining significant recognition in the scientific community as a powerful tool for psychological healing and personal growth. Emerging research indicates that psilocybin can help facilitate therapeutic healing, especially for conditions like depression, anxiety, PTSD, and existential distress. Beyond clinical settings, psilocybin has also been shown to foster a deeper connection with the physical world, enhancing one's sense of interconnectedness with nature and the environment.

Psilocybin in therapeutic settings primarily helps individuals explore their inner psyche and confront unresolved emotional and psychological issues. One of its most significant effects is its ability to reduce activity in the brain's default mode network (DMN), a network of brain regions associated with self-referential thought, ego, and the sense of self. When the DMN is "quieted," individuals often experience a sense of "ego dissolution"—a state in which they feel less separated from others and their environment. This can be especially beneficial for people suffering from depression and anxiety, where rigid, negative patterns of self-focused thinking dominate.

A study published in *The New England Journal of Medicine* showed that psilocybin therapy resulted in a significant reduction in depressive symptoms, comparable to traditional antidepressants but with a faster onset of action and fewer side effects. The therapeutic process often involves the patient taking psilocybin in a controlled environment under the guidance of a trained therapist. This setting allows the patient to confront their emotions and trauma in a safe space, fostering insight and emotional breakthroughs that can be integrated into everyday life. Beyond that psilocybin has been found to enhance emotional openness and cognitive flexibility. By breaking down the rigid thinking patterns associated with mood disorders, psilocybin therapy helps patients reconnect with feelings of love, compassion, and empathy. Research published in *JAMA Psychiatry* found that a single dose of psilocybin, combined with psychotherapy, led to a sustained reduction in anxiety and depression in patients with life-threatening cancer diagnoses, helping them achieve a sense of peace and acceptance.

Developing a Deeper Connection with the Physical World

In addition to its clinical applications, psilocybin is known for fostering a profound sense of connection to the natural world. Users often report feeling a heightened sense of unity with their surroundings, an increased appreciation for nature, and a deeper understanding of their place within the larger ecosystem. This effect is believed to be due to psilocybin's ability to enhance sensory perception and emotional receptivity, making ordinary experiences— the sound of leaves rustling or the sight of a sunset—more vivid, meaningful, and emotionally resonant. Research published in *Ecopsychology* suggests that psilocybin can promote pro-environmental behavior and an increased sense of ecological awareness.

Participants in the study who experienced a psilocybin-induced connection to nature reported greater motivation to engage in environmentally friendly behaviors and a stronger commitment to conservation efforts. This shift in perspective is thought to occur because psilocybin enhances brain plasticity, allowing for new patterns of thinking and feeling to emerge. This can help individuals overcome feelings of disconnection or alienation from the natural world, fostering a sense of belonging and interdependence with the environment. The enhanced sensory experiences and the emotional openness induced by psilocybin can lead to a profound appreciation for life and the interconnectedness of all things. This perspective shift can be especially valuable for individuals who feel isolated, depressed, or disconnected, as it offers a new way of perceiving reality that is filled with wonder, awe, and a renewed sense of purpose.

The therapeutic and transformative potential of psilocybin is heavily influenced by "set and setting,". The mindset should be one of openness, curiosity, and a willingness to explore inner experiences, while the setting should be safe, supportive, and free from distractions. This environment allows the individual to explore emotions, thoughts, and sensations with minimal interference from external stimuli. Psilocybin therapy should only be conducted under the guidance of a licensed professional in a controlled environment to ensure safety and effectiveness. This setting can include a comfortable room, soothing music, and the presence of a trained therapist who can provide support, reassurance, and guidance throughout the experience.

Preparation sessions before the psilocybin journey help set intentions and prepare the participant for what might surface, while integration sessions afterward help process insights gained and incorporate them into daily life. By altering brain activity and enhancing neuroplasticity, psilocybin therapy can facilitate profound emotional and cognitive changes, helping individuals heal from trauma, depression, and anxiety. When used responsibly in the right "set and setting," under professional guidance, psilocybin can be a potent tool for both personal growth and planetary healing.

MDMA

MDMA (3,4-methylenedioxymethamphetamine), commonly known as "ecstasy" or "molly", is increasingly recognized as a powerful tool for treating post-traumatic stress disorder (PTSD) and other traumatic wounds. MDMA-assisted psychotherapy combines the therapeutic effects of MDMA with psychotherapeutic techniques, creating an environment that allows patients to process trauma with reduced fear and emotional distress. Research has shown that this approach can lead to significant and lasting reductions in PTSD symptoms, offering hope to those who have not responded to traditional treatments.

MDMA therapy works by leveraging the drug's unique effects on the brain to facilitate emotional processing and healing. MDMA primarily acts as an empathogen, enhancing feelings of empathy, connection, and trust while reducing fear and anxiety. The substance achieves these effects by influencing several key neurotransmitters.

Increased Serotonin Release: MDMA stimulates the release of serotonin, a neurotransmitter that regulates mood, social behavior, and emotional responses. This surge in serotonin contributes to feelings of well-being, relaxation, and emotional openness, allowing patients to revisit traumatic memories without the overwhelming fear or panic that typically accompanies them.

Boosted Oxytocin and Prolactin Levels: MDMA also increases the release of oxytocin, often referred to as the "love hormone," and prolactin, which are associated with social bonding, trust, and emotional closeness. This hormonal shift promotes a sense of safety and connection between the patient and therapist, fostering a therapeutic environment where deep emotional work can occur..

Reduction of Amygdala Activity: The amygdala, a part of the brain involved in processing fear and threat responses ("fight or flight"), shows decreased activity under the influence of MDMA. This reduction in activity is crucial for individuals with PTSD, as it enables them to revisit traumatic memories without becoming overwhelmed by fear and anxiety. This dampening of the fear response allows for a more productive therapeutic session, where the individual can engage with painful memories and emotions in a controlled and supportive environment.

Enhanced Prefrontal Cortex Function: MDMA increases activity in the prefrontal cortex, the area of the brain associated with decision-making, rational thought, and emotional regulation. By enhancing connectivity between the prefrontal cortex and the hippocampus (responsible for memory), MDMA helps patients process traumatic memories in a more regulated and constructive way, enabling them to integrate these memories into a coherent narrative rather than experiencing them as fragmented, distressing flashbacks.

MDMA therapy's effectiveness lies in its unique ability to create a "window of tolerance"—a mental state where patients can explore traumatic memories without becoming overwhelmed. By reducing fear and enhancing emotional connection, MDMA allows patients to confront and process their trauma in ways that traditional therapies may not achieve. This process can help break the cycle of avoidance and hyperarousal that perpetuates PTSD symptoms, facilitating deeper healing and integration of traumatic experiences. Under the guidance of trained professionals and in a controlled therapeutic environment, MDMA therapy can help patients achieve lasting emotional healing and a renewed sense of well-being.

Ketamine

Ketamine, a dissociative anesthetic that has gained recognition as a rapid-acting antidepressant, offers unique therapeutic potential due to its ability to promote the formation of new neural networks in the brain. Unlike traditional antidepressants, which can take weeks or even months to show results, ketamine often produces immediate effects, sometimes within hours, which is particularly valuable for individuals with treatment-resistant depression. The longer-term efficacy and permanence of the therapeutic work done under the influence of ketamine are closely tied to its effects on neuroplasticity, or the brain's capacity to reorganize itself by forming new neural connections.

Ketamine's primary mechanism of action involves blocking NMDA (N-methyl-D-aspartate) receptors in the brain, which are associated with glutamate, the most abundant excitatory neurotransmitter. By blocking these receptors, triggers a cascade of intracellular events that ultimately increase the production of brain-derived neurotrophic factor (BDNF), a protein that plays a critical role in the growth, survival, and differentiation of neurons. Enhanced BDNF production promotes synaptogenesis—the formation of new synapses or neural connections—and strengthens existing neural circuits. The ability of ketamine to promote rapid neuroplasticity is particularly important for its therapeutic effects. Research published in *Nature* demonstrated that ketamine can induce synaptogenesis within hours, leading to the formation of new neural pathways that help alleviate symptoms of depression. This rapid formation of new connections is believed to help "reset" dysfunctional neural circuits that contribute to mood disorders, allowing for a more adaptive response to stress and emotional stimuli. The insights and emotional breakthroughs that occur during ketamine sessions are often more easily integrated into everyday life due to the substance's effects on the brain's neuroplasticity. By enhancing the brain's ability to form new connections and adapt to new experiences, ketamine creates a more flexible cognitive environment in which individuals can process and reframe traumatic memories, confront unconscious patterns, and establish healthier ways of thinking and behaving.

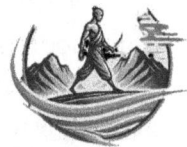

FINAL THOUGHTS

The journey you've embarked on through *The Modern Monk* isn't simply about checking boxes or adopting fleeting wellness trends—it's about tuning into the signals your body continuously sends and responding with intention. The program's aim isn't perfection but awareness and consistent, incremental degrees of improvement. Through the five foundational pillars—sleep, meditation, nutrition, exercise, and neuroplasticity—each small shift you embrace adds to a powerful compounding effect, transforming your health, clarity, and resilience in meaningful and lasting ways.

Whether you've found your entry point with better hydration, practicing meditation, or improved sleep hygiene, each mindful choice creates momentum, steering you toward a brighter, more vibrant version of yourself. Life is a series of moments and choices, each offering a new chance to realign your trajectory towards something greater. Embrace these opportunities, celebrating each small victory along your path. In doing so, you're not just enhancing your own life—you're becoming a beacon, illuminating the path for others.

I sincerely hope that the brief investment of time spent reading this book has inspired you in some way to engage your journey down the path to living a long, healthy, and vibrant life in ways you might not have previously considered.

Over the course of the past decade in my own journey following this path, I have completely healed my gut microbiome, eliminated caffeine intake, returned to sleeping long restful nights (without even getting up even once to go to the bathroom), stabilized my body fat between 10-12%, and am physically the most fit I've been since I was in my 20s. I've got more energy and am producing more creatively than at any point in my life. I am deeply grateful for my health and grateful for the support and presence of my friends and family. Put simply, it feels incredible to be alive (almost) every single day and I owe it all to following the steps outlined in the pages of this book. In writing this, I want that for you too. If you've taken away even just one new practice or idea that you implement, then you have shifted your trajectory by 1° from where you were headed when you first picked up this book. That means you are on course to end up somewhere new and unexpected and that is all I can hope to accomplish in putting these thoughts and ideas into the world for you to consider. No matter where you go or how you choose to get there, may you always travel the path of least resistance.

終了 / 開始
End / Begin

SELECTED BIBLIOGRAPHY

Sleep

The Sleep Solution: Why Your Sleep is Broken and How to Fix It by W. Chris Winter

Why We Sleep by Matthew Walker

The Art of Dreaming by Carlos Casteneda

Mindfulness & Meditation

A New Earth, by Eckhart Tolle

Wherever You Go, There You Are: Mindfulness Meditation in Everyday Life by Jon Kabat-Zinn

The Miracle of Mindfulness: An Introduction to the Practice of Meditation by Thich Nhat Hanh

The Untethered Soul: The Journey Beyond Yourself by Michael A. Singer

Nutrition

The Omnivore's Dilemma: A Natural History of Four Meals by Michael Pollan

Never Be Sick Again: Health Is a Choice, Learn How to Choose It by Kester Cotton and Raymond Francis

The Longevity Diet: Discover the New Science Behind Stem Cell Activation and Regeneration to Slow Aging, Fight Disease, and Optimize Weight by Valter Longo

Exercise & Functional Movement

Born to Run: A Hidden Tribe, Superathletes, and the Greatest Race the World Has Never Seen by Christopher McDougall

Becoming a Supple Leopard: The Ultimate Guide to Resolving Pain, Preventing Injury, and Optimizing Athletic Performance by Dr. Kelly Starrett

Cold Exposure

Uncommon Cold: The Science & Experience of Cold Plunge Therapy by Thomas P. Seager PhD

Winter Swimming: The Nordic Way Towards a Healthier and Happier Life by Susanna Søberg

Recovery

The Wim Hof Method: Activate Your Full Human Potential by Wim Hof

The Sauna Solution: Secrets to Sweating and Staying Fit by Mark Hyman, M.D.

Lifespan: Why We Age—and Why We Don't Have To by David A. Sinclair

Forming Habits

Extreme Ownership: How U.S. Navy SEALs Lead and Win by Jocko Willink

Atomic Habits: An Easy & Proven Way to Build Good Habits & Break Bad Ones by James Clear

Non-Traditional Healing Modalities/Plant Medicines

How to Change Your Mind: What the New Science of Psychedelics Teaches Us About Consciousness, Dying, Addiction, Depression, and Transcendence by Michael Pollan

The Psychedelic Explorer's Guide: Safe, Therapeutic, and Sacred Journeys by James Fadiman

DMT: The Spirit Molecule: A Doctor's Revolutionary Research into the Biology of Near-Death and Mystical Experiences by Rick Strassman MD

Forest of Visions: Ayahuasca, Amazonian Spirituality, and the Santo Daime Tradition by Alex Polari de Alverga

ADDITIONAL RESOURCES

For information and links to all products and resources mentioned in this book, go to: https://subscribepage.io/Resources or scan the QR code below

REFERENCES

n.d. The Ecologist: Home. Accessed October 21, 2021. https://theecologist.org/.

n.d. Consumer Reports: Buy, Own and Live Better. Accessed October 21, 2024. https://www.consumerreports.org/homepage/.

n.d. Environmental Working Group – COMING SOON | Environmental Working Group. Accessed October 21, 2024. https://www.ewg.org/.

n.d. Chicago Tribune - Chicago News, Sports, Weather, Business & Things to Do. Accessed October 21, 2024. https://www.chicagotribune.com/.

"Abnormal menstrual cycle." n.d. National Center for Biotechnology Information. Accessed October 23, 2024. https://www.ncbi.nlm.nih.gov/medgen/534926.

"Anaemia." n.d. World Health Organization (WHO). Accessed October 19, 2024. https://www.who.int/health-topics/anaemia#tab=tab_1.

Anderson, J. W., et al. n.d. "Psyllium fiber reduces serum cholesterol levels in hypercholesterolemic men and women." *American Journal of Clinical Nutrition*. Accessed 2000.

"Anemia - Vitamin B12–Deficiency Anemia." 2022. NHLBI. https://www.nhlbi.nih.gov/health/anemia/vitamin-b12-deficiency-anemia.

Arnold T and Johnston CS. n.d. "An examination of relationships between vitamin B12 status and functional measures of peripheral neuropathy in young adult vegetarians. Front. Nutr." Accessed 2023. 10.3389/fnut.2023.1304134.

Barański, M., et al. 2014. "Higher antioxidant and lower cadmium concentrations and lower incidence of pesticide residues in organically grown crops: a systematic literature review and meta-analyses." *British Journal of Nutrition*.

Bouso, J. C., et al. n.d. "Personality, Psychopathology, Life Attitudes and Neuropsychological Performance among Ritual Users of Ayahuasca: A Longitudinal Study." *Transcultural Psychiatry*. Buford, T. W., et al. n.d. "International Society of Sports Nutrition position stand: creatine supplementation and exercise." *Journal of the International Society of Sports Nutrition*. Accessed 2007.

Byrd, K. B. n.d. "A remote sensing-based model of tidal marsh aboveground carbon stocks for the conterminous United States." *ISPRS Journal of Photogrammetry and Remote Sensing, 139, 255-271*. Accessed 2018.

Carhart-Harris, R. L., et al. n.d. "The effects of MDMA on amygdala activity in healthy volunteers."

Biological Psychiatry. Accessed 2014.

Carhart-Harris, R. L., et al. n.d. "Neural correlates of the psychedelic state as determined by fMRI studies with psilocybin." *Psychopharmacology*. Accessed 2012.

Carhart-Harris, R. L., et al. n.d. "Psychedelics and the essential importance of context." *Frontiers in Psychology*. Accessed 2018.

Carhart-Harris et al. n.d. "rial of psilocybin versus escitalopram for depression." *New England Journal of Medicine*. Accessed 2021.

Centers for Disease Control and Prevention (CDC). n.d. "Antibiotic Resistance Threats in the United States." Accessed 2019.

Claesson, M. J. n.d. "Gut microbiota composition correlates with diet and health in the elderly."

Nature. Accessed 2012.

Clark, K. L., et al. n.d. "24-Week study on the use of collagen hydrolysate as a dietary supplement in athletes with activity-related joint pain." *Current Medical Research and Opinion.* Accessed 2008.

Clarke, G. n.d. "The microbiome-gut-brain axis during early-life regulates the hippocampal serotonergic system in a sex-dependent manner." *Molecular Psychiatry.* Accessed 2014.

Creswell, J. W. n.d. "Educational research: Planning, conducting, and evaluating quantitative and qualitative research (4th ed.)." *Boston, MA: Pearson.* Accessed 2012.

Creswell et al. 2014. "Mindfulness-Based Stress Reduction training reduces loneliness and pro-inflammatory gene expression in older adults: A small randomized controlled trial." *Brain, Behavior, and Immunity* 28:88-92. 10.1016/j.bbi.2012.04.009.

Cryan, J. F., & Dinan, T. G. n.d. "Mind-altering microorganisms: the impact of the gut microbiota on brain and behaviour." *Nature Reviews Neuroscience.* Accessed 2012.

"Cycle-menstrual-data." n.d. National Center for Biotechnology Information. Accessed October 23, 2024. https://www.ncbi.nlm.nih.gov/medgen/604457.

"The Dangers of Trans Fats." n.d.

https://www.health.harvard.edu/staying-healthy/the-dangers-of-trans-fats.

"Dietary Reference Intakes (DRIs)." n.d. The National Academies Press. Accessed October 19, 2024. https://www.nap.edu/.

Duman, R. S., & Aghajanian, G. K. n.d. "Synaptic Dysfunction in Depression: Potential Therapeutic Targets." *Science.* Accessed 2019.

"EWG's 2024 Shopper's Guide to Pesticides in Produce | Dirty Dozen." n.d. Environmental Working Group. Accessed October 23, 2024. https://www.ewg.org/foodnews/dirty-dozen.php.

Feduccia, A. A., et al. n.d. "MDMA-assisted psychotherapy for PTSD: A promising novel therapy." *Current Psychiatry Reports*. Accessed 2018.

Feinberg, I., et al. 1975. "Effects of High Dosage Delta-9-Tetrahydrocannabinol on Sleep Patterns in Man." *Clinical Pharmacology & Therapeutics* 17 (6): 541-549.

"Finding of regularity of menstrual cycle." n.d. National Center for Biotechnology Information. Accessed October 23, 2024. https://www.ncbi.nlm.nih.gov/medgen/604465.

"FoodData Central Search Results." n.d. FoodData Central. Accessed October 19, 2024. https://fdc.nal.usda.gov/fdc-app.html#/food-details/170414/nutrients.

"FoodData Central Search Results." n.d. FoodData Central. Accessed October 19, 2024. https://fdc.nal.usda.gov/fdc-app.html#/food-details/168507/nutrients.

"FoodData Central Search Results." n.d. FoodData Central. Accessed October 19, 2024. https://fdc.nal.usda.gov/fdc-app.html#/food-details/169126/nutrients.

"FoodData Central Search Results." n.d. FoodData Central. Accessed October 19, 2024. https://fdc.nal.usda.gov/fdc-app.html#/food-details/169910/nutrients.

"FoodData Central Search Results." n.d. FoodData Central. Accessed October 19, 2024. https://fdc.nal.usda.gov/fdc-app.html#/food-details/168460/nutrients.

"Food Dyes: A Rainbow of Risks." n.d. Center for Science in the Public Interest. https://cspinet.org/eating-healthy/chemical-cuisine/food-dyes-rainbow-risks.

Forstmann, M., & Sagioglou, C. n.d. "Lifetime experience with (classic) psychedelics predicts pro-environmental behavior through an increase in nature relatedness." *Journal of Psychopharmacology*. Accessed 2017.

Francino, M. P. n.d. "Antibiotics and the Human Gut Microbiome: Dysbioses and Accumulation of Resistances." *Journal of Clinical Investigation*. Accessed 2016.

Fredrickson et al. 2008. "Open hearts build lives: Positive emotions, induced through

loving-kindness meditation, build consequential personal resources." *Journal of Positive Psychology*

3 (3): 175-187. 10.1080/17439760801999445.

Griffiths, R. R., et al. n.d. "Psilocybin produces substantial and sustained decreases in depression and anxiety in patients with life-threatening cancer: A randomized double-blind trial." *The Journal of Psychopharmacology*. Accessed 2016.

Harvard T.H. Chan School of Public Health. n.d. "Omega-3 Fatty Acids: An Essential Contribution." Accessed 2019.

Hempel, S., et al. n.d. "Probiotics for the Prevention and Treatment of Antibiotic-Associated Diarrhea: A Systematic Review and Meta-analysis." *JAMA*. Accessed 2012.

Hölzel et al. 2011. "Mindfulness practice leads to increases in regional brain gray matter density."

Psychiatry Research: Neuroimaging 191 (1): 36-43. 10.1016/j.pscychresns.2010.08.006. Jerome, L., et al. n.d. "Clinical potential of MDMA-assisted psychotherapy." *Journal of Psychopharmacology*. Accessed 2020.

Johnson, M. W., Richards, W. A., & Griffiths, R. R. n.d. "Human hallucinogen research: guidelines for safety." *The Journal of Psychopharmacology*. Accessed 2008.

Lan, J., et al. n.d. "Skin damage among health care workers managing coronavirus disease-2019." *Journal of the American Academy of Dermatology*. Accessed 2020.

Leyer, G. J., et al. n.d. "Probiotic effects on cold and influenza-like symptom incidence and duration in children." *Pediatrics*. Accessed 2009.

Li, N., et al. n.d. "mTOR-dependent synapse formation underlies the rapid antidepressant effects of NMDA antagonists." *Nature*. Accessed 2010.

Luna, L. E. n.d. "The Concept of Plants as Teachers among Four Mestizo Shamans of Iquitos, Northeastern Peru." *Journal of Ethnopharmacology*. Accessed 1984.

Madsen, K. L. n.d. "The effect of probiotics on the intestinal microbiota in humans." *Journal of Applied Microbiology*. Accessed 2001.

Mithoefer, M. C., et al. n.d. "MDMA-assisted psychotherapy for PTSD: A Phase 3 trial." *The Lancet Psychiatry*. Accessed 2018.

Moayyedi, P., et al. n.d. "The efficacy of probiotics in the treatment of irritable bowel syndrome: a systematic review." *Gut*. Accessed 2010.

Palhano-Fontes, F., et al. n.d. "The Therapeutic Potential of Ayahuasca in the Treatment of Depression." *Frontiers in Pharmacology*. Accessed 2018.

Proksch, E., et al. n.d. "Oral intake of specific bioactive collagen peptides reduces skin wrinkles and increases dermal matrix synthesis." *Journal of Cosmetic Dermatology*. Accessed 2014.

Rae, C., et al. n.d. "Oral creatine monohydrate supplementation improves brain performance: a double-blind, placebo-controlled, cross-over trial." *Psychopharmacology*. Accessed 2003.

Roenneberg, Till. 2012. *Internal Time: Chronotypes, Social Jet Lag, and Why You're So Tired.* N.p.: Harvard University Press.

Rosekind, M. R., et al. 1994. "Alertness management: Strategic naps in operational settings." *Journal of Sleep Research* 3 (4): 229-241. 10.1111/j.1365-2869.1994.tb00135.x.

Santos, R. G., et al. n.d. "Effects of Ayahuasca on Psychopathology, Neuropsychology, and Brain Function in Healthy Volunteers: A Preliminary Report." *Journal of Psychopharmacology.* Accessed 2016.

Sessa, B. n.d. "MDMA and PTSD treatment: 'PTSD: From novel pathophysiology to innovative therapeutics.'" *Neuropharmacology.* Accessed 2017.

Shannon, Lewis S., H. N. Lee, and S. Hughes. 2019. "Cannabidiol in Anxiety and Sleep: A Large Case Series." *The Permanente Journal* 23 (1). 10.7812/TPP/18-041.

Sorensen, H. n.d. "Inside the Mind of the Shopper: The Science of Retailing." *Journal of Retailing.* Accessed 200.

"Sustainable Pulse." n.d. Sustainable Pulse. Accessed October 21, 2021. https://sustainablepulse.com/.

Tremaroli, V., & Bäckhed, F. n.d. "Functional interactions between the gut microbiota and host metabolism." *Nature.* Accessed 2012.

Turnbaugh, P. J. n.d. "A core gut microbiome in obese and lean twins." *Nature.* Accessed 2009. "Vitamin B12 - Consumer." 2023. NIH Office of Dietary Supplements. https://ods.od.nih.gov/factsheets/VitaminB12-Consumer/.

Walker, Matthew. 2017. *Why We Sleep: Unlocking the Power of Sleep and Dreams.* N.p.: Scribner. Wang, A., et al. n.d. "Triclosan exposure and its effects on human endocrine function." *Environmental Health Perspectives.* Accessed 2018.

Winter, W. C. 2018. *The Sleep Solution: Why Your Sleep is Broken and How to Fix It*. N.p.: Penguin Publishing Group.

- Winter, C. K., & Davis. n.d. "Organic foods." *Journal of Food Science*. Accessed 2006.

Zhang, C., et al. n.d. "Antimicrobial resistance and environmental persistence of triclosan and triclocarban." *Environmental Science & Technology*. Accessed 2019.

THANK YOU FOR READING MY BOOK!

I really appreciate all of your feedback and
I love hearing what you have to say.

I need your input to make the next version of this
book (and my future books) better.

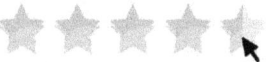

Please take two minutes now to leave a helpful review on
Amazon letting me know what you thought of the book.

Thanks so much!

- Hayden

Book Error Submission Form

Thank you for helping improve the accuracy and quality of this book. If you find a typo, factual error, or inconsistency, I'd love to know about it.

Submit your findings at:

subscribepage.io/errorcapture

www.ingramcontent.com/pod-product-compliance
Lightning Source LLC
Chambersburg PA
CBHW060455030426
42337CB00015B/1600